LIPOSOMES
in
GENE
DELIVERY

LIPOSOMES
in
GENE
DELIVERY

Danilo D. Lasic

CRC Press
Boca Raton   New York

COVER: Artistic impression of liposome DNA complex: double helix of DNA interactingwith liposomes (violet) in context of cells (green).

Technique: Water colors
Artist: Alenka Dvorak Lasic, Spring 1994

Acquiring Editor: Paul Petralia
Project Editor: Carrie L. Unger
Editorial Assistant: Norina Frabotta
Marketing Manager: Susie Carlisle
Direct Marketing Manager: Becky McEldowney
Cover design: Dawn Boyd
PrePress: Kevin Luong
Manufacturing: Sheri Schwartz

Library of Congress Cataloging-in-Publication Data

Lasic, D. D.
    Liposomes in gene delivery / Danilo D. Lasic.
        p.   cm.
    Includes bibliographical references and index.
    ISBN 0-8493-3109-0
    1. Gene therapy. 2. Liposomes.   3. Gene Therapy   I. Title.
    [DNLM: 1. Liposomes.   2. Liposomes.   3. Gene Therapy.   4. Drug Delivery Systems
RB155.8.L38   1997
616'.042—dc20
DNLM/DLC
for Library of Congress
                                                                        96-35300
                                                                        CIP

DEDICATION

To my parents

THE AUTHOR

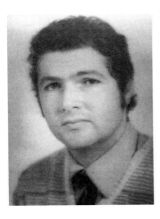

Danilo D. Lasic, Ph.D., is a liposome (drug and gene delivery) consultant in Newark, California. Beforehand, he was at MegaBios Corp., where he worked with cationic liposomes, DNA-lipid complexation, and scale-up. Previously, he was a Senior Scientist at Liposome Technology, Inc., (now Sequus), where he led studies for theoretical understanding of long circulating liposomes. He also developed the first formulations for preclinical studies. In addition, he also actively participated in the scale-up of the preparation of stealth liposomes laden with the anticancer agent doxorubicin, which became the first FDA-approved liposome formulation and has been commercially available since 1995. Dr. Lasic graduated from the University of Ljubljana in 1975 with a degree in physical chemistry. He received his M.S. in 1977 from the University of Ljubljana. He obtained his Ph.D. at the Institute J. Stefan, Solid State Physics Department, Ljubljana, in 1979. After doing his post doctoral work with Dr. Charles Tanford at Duke University, North Carolina, and Dr. Helmut Hauser at ETH Zurich, he was a research fellow at the Institute J. Stefan, a visiting lecturer in the Department of Chemistry, and a visiting scientist in the Department of Physics at the University of Waterloo in Canada. Dr. Lasic then joined Liposome Technology, Inc., Menlo Park, California, where he studied cationic liposomes, DNA-liposome interactions, and DNA-complexes for gene delivery and gene therapy. Dr. Lasic has published more than 150 papers as well as authored a monograph on liposomes, *Liposomes: From Physics to Applications* (Elsevier, 1993). co-edited a book, *Stealth Liposomes* (CRC Press, 1995, and co-edited a series of four books, *Nonmedical Application of Liposomes* (CRC Press, 1996). His best known papers are those that deal with thermodynamics and the mechanism of vesicle formation, the stability of liposomes, the origin of liposome stability in biological environments, and the applications of drug-laden liposomes.

■ PREFACE

The extremely rapid development of molecular biology has resulted in applications well beyond the scope of biology, and in order to solve complex problems, this technology has had to combine its efforts with many other sciences. In gene therapy, for instance, only the synergistic action of basic medical research, recombinant DNA technology, and drug delivery techniques can give rise to successful medical applications leading to superior disease treatments at reduced risk, patient discomfort, and cost. The seemingly unlimited potential of these treatments has attracted the attention of the general public as well. Furthermore, direct intervention of humans with nature, or God for some, will require that not only numerous scientific, but also philosophical, ethical, moral, and social problems, to be solved. As a result of this multidisciplinary research, not many scientists are familiar with all the aspects of this complex field. In nonviral gene delivery, which is emerging as a major technology, for instance, researchers should understand the principles and potential of molecular biology as well as of drug delivery. Among the delivery systems, lipid-based formulations seem to be the leading candidate for an efficient and safe gene delivery system. Not many specialists seem to be familiar with both, various aspects of drug delivery and molecular biology of DNA vectors. Nor do any comprehensive monographs or reviews exist. The aim of this monograph is therefore to fill this gap. I hope that molecular biologists, who can skip the DNA part, will be able to obtain sufficient basic knowledge of lipids, liposomes, and some other gene delivery vehicles, and that on the other side, pharmacologists and lipid and drug delivery scientists will gain knowledge of DNA, molecular biology, and DNA manipulation. In the future I also envisage a greater impact of theory, and I hope that theoreticians will get an idea of some experimental designs and data, and vice versa. Of course, I encourage specialists to skip appropriate parts. This book is also aimed at physicians and students as an introductory course in this interdisciplinary field. The problems are more complex than most people imagine, and I hope that after reading this volume, readers will obtain a more critical relationship to the field. Too often I have become aware of too naive scenarios and misinterpretation of the data as a result of nonspecific effects. A typical example would be treatment of cancer in a particular tissue by only using cationic liposomes and a tissue specific promoter or attribution of anticancer activity of the formulation to specific effects instead of simply to the toxicity of lipids and especially of degraded lipids.

I hope that this book will explain some of these issues and prepare readers to perform well-controlled experiments with appropriate controls. At present, there is not a single DNA carrier system which has a promising therapeutic application and a viable commercial future, and I shall make it clear that such a system has yet to be discovered and assembled. It will be based on the ideas and approaches reviewed and presented in this volume. All the efforts of human genome characterization and studies of the functionality of discovered genes are leading undoubtedly to medical treatments on the genetic level. However, the time scale may be longer than the one which can be inferred from reading articles, press releases, and business reports. My goal has been to provide an introductory text for nonspecialists in nonviral gene therapy. Upon introducing the subject and some examples of the diseases which can be treated with this technology, nucleic acids are introduced. I have also added a short section on theoretical description of DNA which is followed by a brief description of recombinant technology. As it seems now, the major effort in nonviral gene delivery involves lipids. Therefore, lipids and liposomes are introduced. Their stability and interaction properties are described, and a chapter on their complexation with DNA plasmids follows. The DNA-lipid particles formed are called genosomes, and they may include complexes of cationic liposomes and DNA, encapsulated DNA in conventional liposomes, or in a broader sense, any colloidal suspension of DNA interacting with some agent. The next chapter describes gene expression of genosomes in various models. A review of data is followed by a chapter on structure–activity relationships, and a chapter on transfection models discusses the mechanisms involved in the process. Here practically no data exist and I have tried to establish some models based on scarce experimental data and appropriate Gedanken experiments. Definitively, I disagree with a majority of workers in the field who claim that there is, for instance, no correlation hetween *in vivo* and *in vitro* results. I believe that our limited understanding is due to our lack of knowledge of the mechanisms involved and not to the existence of two different processes. Based on the models presented in the book, I shall try to explain the differences. I am aware that the models are based on few published data. The problem in the field is that people have mostly changed primary experimental parameters and followed gene expression and have not measured the physicochemical properties of the complexes and their biological interactions following the administration. I am also well aware that the models proposed may be too simplified and inconsistent with some experimental data, which are often inconsistent among various studies as well. But I also hope that such models will stimulate further mechanistic studies and modeling which will ultimately result in improved understanding, successful applications, and commercial products. In addition to urging scientists to do more basic studies on the properties, stability, and interaction characteristics of various systems, I also propose more serious safety tests.

Sometimes I have a feeling that the field of gene therapy in general and lipid-based gene delivery in particular follows the thorny path of liposomes in medical applications. Quite a few scientists, often due to nonscientific reasons, publish irreproducible and even artifactual data. In the long run this may and probably will have negative consequences, exactly as has happened with liposomes. In this case, papers in the mid 1970s and early 1980s promised practically unlimited and very quick applications. In reality, however, no products were forthcoming, and only after several years of complete skepticism and pessimism did a few products appear. It was only the increased understanding of basic science, mostly the stability and interaction characteristics of liposomes and its successful coupling with engineers, that stimulated this development and not opportune talk, unrealistic reviews, and the unfulfilled promises of some scientists and people in the business world a decade before. The appearance of manipulations on the molecular and genetic level coincides with rapid development in a few other scientific disciplines, such as supramolecular chemistry, artificial self-assembly, nanotechnology, and computer-aided automated systems. While some of these disciplines already have had some impact in gene therapy, it will take years before our understanding and control of these processes will allow us to couple all these technologies synergistically. Therefore, we must look at these interconnections *con grano salis*. Namely, recently self-assembled systems and supramolecular chemistry have become very popular, and in several presentations I have noticed that people use these terms rather loosely. So, briefly, the liposome itself is a self-assembled system because it is composed of self-assembled lipid bilayers. Similarly, DNA condensation itself is a supramolecular phenomenon which depends on specific inter-action with cationic substances. It is well known that univalent cations cannot condense DNA. However, we show that a self-organized assembly of them, such as a lipid bilayer or liposome(s), can do that. This is an example of supramolecular chemistry. So may be assembled lipid, poly-mer, and protein systems which in concord perform some function. With newly emerging nanotechnologies, however, it may even become possible to build these complexes in a small, well-defined space using the power of self-assembly and nanotechnology. Ultimately, such systems may even deliver them. At present, however, these processes are still quite random and based on colloidal interactions rather than on two dimensional surface build-up, and drug and gene delivery has to comply with biological laws in the body. However, after the ups and downs of gene delivery, the introduction of nanotechnology and other modern techniques may one day revolutionize our current drug and gene delivery, and my hope is that this book can serve as a modest beginning of this quest. To com-mence, though, let us go back to the reality, i.e., DNA, lipids, liposomes, and their interactions, and the stability and interaction characteristics of their mixtures.

CONTENTS

ACKNOWLEDGMENTS

The field is really quite broad and difficult to cover by an individual. Having some experiences with lipids and liposomes, I relied on the help and advice of molecular biologists. The improvement of the text in these parts is due to Drs. Teni Boulikas, Nancy Smyth-Templeton, and David Ruff. For help in the physical aspects of DNA, I am thankful to Dr. Rudi Podgornik, while Dr. Peter M. Frederik supplied me with exceptional micrographs. I also appreciate the help of Dr. Joe Vallner and Lee Pedersen from Sequus Pharmaceuticals, Inc., and William L. Brown who generously helped me with some technical issues. I am deeply indebted to Stanley E. Hansen who for his love of computers and science spent numerous evenings and weekends preparing computer graphics, with some of the pictures so large that they had to be printed over the weekend. Last, I must thank my family for their full support of my extracurricular activities, especially little Eva who missed many evening stories because of this book and my wife Alenka who, additionally, illustrated the cover.

INTRODUCTION

1

Genetics is one of the oldest scientific endeavors of humans. People have selectively bred various plants and animals since the Stone Age. But it was only in the mid 1940s, long after the work of Mendel (1860), the discovery of nucleic acids by Miescher (1869), and many other important findings, such as the search for transforming factors (Griffith, 1928; Avery, 1944) and chemical analysis of DNA (Chargaff in the 1940s), that it was realized that genetic information is transferred via DNA and not by, say, genetic proteins or complex polysaccharides. The double-helical structure of DNA and the mechanism of its replication were explained by Watson and Crick in 1953. In the decades that followed, the understanding of nucleic acids, their manipulation, as well as the structure and function of genes and the origin of diseases on the molecular level was rapidly improving, resulting in many new applications. One of them is gene therapy. Its aim is to improve or correct the conditions of the sickness on the molecular level. This would not only alleviate the symptoms but also eliminate the cause of the disease as well.

From the daily press we are aware of genetically altered plants, which are immune to some pesticides or extreme weather conditions, and microbes, which can survive by digesting ecologically damaging debris into useful products, as well as of almost weekly discoveries of genes responsible for various disorders, from cancers to obesity and, of course, of the human genome project. When completed, early in the next millennium (2002/3), the project will yield the detailed sequence of around 3 billion base pairs of the human genome. It is hoped that parallel studies of the function of these genes will give invaluable tools in the treatment of hereditary and acquired diseases.

Very rapid developments in recombinant DNA technology, in understanding of the genetic basis of many diseases on the molecular level, as well as in sequencing and mapping of the human genome coupled with functional characterization, have therefore opened the possibility of medical therapy on the genetic level. While recombinant DNA techniques have permitted preparation of larger quantities of therapeutic proteins, the aim of gene therapy is the synthesis of these proteins *in situ,* ideally in the appropriate cells of the patient. Gene therapy therefore requires, after diagnosis of the problem and construction of appropriate plasmids, effective and safe transfection and gene expression. Transfection describes the transfer of genetic material into the cell nucleus, and gene expression indicates the subsequent synthesis of the encoded protein by the cell machinery.

The delivery of the gene with the encoded sequence for a particular protein into appropriate cells, preferably *in vivo*, currently seems to be the largest obstacle in this field. The next hurdle is the duration of the expression. While many researchers use viral vectors, the concerns with safety, strong immune response, large-scale noncontaminated production, and cost are putting more and more emphasis on nonviral DNA carriers. Currently, the largest emphasis is in the use of cationic liposomes as DNA-complexing agents. From the point of view of safety and of the ability to control the biological fate of complexes, noncationic lipids are also becoming interesting as gene delivery systems. Not much of the data on these systems is published, and therefore we shall concentrate mostly on cationic lipids for gene transfection.

Liposomes and lipid-based systems are, because of their self-assembling properties, their ability to interact with DNA in a controllable manner, and the enhanced delivery of the complex into the cells, as well as their potential biocompatibility, emerging as prime candidates for the formulation of gene delivery systems.

In this book we shall review nucleic acids, liposomes, their complexes, and their applications in *in vitro* and *in vivo* transfection and gene expression, including clinical trials in humans. We shall follow with physicochemical characterization of the complexes, models of *in vitro* and *in vivo* transfections, and structure–activity relationships. We shall conclude with other gene-carrying particles, delivery of antisense oligonucleotides and ribozymes, future directions, and possible optimization of transfection.

ADDITIONAL READING

Anderson, W. F., Human gene therapy, *Science,* 256, 808–813, 1992.
Lasic, D. D., *Liposomes: From Physics to Applications,* Elsevier, Amsterdam, 1993.
Watson, J. D., Toose, J., Kurtz, D.T., *Recombinant DNA,* Scientific American Books, New York, 1983.

GENE THERAPY

2

Medicine has passed in its history through several breakthroughs, from Galen and Pasteur to the introduction of anesthesia, surgery, vaccines, antibiotics, novel imaging techniques, lasers, and remote operating devices. Direct treatment on the molecular level of diseases themselves and not their symptoms may be the next important development in human therapy.

Gene therapy is emerging as a new modality as well as a technology in medical practice. It offers the potential to cure disease on its most basic level and has therefore captured the imagination of scientific and popular media. The therapy requires the insertion of a functional gene or other molecule with an information sequence into a cell to achieve a therapeutic effect, and the gene therefore serves as a drug (Anderson, 1992; Miller, 1992; Mulligan, 1993; Goldspiel et al., 1993).

All the organisms of a particular species have an identical number and type of genes. Obviously, because we are not absolutely identical, small variations among genes exist within the species. While most of these polymorphisms have no effect on the protein function and some of them bring only innocuous variations in physical appearance, such as the color of eyes or hair, some of them produce serious inherited disorders. These disorders can be apparent immediately after birth or can develop only later in the life span; they can also make some individuals more susceptible to environmental factors. It is anticipated that gene therapy can handle or eliminate such problems.

STRATEGIES IN GENE DELIVERY

Several thousand diseases can be traced to defective or missing functional genes, and it is hoped that by delivering the appropriate gene into the appropriate cells, the mutated or missing proteins can be synthesized and the signs of the disease alleviated. In the majority of cases the mutation is in the coding region of the gene. This can result in an amino acid substitution, and if this happens in an important domain of the protein, it may not be functional. On the other hand, mutations in the regulatory regions or in the DNA-binding or transactivation domains of transcription factors normally result in downregulation of gene expression.

3

One can use several different modes of action to repair these defects. The so-called gene replacement therapy aims to deliver the appropriate gene into cells with nonfunctional genes and via novel synthesis of the nonfunctional or missing proteins to improve the patient's health. Examples are cystic fibrosis, in which the transregulatory protein (CFTR) does not function from birth, and cancer, in which genes such as tumor suppressor genes become damaged with time.

Gene therapy in a broader sense also encompasses enhancement of the immune system, tagging neoplastic cells for autoimmune destruction, and vaccination in which the body itself produces antigens to induce an immune response. Low levels of antigens can be produced constantly, or they can be produced upon a specific trigger. Infected patients can be treated with genes of pathogens and this may boost their own immune response. T cells are critical mediators of tumor specificity, and appropriate peptides can upon association with major histocompatibility complex class I (MHC) stimulate cytotoxic (CD8+) T cells, resulting in cancer immunotherapy. The origin of genetic vaccination, however, and the fact that it works in the absence of adjuvants (is it DNA or cell surfaces?), is still not understood. Furthermore, other possibilities of gene therapy include infectious diseases, inflammation states, or cancer, in which one can stimulate the immune system to produce and secrete more cytokines, such as various colony-stimulating factors, interferons, interleukins (IL), and tumor necrosis factor, and, via enhanced cytotoxicity and/or enhanced number of killer cells, alleviate the diseased state. This can also be done by inserting genes for the synthesis of cytokines which potentiate the immune system response. Alternatively, by direct injection into tumors one can force tumor cells to express highly immunogenic genes which makes them highly visible and susceptible to the attack of the immune system. Such therapy, however, requires a high percentage of cells to be transfected, and we shall discuss some of these implications below. Similarly, suicide genes can sensitize transfected cells to conventional drugs. For instance, transfer of the herpes virus simplex thymidine kinase gene *(HSVtk)* makes cells susceptible to the drug ganciclovir. Human thymidine kinase cannot use ganciclovir as a substrate for phosphorylation and subsequent incorporation into DNA, and thus cells not transfected with the gene are not damaged. Alternatively, in anticancer therapy the nonfunctional tumor suppressor genes can be enhanced or oncogenes can be inactivated.

Another variation would be protection of patient cells during chemotherapy. Currently, the dose-limiting factor is normally leukopenia, and white blood cell count is stimulated by addition of various stimulating factors, such as granulocyte/macrophage colony-stimulating factor (GMCSF). The multidrug resistance protein (glycoprotein P), for instance, which excretes drug molecules and severely compromises drug activity, can be synthesized in the bone marrow cells of the patient, thus rendering white blood cell precursors resistant to chemotherapy (Culver and Blaese, 1994). Similarly, other drug-resistance mechanisms, such as the introduction of drug-degrading enzymes, can be used.

Some of these concepts require that all the cells be transfected, while in some cases, such as in cystic fibrosis, gene expression in only a fraction, such as 10%, of the cells may be enough. In cancer, for instance, a single surviving cell can start the tumor growth anew. It is hoped, however, that the so-called bystander effect can eradicate all the affected cells. In such a case, synthesized proteins would diffuse into surroundings and stop the cell growth. Another example is selective activation of a prodrug: if vectors containing the cytosine deaminase gene driven by the carcino-embryonic antigen (CEA) promoter to colorectal carcinoma cells become expressed, these cells can activate prodrug 5-fluorocytosine into toxic 5-fluoracil which can diffuse in the surrounding tumor cells (Huber et al., 1994).

In addition to a "turn-on" concept as described above, a therapy is also possible for switching genes off. According to antisense technology, a short, normally single-strand oligonucleotide complementary to a part of the target gene or messenger RNA is delivered and stops processes such as cancer, scar tissue, or other undesired cell growth by halting the information readout. A similar concept is also being tried by the use of short sequences which permit triple helix formation and adsorption of special proteins to complex nucleic acids (Cohen and Hogan, 1994). The purpose of this technology is to diminish or eliminate the expression of gene at the genome or RNA level.

Table 2-1 summarizes some of the modalities of gene therapy and their possible applications.

TABLE 2-1

MODES OF ACTION OF GENE THERAPEUTICALS

Gene replacement	Cystic fibrosis, cancer
Immune system activation	Cancer, infections
Suicide gene	Cancer
Bone marrow protection	Cancer
Vaccination	Viral infections, cancer
Gene downregulation	Cancer

At present, gene therapy approaches are targeted toward somatic cells, i.e., they would affect only nonreproductive cells. Germ cell therapy, involving transfection of ova and sperm cells, however, brings about, in addition to scientific problems, a variety of ethical, social, and philosoph-ical issues which will have to be solved before we may continue with applications of this research. Therefore, in vivo gene therapy, as a logical development of ex vivo treatments (i.e., direct injection instead of collec-tion of some cells, transfection in the test tube, and reinjection), envisages targeting of tissues or cells of certain organs, such as heart, lung, blood, vascular endothelium, liver (hepatocytes or macrophages), spleen, lymph nodes, muscle, pancreas and other glands, muscle (fibroblasts), potentially brain and nerve cells, skin, thymus, and others upon systemic or local application. Among hundreds of different cells in various tissues, macrophages and monocytes, vascular endothelium, hepatocytes, lung epithelium, neural muscle, stem and mucosal cells, and adipocytes seem to be the primary targets.

Currently, in addition to efficient and safe gene delivery, the duration of expression, especially in the case of nonviral vectors, seems to be the largest unsolved problem. In principle, depending on the disease, a short-term transient expression or a long-term sustained expression can be designed by using appropriate DNA cassettes. DNA sequences can regulate rate, duration, and location of expression. While current nonviral delivery systems aim for episomal delivery (i.e., not integrating into the chromosome), the next generation of plasmids may contain sequences for adhesion to the nucleus and self-replication. They may also contain peptide stretches specifying nuclear localization (Boulikas, 1995; 1996), site-specific chromosome integration, and possibly homologous recombination.

Cells are transfected with genes which are inserted into altered viruses or inserted into plasmids. These are circular or linear DNA constructs which flank the gene (cDNA) with segments having different functions. A cDNA copy of the gene of interest can be inserted into an adenovirus, retrovirus, or plasmid vector under the control of viral or cellular promoter and enhancer regulatory elements. Depending on the delivery system, a gene can be inserted into the host genome (chromosome) or simply localized in the cell nucleus replicating as an extrachromosomal nonintegrated plasmid. This is referred to as episomal location. Because at present the site of chromosomal insertion cannot be controlled, episomal delivery is preferred. It does not permanently alter the host genome and increases safety by avoiding possible side effects such as the highly unlikely event of cancer or viral infection. However, this approach therefore requires either frequent dosing or development of self-replicating plasmids that replicate and persist in the cell nucleus during cell division.

In the following we shall discuss the major technical challenges to gene therapy. They can be listed as

- Identification of the disease
- Identification of the genetic defect
- Construction of the appropriate plasmid or viral vector
- Design of delivery system and its optimization
- Efficiency of gene transfection
- Number of cells transfected
- Cell type, tissue, or organ specificity
- Duration of expression

- Expression possibility in dividing or nondividing cells

- Inflammatory and/or immune response

- Short-term toxicity

- Long-term toxicity

- Formulation scaleup, quality control, sterility, and stability

- Preclinical data

- Clinical results

    Phase I: determine safety and dosage (maximal tolerated dose)

    Phase II: evaluate effectiveness and check side effects

    Phase III: verify effectiveness, monitor adverse reactions from long-term use

    Phase IV: (possibly/likely for a new modality in therapeutics) additional postmarketing testing

- Regular affairs and patent issues

- Marketing, sales, and public awareness and education

An ideal disease candidate should have been caused by a single mutation in only one gene, which should have been cloned and the mutation identified. The expression of the healthy copy (wild-type) should reverse the physiological defect also in the case when only a small proportion of cells was transfected and in the presence of a mutant. The expression of the gene should follow a simple on–off regulation and not, say, a complex temporal and quantitative regulation of expression in particular cells (Ville, 1996). Finally, the new protein should be recognized as "self" and therefore not be attacked by the body's immune system.

At this stage, we shall assume that the majority of these issues is already solved, and we shall concentrate mostly on achieving efficient gene expression in particular cell types. Only biological response studies will tell if adequate expression was obtained. While it seems that functional plasmids with cell-specific promoters can be now routinely constructed, their delivery, not only *in vitro* and *ex vivo,* but especially *in vivo,* presents the largest challenge. Currently, in most therapies appropriate cells are removed and, after transfection *ex vivo,* injected back into the patient.

Ex vivo approaches are rather complex procedures in which cells, most frequently from bone marrow, are removed from the patient, cultured, transfected with genes which potentiate a function (*MDR1* — resistance to the drug adriamycin and other drugs) or their ability to attack malignant cells (*IL2* gene — tumor-infiltrating lymphocytes), and reintroduced into the patient. Despite some advantages, such as better control and efficiency of transfection and safety due to the possible avoidance of the use of delivery vectors, its drawbacks are the limited number of accessible cells as well as the fact that it is a labor- and time-intensive procedure.

Obviously, the ideal treatment is *in vivo* administration of appropriate plasmids or their constructs with various carriers. Because naked DNA is chemically not stable in contact with various body fluids and because due to its size and charge, it is unlikely to enter into cells and their nuclei, it is normally packaged with appropriate delivery vehicles into colloidal particles.

The major diseases that are being treated in experimental phases by administering genes for defective (mutated) or missing proteins are various types of cancer, cystic fibrosis, cardiovascular disorders, and some neurological diseases.

■ DISEASE APPLICATIONS OF GENE THERAPY

In this part we shall briefly discuss some diseases that are the prime candidates for genetic therapy. We shall divide them into genetic diseases, cancer, neurological, infectious, and cardiovascular diseases, and others.

Genetic Diseases

Although these diseases are rather rare, existing treatments can only reduce symptoms and improve and possibly prolong life without addressing the cause of the disease.

Cystic fibrosis is an autosomal-recessive disease. This means that both parents must carry the bad copy of the gene for cystic fibrosis transmembrane conductance regulator (CFTR) protein which regulates the transport of chloride ions across the cell membrane in the mucosal surface of epithelial cells lining the airway and intestinal tract; what results is the accumulation of mucus in the lung and concomitant infection which is normally fatal. Treatments mostly postpone the time schedule of the events. This is the most common genetic disease among Caucasians and occurs in approximately 1 in 2000 newborns (Caplen and Alton, 1996). It is hoped that the disease can be alleviated by introduction of the *CFTR* gene in the epithelial cells lining the airways of the lung by inhalation of an appropriate aerosol. The *CF* gene was found on chromosome 7 and was identified in 1989. Despite its genetic simplicity as well as many clinical trials, it is by no means an easy model. While there is still a dispute about which cells are getting and/or have to be transfected by various delivery systems, one must also keep in mind the physical inaccessibility of cells covered with thick mucus. Similarly, in *Gaucher's disease* patients have a nonfunctional enzyme glucocerebrosidase resulting in improper carbohydrate metabolism. The cure is sought in delivering the glucocerebrosidase gene into stem cells. *Sickle cell anemia* occurs at the rate 1 in 500 newborns and is the most frequent genetic disease among blacks. An abnormal type of hemoglobin causes insufficient oxygenation of tissues because red blood cells collapse and the sickle-shaped erythrocytes have difficulty passing through small capillaries. Also caused by a hemoglobin dysfunction, but more life threatening, is *thalassemia*. This is an autosomal-dominant disease that affects 1 in 2000 individuals of Mediterranean descent. Delivery of globin genes is being studied as a treatment in both diseases. One sex-linked illness is *hemophilia;* the gene for protein Factor VIII (or IX, in hemophilia A and B, respectively) is carried on the chromosome X and 1 in 15,000 males (hemophilia A and 1 in 30,000 for hemophilia B) lacks the ability to clot blood because this protein is involved in the clotting cascade. Factor VIII is secreted from many different types of somatic cells, including hepatocytes, capillary endothelium, spleen cells, lymph nodes, and kidney cells, and it seems therefore that because of the systemic accessibility the therapeutic approach should be straightforward. Patients with *familial hypercholesterolemia* lack a receptor for low-density lipoproteins (LDL), and cholesterol builds atherosclerotic plaques on blood vessel walls at an accelerated rate. Transfection of liver cells with a gene for the LDL receptor is thought to be capable of improving the condition of this autosomal-dominant disease. Experiments with hyperlipidemic rabbit model have been successful, and this approach has entered a clinical trial.

Cancer

In contrast to other genetic diseases, the real aim in most approaches in cancer gene therapy is not to correct the genetic defect, which is mutation in genes such as *ras, p53, myc,* or *myb,* but to kill the target cells as efficiently as possible, with minimal side effects (Culver and Blaese, 1994; Ville, 1996).

There are several different ways in which cancer can be treated using gene therapy. One can stimulate the body's immune system against cancer antigens or sensitize cancer cells to a cytotoxic drug. Cancer genesis often originates from a mutation in a protein in one of the two classes of proteins that regulate cell growth. Normally, it is sustained and controlled by the balance between oncogenes and tumor suppressor genes. In some individuals who have, as a result of mutations, lost the functional activity of tumor suppressive genes, such as *Rb, p53*, or the recently discovered *FHIT* gene, which control the growth of cells, the function of such genes in cancer cells is tried to be restored. Recently, researchers have shown evidence that the gene *BRCA1* suppresses tumor growth in breast and ovarian cancers and that when the gene is defective women are more susceptible to these cancers. Alternatively, the synthesis of oncogenes can be blocked by oligonucleotides, as will be discussed more in Chapter 12.

It is believed that mutations in the *p53* gene and consequent loss of the growth inhibition exerted by this gene play a major role in cancer; mutations in this gene occur in over one half of human cancers. The mechanism is still unknown, but it is believed that the protein coded for by *p53* is a transcription factor that stimulates production of a second protein which inhibits key enzymes needed to drive cells through the cell cycle and into cell growth and which normally can suppress cell growth. These mechanisms are very complex and can in several steps, via specific inhibitions of phosphorylation, interfere with cell division and function of DNA polymerases (Boulikas, 1996).

Another important protein is Ras which is a molecular switch and which controls the decision of a cell to differentiate or to grow. *ras* is GTPase which is a sensitive sensor and its activation may result in either proliferation or differentiation by increasing the activity of cytoplasmic kinases. Because activated *ras* oncogenes were identified in human cancers, the suppression of these oncogenes may be important in cancer therapy.

One alternative is also to protect normal cells against damage from chemotherapy or to increase the number of lymphocytes, as discussed before. Antiangiogenesis, the blockage of new capillary beds or the stoppage of their proliferation/growth before they are established, on a molecular level is another possible approach.

Malignant cells can be destroyed by white blood cells including natural killer (NK) cells, lymphokine-activated tumor cells (LAK), cytotoxic T lymphocytes (CTL), tumor-infiltrating lymphocytes (TIL), and activated macrophages. The immunogenicity of tumor cells can be increased by the expression of (MHC) antigen or by increasing local production of cytokines. The immune system can therefore be stimulated by transfecting tumor cells with genes for antigens that control rejection of the transplants, such as *HLA-B7*. If transfected cells express this antigen, the cytotoxic T cells can destroy the tumor. CTL cells can be activated also by GMCSF, interferons, and interleukins (IL-2), and genes for these cytokines are being used for transfection and consecutive stimulation of the immune response.

Tumor cells can be also sensitized to become more susceptible to conventional chemotherapy. Ganciclovir is a very effective drug for herpes viruses, and expressing herpes virus *TK* gene in tumor cells can make them sensitive to this drug. An opposite case was also reported: cisplatin-resistant tumor cells have shown enhanced liposome-mediated transfection of marker genes in the presence of the drug. The mechanism that is cisplatin specific is still not understood, but the effect may offer a sequential therapy; i.e., cells remaining after cisplatin treatment can be eradicated by gene therapy (Son and Huang, 1994).

While most of the current preclinical and clinical studies concentrate on melanoma and other easily accessible tumors for direct injection, in the long run experts expect that major applications will be in breast, colorectal, bladder, lung, ovarian, and renal cancer. Expression of the *p53* gene in the lung can, in principle, be used in a preventive way in populations at high risk of acquiring lung cancer.

The following list summarizes some of the potential strategies for cancer gene therapy:

- Enhancing the immunogenicity of the tumor (introducing genes for foreign antigens)

- Enhancing activity of immune cells (by introducing genes for cytokines)

- Inserting a suicide gene into the tumor *(HSVtk)*

- Inserting a tumor suppressor gene (wild-type *p53*)

- Blocking the expression of genes (introducing genes that encode antisense message, ribozymes, or antisense oligonucleotides)

- Protecting stem cells (introducing drug-resistance genes)

- Killing tumor cells by inserting toxin genes under tumor-specific promoters

In general, cell proliferation is an extremely complex process which on the one side offers many different strategies, but on the other makes attack on one single reaction in this very complex scheme of dozens of coupled reactions unlikely to accomplish the goal.

Infectious Diseases

While antibiotics are very effective drugs in bacterial infections, viral infections are very difficult to treat. In addition, most chemotherapeutic agents quickly lose potency because viruses rapidly develop resistance due to mutations in transcriptase and protease genes. It is hoped that gene therapy will be able to provide new means to treat these illnesses (Gilboa and Smith, 1994).

Two strategies can be employed to use gene therapy for the treatment of *AIDS*. The immune system may be stimulated to destroy infected cells and one can try to stop viral replication inside the cell. HIV selectively destroys the CD4 population of white blood cells. These cells orchestrate the response to infection by secreting a number of regulatory cytokines. CD4 cells also activate CD8 cells to become cytotoxic T lymphocytes (CTLs) and acquire specificity for viral proteins expressed on the membranes of infected cells. One way of achieving increased immune response is to transfect CD8 cells with the gene for IL-2. HIV antigen triggers secretion of IL-2 and concomitant proliferation of CTL.

Intracellular approaches are searching for proteins that interfere with viral production and transfecting cells with appropriate genes. None of these tactics can eradicate the virus, but it is hoped that they can reduce its numbers and the number of infected cells to levels sufficient to postpone the disease. Vaccines also use the HIV envelope gene. The problem is that the envelope protein mutates very frequently and is thus highly unstable, and vaccines based on the envelope protein may quickly become irrelevant. Similar strategies are used also in the treatment of cytomegalovirus, hepatitis B, and herpes simplex virus (HSV) infections.

A new approach is "intracellular immunization" in which intracellular antibodies can block viral replication at various steps. Single-chain antibody sequences can be inserted into artificial genes and their expression in the hematopoietic stem or progenitor cells or differentiated mononu-clear cells can inhibit viral replication.

Neurological Diseases

After early skepticism regarding the feasibility of gene therapy for neu-rological diseases and disorders due to the high compartmentalization of the neural system, the tight blood–brain barrier, and the physical inac-cessibility of the central nervous system (CNS), there is optimism that these disorders and defects in the CNS and in the peripheral nervous system may become amenable to genetic therapy (Friedmann, 1994).

Progressive decrease of the secretion of dopamine, an important neurotransmitter, due to the degeneration of neurons in the *substantia nigra* causes *Parkinson's disease* which is characterized by tremors and muscular rigidity. A potential treatment is the implantation of the fibro-blast-containing gene for tyrosine hydroxylase which produces dopamine in the brain. Neuron degeneration is the cause of *Alzheimer's disease,* and one possibility for therapy is to use growth factors to reduce the rate of this degradation. Since brain cells are nondividing, retroviral vectors are not effective. To circumvent *ex vivo* treatments, gene formu-lations can be directly injected into the CNS (brain and spinal cord).

Cardiovascular Diseases

Despite the fact that cardiovascular diseases remain the leading cause of mortality among adults no particulate drug delivery vehicle has made any impact on clinical practice yet. Practically all treatments rely on oral or parenteral application of small-molecular-weight drug molecules. It is hoped that localized introduction of genes encoding proteins which can inhibit cell proliferation or thrombogenesis into vascular cells will be a promising approach to the therapy of *atherosclerosis, restenosis,* and *thrombosis.* Vascular muscle cells can be transfected in localized segments of peripheral or coronary arteries by using double-balloon catheters. The blood flow is stopped for 20 to 30 min and plasmid formulation is instilled into the area through a central port (Plautz et al., 1993).

We have already mentioned *familial hypercholesterolemia, blood clot-ting disorders,* and *sickle cell anemia.* Restenosis is a growth of smooth muscle cells in blood vessels which often follows injury or angioplasty. By blocking the synthesis of vital proteins by antisense molecules this proliferation can be halted.

Anemia is successfully treated by supplying the genetically engineered blood hormone erythropoietin. From the point of view of gene therapy, cells in the body can produce this protein itself if transfected with an appropriate gene. In principle, it can be delivered either systemically in the hope that vascular endothelium will be transfected and will secrete protein or via implants of *ex vivo* transfected fibroblasts. *Heart ischemia* and reperfusion result in necrosis and cardiomyocyte death, and preven-tion of apoptosis, the self-programmed death of these cells, may be an important approach to treat heart diseases. One possibility is the transfer of vascular endothelial growth factor *(VEGF)* gene to the arteries and heart muscle.

Other Diseases

Antagonists to inflammatory mediators, such as cytokines and others, can be used also in the treatment of *arthritis* and *asthma*. Destruction of cells in the pancreas that produce insulin causes *diabetes*, and the genetic therapy approach is to transfect fibroblasts with the insulin gene followed by their reimplantation. The problem, however, is the correlation of insulin release with food intake. The gene for calcitonin, a protein which regulates bone metabolism, is being studied in prevention of *osteoporosis*.

Aging is often explained as free radical and oxidative damage to proteins, lipids, and DNA. Overexpressing antioxidant enzymes, such as heme oxygenase, catalase, and superoxide dismutase, may reduce the oxidative damage.

In principle, beyond the treatment of diseases there is a possibility that some individuals may benefit from preventive therapy; for instance, humans do not have enzymes to degrade uric acid which can result in kidney stones. Carnivorous animals, such as dogs, however, can digest uric acid and introduction of genes encoding for such enzymes may be beneficial to people with high risk of developing diseases correlated with high levels of uric acid, including gout.

■ SUMMARY

In this chapter several different strategies in gene therapy as well as the most studied diseases were described. Blockage of cell or vital growth by binding antisequences nucleic acids will be discussed in Chapter 12. For more information, an interested reader is referred to the list of general and specific references.

Many diseases originate in mutations of genes. Gene therapy is a medical treatment that is trying to correct the disease or disorder on a molecular level. If the correct gene can be inserted or a mutant gene turned off, the disease as well as its cause may be eliminated.

■ ADDITIONAL READING

Boulikas, T., The phosphorylation connection to cancer, *Int. J. Oncol.*, 6, 271–278, 1995.

Levine, F., Friedmann T., Gene therapy, *AJDC*, 147, 1167–1174, 1993.

Many authors in a series of papers in *Trends in Genetics (TIG)*, 10, in April, May, and June issues of 1994.

Morsy, M.A., Mitani, K., Clemens, P., Caskey, T., Progress toward human gene therapy, *JAMA*, 270, 2338–2345, 1993.

Silverman, E., *Gene Therapy: An Investors Guide*, Prime Charter Ltd., New York, 1994.

NUCLEIC ACIDS

3

Nucleic acids are macromolecules that store and carry genetic information. Deoxyribonucleic acid (DNA) contains the complete genetic information that specifies the structure of all the proteins and ribonucleic acids of the organism. It determines in space and time the biosynthesis, activity, and individuality of a given organism during its life. Ribonucleic acid (RNA) normally carries information stored in DNA to the protein production sites. Genetic information is coded in the sequence of four different bases attached to the molecular backbone in a specific order.

Genetic information is conserved by replication of DNA, which maintains this information, and by transcription and translation, which via RNA results in the synthesis of the encoded proteins (Figure 3-1).

The size of a genome can vary from small chromosomes of a virus containing around 5000 base pairs (bp), to around 4 million for *Escherichia coli,* while the 46 human chromosomes contain coding for almost 10^5 different proteins encoded in about 3 billion bp. It is estimated that approximately 10 trillion cells of the human body contain about 100,000 genes each. Differential transcription of genes during embriogenesis and between different cell types and organs is responsible for maintaining the specialization of the cell types. However, in humans around 97% of the DNA does not code for any proteins. It is likely that this DNA, which is often called junk DNA, is not (completely) wasteful and that it contains important information about temporal and structural events, such as regulation of gene expression. Some of it forms telomers which protect the ends of chromosomes and centromers which are attachment sites for spindles. Gene regulators turn on the right genes, at the right places, at the right times and allow, in addition, genes to be switched on and off by some environmental factors, such as concentration changes of some peptides, proteins, hormones, or simple molecules, like sugars. Some of the DNA stretches may act as membrane (nuclear matrix) attachment sites, while others may be important in DNA packaging. The length of the junk DNA varies from species to species. For instance, salamanders have 40 times longer DNA than humans while puffin fish have an eight-fold shorter genome than similar vertebrates (Holmes, 1995).

In gene therapy, the major interest is in DNA and cDNA (complementary DNA which is sequences of DNA that encode particular proteins). Therefore, we shall briefly introduce DNA, from its biological, chemical,

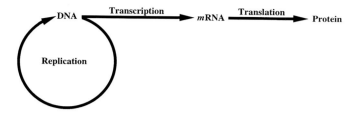

Figure 3-1   Transcription describes a process in which a particular RNA complementary to the DNA template is synthesized from nucleotides with the help of enzymes and energy from ATP. In the translation process amino acids are linked into proteins in ribosomes with the help of enzymes and according to the RNA code. Replication produces daughter DNA molecules with the same structure. Very complex enzymes ensure extraordinary fidelity of the transmission of genetic information to offspring. It is estimated that spontaneous mutations occur at a rate of less than 1 per billion base pairs per division. The great accuracy of replication is based on several levels of control, from nonpolymerization of improper base, excision nucleases, and by heteroduplex repair. (Adapted from Kunkel, T., *J. Biol. Chem.*, 267, 18251–18254, 1992. Figure courtesy of Stan Hansen.)

and physical viewpoint which will enable us to appreciate the complexity of genosomes as well as the thermodynamics and kinetics of DNA interactions with liposomes.

DNA STRUCTURE AND CONFORMATION

Nucleotides are molecules that contain a nitrogenous base, a pentose, and phosphoric acid. Bases can be purines or pyrimidines. The sugar group in DNA is deoxyribose and is ribose in RNA, as shown in Figure 3-2. DNA contains two purines, adenine (A) and guanine (G), and two pyrimidines, cytosine (C) and thymine (T), while RNA contains uracil (U) instead of thymine. DNA is composed of a linear sequence of nucleotides that are joined together through phosphodiester linkages spanning the 5′-hydroxyl group of pentose with the 3′-hydroxyl group of the pentose of the next nucleoside. Alternating phosphate and pentose groups form the covalent backbone on which the bases are attached as side groups. Figure 3-3 shows three different presentations of the chemical structure of DNA. This linear polymer is in the helical conformation and matches with a complementary helix into a double helix, which is bound together via hydrogen bonds between bases: adenine forms two hydrogen bonds with thymine and guanine forms three with cytosine. Figure 3-4 shows the chemical structures of the four bases as well as their pairing via hydrogen bonds. Because different DNA molecules have different proportions of G≡C and A=T pairs, their physical properties differ. For instance, temperature of denaturation can vary from 60 to 95°C and

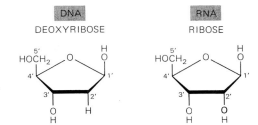

Figure 3-2 Chemical structures of deoxyribose and ribose, the building blocks of DNA and RNA, respectively.

increases with GC content. In pure polynucleotides (polyA, for example) the transition is very sharp (about 1°), while long DNA can exhibit gradual melting, with some parts of molecules being separated and others not.

$$\text{double strand} \xleftrightarrow{\;T_m\;} 2 \text{ single strands} \qquad (3\text{-}1)$$

As in the case of proteins, we can distinguish several levels of structural characterizations. The *primary structure* is the sequence of bases and is simply denoted as a train of bases, i.e., A, C, G, and T bases in a particular sequence that forms a code for a specific amino acid sequence. Three consecutive bases form a code for a particular amino acid (at $3^4 = 64$ possibilities there are enough codes for 20 amino acids). Figure 3-5 shows a model presentation of DNA and its dimensions. Work with concentrated solutions can be different due to adsorption, viscosity and its macroscopic character as is shown in solution (Figure 3-5) where DNA molecules are spooled around a pipette.

The *secondary structure* describes the structure of the entire DNA molecule. Normally, this is a double helix, in which pairs of bases lie flat and are stacked one on top of the other and a "helical staircase" is formed between the two helical strands. On the outside, however, two helical grooves are formed: the wider one is called the major groove and the smaller one the minor groove. The two chains have different polarities because one strand of the internucleotide linkage is $3' \rightarrow 5'$ and the opposite in the other one. The structure of the helix can vary. In normal solutions, as well as in *in vivo* conditions, the bases are more or less perpendicular to the backbone helix. The pitch of the helix contains approximately 10 bp and is, at segment length of 0.34 nm, 3.4 nm long (because each segment is 0.34 nm long). The twist along the helical direction is 36°/bp as schematically shown in Figure 3-5. This is called the B structure and is normally present in solutions. At higher ionic strengths and lower humidities DNA forms A and C structures in which the inclination of base pairs against the helix director changes from the perpendicular. The pitch length is normally shorter and can contain 11 residues per turn. In the A structure the tilt angle is 20° and the structure has a cylindrical hole, parallel to the direction of the helical strands, in its interior. The tilted structure has a shorter longitudinal

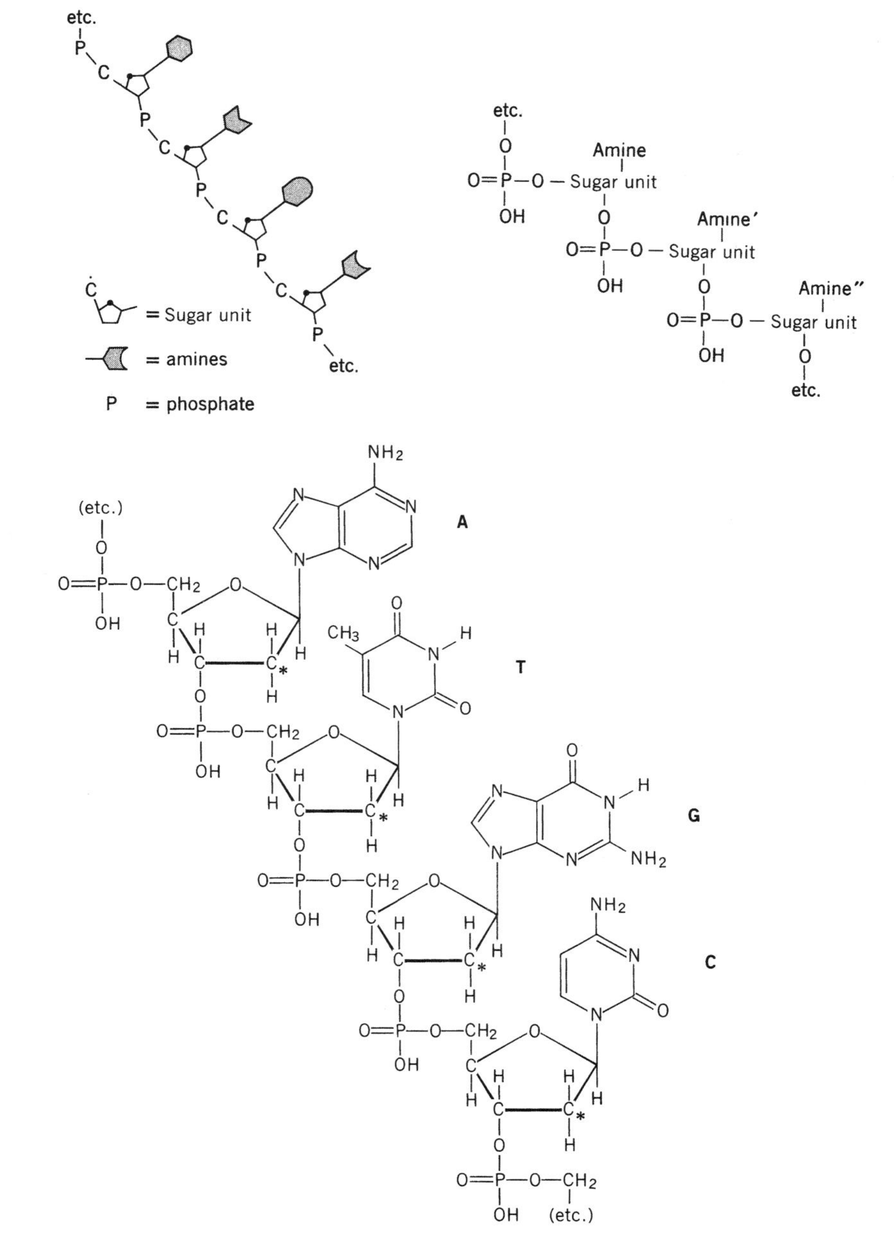

Figure 3-3 DNA in schematic and chemical structure presentation.

dimension per base pair and an intrinsic cavity in the helix. The diameter of the C structure is around 2.5 nm, while in normal B conformation it is around 2 nm. These structures, including another tilted C configuration (tilt 6°), are not very important in the biochemistry of life but may be

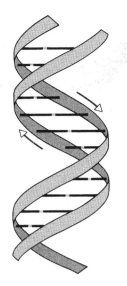

Figure 3-4   Chemical structures of the four bases and their pairing via hydrogen bonds and organization in a double helix.

important in the complexation with cationic lipids where strong electrostatic interactions may cause dehydration and lead to conformational changes.

A, B, and C structures are right-handed. In addition, a left-handed helix was discovered (for instance, polyGC in high salt) and was termed the Z configuration. It forms a wider major groove and has a zigzag helix, which is narrower (1.8 nm) and contains 12 bp/turn. One possible biological role of left-handedness may be to relieve the strain in supercoiled DNA, in a similar way as do single-stranded regions (palindromes), and can serve as sites for recombination. An important difference in these formulations is the dimensions of major and minor grooves which may significantly affect interactions as well as influence supercoiling properties. Recent spectroscopic observations indicate that DNA is not a static structure but that it is in a continuous dynamic equilibrium with deformations such as twisting, bending, and internal distortions. This is in line with the opinion that alternative structures to the right-handed double helix, such as left-handed DNA, triple-helical DNA, cruciform structures, and quadruplex DNA are transiently present in all mammalian cells and support important regulatory functions.

In the beginning, researchers considered that hydrogen bonds between base pairs are by far the dominant interaction determining the structure of DNA. Current opinion is that hydrophobic forces between base pairs and hydration forces are more important than previously thought. Other forces important in these systems on a colloidal level are osmotic, electrostatic, electrodynamic (ion correlation attraction), and,

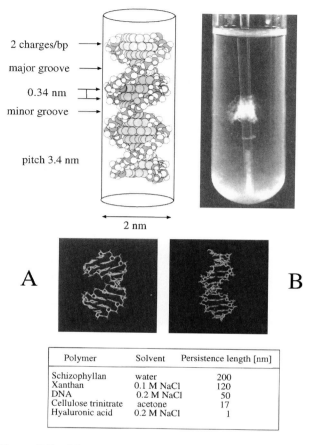

2 charges/bp

major groove

0.34 nm

minor groove

pitch 3.4 nm

2 nm

A

B

Polymer	Solvent	Persistence length [nm]
Schizophyllan	water	200
Xanthan	0.1 M NaCl	120
DNA	0.2 M NaCl	50
Cellulose trinitrate	acetone	17
Hyaluronic acid	0.2 M NaCl	1

Figure 3-5 Schematic presentation of DNA double helix with dimensions. On the right, spooling of a very long DNA condensed with ethanol around a Pasteur pipette is shown. Threads of condensed DNA can be observed and the milky appearance indicates light scattering due to invisible colloidal ribbons. Below, two different conformations are shown. The rigidity of DNA is compared with some other polymers in the table on the bottom.

possibly, undulation forces. In the presence of other colloidal particles van der Waals attraction, attractive or repulsive electrostatic forces, as well as specific interactions (intercalation, steric interactions), are also important.

The *tertiary structure* distinguishes between linear and cyclic forms. Open or linear forms are produced by double-strand breaks, while nicked DNA is cyclic with one strand broken. Cyclic forms can have a supercoiled (superhelical) conformation. Catenated circles are linked dimers or trimers in which closed rings are interlocked. Large-scale conformational properties also include supercoiling, looping, catenation, and knotting and strongly depend on ionic conditions in the solution. Additionally,

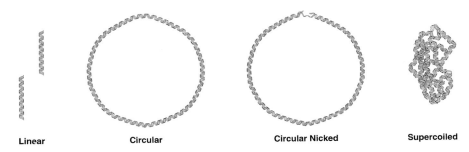

| Linear | Circular | Circular Nicked | Supercoiled |

Figure 3-6   Several different forms of DNA: linear, circular, nicked (closed and relaxed with a nick), and supercoiled. (Courtesy of Stan Hansen.)

supercoiling causes twist (sometimes called writhe and twist) which can lead to the formation of sequence-specific binding sites for various proteins (Trifonov, 1991). While the majority of the extrachromosomal DNA in living cells is circular, some viruses have linear plasmids typically ~2000 bp in length. Figure 3-6 shows some of the possible DNA forms in solution.

Satellite DNA contains very short sequences which are repeats or inverted repeats. They form circular molecules and hairpin loops (palindromes) which may also be important for organization of DNA within chromosomes and for maintaining its structural integrity.

Palindromes are specific regions in eukaryotic DNA containing inverse repetitions of base sequences (palindrome means a sentence or phrase which is the same if read backward, such as "a toyota"). They pair and form various loops, such as cruciforms (crosslike loops) and similar structures. They may be regulatory/packing or attachment sequences.

DNA exists in aqueous solutions in linear, circular (closed or relaxed with a nick), or supercoiled conformation which can be approximated, depending on the length, by a random coil structure or a rigid wormlike structure. Thermodynamic properties of DNA in solution can be approximated by relatively simple polyelectrolyte theories. Due to complete ionization at physiological pH, DNA is a semirigid rodlike polymer because this conformation maximizes the charge separation.

For molecules shorter than about 1 kb, we can imagine DNA as a flexible rod while longer molecules resemble stiff wormlike coils (random coil of semirigid polymer with excluded volume effects). Persistence length, i.e., the length in which DNA can bend for half a turn at energy of 1 kT (k is Boltzmann constant, T temperature) is, at low ionic strengths, about 50 to 70 nm and about 35 nm at higher ionic strengths. For specific anisotropic charge neutralization the turns may be even sharper. Persistence length (l_p) of DNA that indicates the stiffness of the polymer in good solvent is characteristic of a semirigid polymer. Rigid polymers, such as schizophyllan and xanthan have persistence lengths around 200 and 120 nm, while very flexible hyaluronic acid is characterized by l_p of 1 nm (Podgornik et al., 1995).

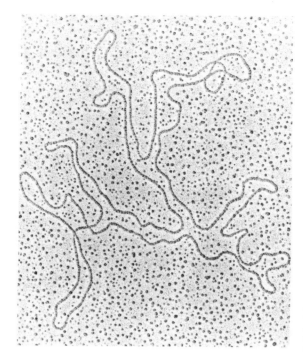

Figure 3-7 Electron micrograph of a bacterial plasmid. Contour length is around 17 μm.

It was shown that upon neutralization or shielding of this charge DNA collapses into a condensed particle, as will be discussed below.

To get the idea of the size of DNA we shall use the numbers presented above to make some estimates of the DNA size. Lambda DNA is a typical viral DNA and is about 50 kb long. Fully extended this yields ~170 μm linear plasmid or circular plasmid with radius of <30,000 nm. Figure 3-7 shows a bacterial plasmid. *E. coli* genome is at about 4 million nucleotide pairs, which encode approximately 3000 genes, around 1.4 mm long. Human genome is at 3×10^9 bp at 0.34 nm each around a meter in length, if extended. Yet all this material fits into a cell nucleus which is between 5 and 8 μm in diameter. Considering that we have approximately 10^{13} cells which carry the genome we can estimate that the length of DNA in our bodies equals 60 times the distance from Earth to the Sun.

■ DNA STABILITY AND INTERACTIONS

In general, on the chemical level, DNA molecules are, in contrast to RNA, rather stable chemically. DNA (especially longer-chain molecules) can be physically damaged by pipetting, (vigorous) mixing, agitation, freeze-thawing, and so on. For plasmids below 15 MDa and at concentrations used in gene therapy, DNA is rather robust and does not break upon stirring (Hershey and Burgi, 1960). At concentrations above few micromolar it is more stable and exhibits the so-called self-protecting effect.

In biological samples one must be careful to inhibit DNA degradative enzymes, while, with respect to temperature stability, oxidation, and reduction, careful work within normal T and pH ranges normally suffices. Systemically injected DNA and extracellular DNA are rapidly cleaved by DNases present in the bloodstream. RNA is much less stable.

DNA molecules are well hydrated. At least nine to ten water molecules are associated with each nucleotide in the first hydration shell. Water molecules form a helical spine in the narrower minor groove, while in the major groove no structured water networks are present because of large hydrophobic thymine methyl groups. Ribbons of water molecules, however, were found in the major groove in crystalline DNA as well as in solution (B conformation). Now it is believed that well-ordered water molecules are an integral part of DNA structure and can also mediate interactions. The dehydration energy also reduces the negative enthalpy associated with site-specific electrostatic interactions. Counterions can form an ionic atmosphere around the negatively charged DNA cylinders rather than bind to singular charges.

Small molecules can interact with DNA either electrostatically, via hydrophobic interaction, hydrogen bonding, or sterically. The latter includes intercalation, binding to the minor or major groove, and any combination of these. Cross-linking and covalent bonding is also possible upon nucleophilic interaction. This can be very useful for labeling DNA if covalent bonding can be induced by a laser pulse. Some of these interactions are nonspecific, while some others can be very specific. Many anticancer drugs, antibiotics and some other drug molecules function by binding to DNA by one of those mechanisms and at the level of replication, transcription, or translation halt the information readout, as will be briefly discussed below.

A very important area in medicinal chemistry is the interaction of DNA with drugs. Four major groups of drugs as determined by their interactions with DNA can be identified: (1) alkylating agents (mitomycin C, cisplatin), (2) DNA strand-breaking compounds (bleomycin), (3) intercalating agents (doxorubicin, actinomycin D), and (4) drugs that modify DNA in the minor groove. The detailed mechanism of these interactions is still not understood. For instance, the intercalation mechanism of doxorubicin was confirmed by X-ray structure analysis, but was on the other hand never fully supported by structure–activity relationships. Differences were explained by other effects such as the effect on cell membrane and the oxidative DNA damage mechanism. It is also likely that localization in the DNA helix becomes important only at certain steps, such as in topological processing of DNA (Hurley, 1989).

It is expected, however, that new methods in structural analysis (high-resolution X-rays and synchrotron radiation, high-field multidimensional NMR), computational chemistry, and molecular biology (DNA sequencing, cloning) will improve understanding of the interactions leading to novel drugs.

In biological systems, DNA molecules interact with a variety of proteins. Regulatory proteins bind to highly specific sequences and control the expression of a particular gene. Other regulatory proteins perform more-general tasks, such as initiation of transcription, by binding to the specific sequence of the promoter. Repair proteins can excise damaged DNA and join breaks, while structural proteins maintain the integrity of folding. Additionally, some special DNA sequences allow for bending. For instance, the A_6 tract (six repetitive adenine bases) can bend DNA for 20° at a length of approximately 2 nm, as compared with a persistence length of 50 nm. Some proteins, such as transcription activator proteins, can induce high curvature turns via interactions with phosphate groups. Binding energies between protein and DNA can be sufficient to overcome a barrier to local DNA deformation. Processing proteins, like polymerases, can control secondary structure.

Macromolecules and polymers interact with nucleic acids in a similar way. Formation of triple and quadruple helices is also possible. In addition, other colloidal forces may play a role, such as bridging and van der Waals forces, which often precipitate such macromolecular solutions. Excluded volume effects can separate a DNA solution from a solution of neutral polymer, such as polyethylene oxide, as well as anionic polyelectrolyte.

Interactions with cationic detergents have been studied since the early 1960s. At low detergent concentrations the binding of DDAB and TDAB to DNA was found to be highly cooperative (Hagakawa et al., 1983). Longer hydrocarbon chains exhibited higher binding constants in the presence and absence of salt (5400 vs. 1600 M^{-1} in salt-free and 80 vs. 20 M^{-1} in 0.01 M NaCl). At higher concentrations of cationic detergents, ordered structures, consisting of interlocked hexagonal lattices of DNA and rodlike micelles, were observed (Ghirlando, 1991). In the case of some other detergents, amorphous precipitates result.

Mixtures of DNA and oppositely charged micelles or colloidal particles exhibit solubility gaps at particular ratios, normally at equal charges, i.e., when concentrations of negative and positive charges are balanced (Li et al., 1994; 1995). This is a rather general phenomenon and was also observed, for instance, in the mixtures of anionic and cationic liposomes (Lasic, unpublished).

In contrast to highly specific interactions of DNA with functional proteins, which are based also on steric forces and hydrogen bonding, in the genosome formation the interactions seem to be nonspecific. Because the major interaction is electrostatic, there is not much interaction between DNA and nonionic or neutral liposomes. Typically, upon mixing solutions no changes in turbidity or particle sizes can be detected, while after several tens of hours a precipitate is observed. Even dilute solutions of DNA and neutral liposomes eventually flocculate indicating some other weak attractive force, perhaps hydrophobic attraction.

By adding some metal ions, polyamines, or cationic polyelectrolytes which can act as bridging agents between negatively charged DNA and negatively charged liposomes, one can bind, and eventually entrap, DNA into colloidal particles. For instance, DNA has been shown to interact with neutral lecithin liposomes. Simple hydration of thin lecithin films with a DNA solution (10 kb) resulted in partial DNA encapsulation (Hoffman et al., 1978). Although lecithin vesicles are zwitterionic, higher salt concentration dissociated the complex indicating the presence of electrostatic or electrodynamic forces. At a weight ratio of lecithin to DNA above 500, 90% of DNA was associated with liposomes and protected against the action of DNase. Higher encapsulation efficiencies were achieved when divalent cations were present. The efficiency of DNA binding decreased in the order Mn > Ca > Mg, as well as with decreasing DNA length. Magnetic resonance studies indicated that cations bridged phosphate groups on DNA and liposomes (Bichenikov et al., 1988). Increasing lipid concentrations caused DNA encapsulation in the complex. Venanzi and co-workers (1993) also reported that preincubation of phosphatidylcholine or sphingomyelin with supercoiled DNA followed by addition of Mg^{2+} (50 mM) ions could efficiently entrap DNA, especially at higher lipid-to-DNA (50:1 w/w) ratios.

Similarly, triple complexes using negatively charged liposomes, DNA, and polyvalent cations or polycations were prepared. At special ratios stable colloidal solutions could be obtained (Lasic and Leung, unpublished). While these complexes possibly can have low biological toxicity, their large size and instability upon dilution/administration may limit their potential as gene delivery systems.

Interestingly, there are practically no van der Waals attractive forces between DNA molecules. This suggests that one can also prepare rather high concentrations of these molecules in salt solutions. At higher concentrations, when the excluded volume effects, combined with electrostatic and hydration repulsion, become important, this causes orientation of molecules in a fluid phase and formation of liquid crystals. At still higher concentrations DNA crystallizes as is schematically shown in Figure 3-8.

Typically, isotropic solutions of long-fragment DNA (approximately >1 μm in length) change at concentration c >15 to 20 mg/mL into a cholesteric liquid crystalline phase, which at lower water content transforms into a columnar hexagonal phase (Leforestier and Livolant, 1996). Both of these phases have been observed in some chromosomes and bacteriophages and in some sperm heads, respectively. For short-fragment DNA (nucleosomal DNA = 146 bp or about 50 nm) the same transition occurs at 160 mg/mL. Short-fragment DNA transforms upon dehydration into a hexagonal columnar crystal and then into an orthorhombic three-dimensional crystal. It stays in the B conformation all the time. Long-fragment DNA makes a B-to-A transition before transforming into a three-dimensional lattice. The sequence of mesophases in long DNA appears to be different that the one in short DNA (Podgornik et al., 1995).

Recently, small-angle X-ray diffraction and polarizing optical microscopy studies have revealed that bacterial plasmids form liquid crystalline

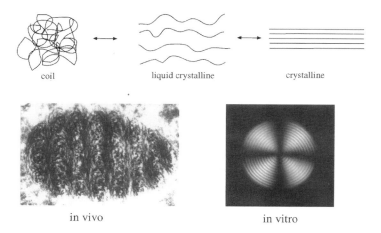

coil   liquid crystalline   crystalline

in vivo   in vitro

Figure 3-8   Upon increasing the concentration, random coils of DNA align into liquid crystalline phases which at lower water content crystallize. Below, DNA can form ordered structures *in vivo* and *in vitro*. (Courtesy of R. Podgornik.)

mesophases in bacteria (Reich et al., 1994). Bacteria may contain over 1000 plasmids which may exceed the amount of DNA in chromosomes. Efficient packing is therefore a necessity. A segregation of supercoiled plasmids was found, and dense clusters have shown a long-range order of 5.15 nm. This indicates liquid crystalline organization at local DNA concentrations about 20 mg/mL. It was shown that supercoiled DNA exhibits this transition to a cholesteric liquid crystalline phase at much lower concentrations, and it is possible that DNA supercoiling promotes DNA segregation and supramolecular packing in analogy with liquid crytalline phases where chirality of molecules determines the density of cholesteric mesophases. Native closed circular DNA exhibits negative, right-handed supercoiling which upon temperature increase or pH-induced partial melting decreases twist, which results in a significant increase of plasmid diameter which, in turn, affects plasmid packing.

■■■ THEORETICAL DESCRIPTION OF DNA

Several different theories have been proposed to explain the behavior of DNA. They range from polymer and polyelectrolyte theories to statistical mechanics and computer simulations.

Statistical Thermodynamic Models and Molecular Dynamics

Currently, molecular dynamics simulations are frequently used to describe polymer behavior. The movements of atoms are described by Newton dynamics in a potential energy surface determined by a particular model. Typical approach is a grand canonical Monte Carlo simulation (Olmsted et al., 1989). Due to long computational times, oligonucleotides are normally modeled. The dodecane duplex (d(CGCGAATTCGCG)$_2$) is the most studied oligonucleotide, both theoretically and experimentally (NMR, X-ray scattering, other spectroscopic and diffraction techniques). Initial structure is often taken from crystallographic data, and its energy is minimized (relaxed) in a given potential field. In addition to spatial and temporal profile of the distribution of DNA and solvent atoms, interactions with ions, molecules or drugs are studied in such conditions. Additionally, molecular deformations, and from them bending and torsion moduli can be determined (Beveridge and Gashinekar, 1994).

A typical result are stereoviews of a section of DNA with water molecules and counterions. These images of structure and ion and solvent distribution can be studied in time to elucidate dynamical properties of the system, such as torsional and angular flexibility, motion of solvent molecules and similar. Additionally, parameters such as translational and rotational diffusion coefficients, persistance length, or bending modulus can be modeled and compared to experimental and theoretical results. One has to be aware, however, that despite very long calculation times, for 5 bp oligonucleotide with several hundred water molecules and counterions almost a day of Cray time is needed (what corresponds to 6 months of calculation on a VAX machine), many assumptions have to be made in describing potentials and interactions (Seibel et al., 1985). Topological properties of DNA, especially its supercoiling and knotting, are also very interesting. Theoretical models from biomolecular folding were used to investigate supercoiling of DNA and its knotting. Computer simulations find minimal energy conformations and can give insight into kinetics of their transformations. The knotting seems to be related to collective bending and twisting modes of the molecule (Schlick and Olson, 1992).

These methods, which treat the system as an ensemble of DNA, small ions and water molecules and all its complexity by Monte Carlo or molecular dynamics methods, therefore require extremely powerful computers and can be useful to investigate fine structural details of DNA and its surroundings under fixed conditions. For calculating free energy of the system, however, such methods are not realistic at present. For instance, a conformational study showed that electrostatic effects which influence the B-Z form transition are of the order of hundredths of kT per base pair and obviously such accuracy cannot be obtained by first principles (Frank-Kamenitskii et al., 1987). For macroscopic description of these systems, therefore, thermodynamic models based on electrostatic interactions, which can be described by Poisson equation, are used and if proper approximations are used, give surprisingly good agreements with experimental data.

Polyelectrolyte Models

Polyelectrolyte theories, one of which we shall briefly present below, were very popular to describe the structure and behavior of DNA in solution. The aim of such theories is to present a model of DNA based on molecular level assumptions and *a priori* to predict results of certain measurements, such as activity and osmotic coefficients of counterions, enthalpies of mixing and other thermodynamic parameters. It turned out that a rather simple concept, namely phase and conformational transitions of a linear, rigid (persistence length ≫ Debye length) array of charges and surrounded by a cloud of counterions which relieve part of the electrostatic stress on the chain, as introduced by Manning (1978), could describe properties with 30 to 50% accuracy, a rather good agreement for its simplicity. More complex models, such as a cell model of poly-electrolytes, did not add further improvements, possibly due to the fact that some errors cancelled in the simple model. In contrast to these models which assume that electrostatic interactions are predominant and are the only ones taken into account, it is becoming clear that other interactions are also important. Realistic solution theory should encompass interactions of all ions with the solvent as well as van der Waals inter-actions and hydrogen bonding and hydrophobic effect. This brings about very complex models and because each system would have to be modeled separately we are not aware of general models that could be useful for describing DNA in solution more precisely.

As in other polyelectrolyte solutions, counterions that shield the linear array of negative charges with a valency z separated by d can bind site specifically or form an ionic atmosphere. None of the simple models include site specific binding and they treat counterion condensation as a free movement of counterions in a bound volume. Thermodynamic properties and interactions depend on this phenomenon and a dimen-sionless parameter ξ, defined as

$$\xi = z^2 e^2 / \varepsilon \, kTd .\qquad\qquad (3-2)$$

where z is the valence of counterion and ε is solvent dielectric constant can describe counterion capture into ionic atmosphere. Manning (1978) showed that there is counterion condensation only for $\xi > 1$. Interestingly, the amount of condensation does not depend on the ionic strength. From DNA at 25°C ξ = 0.714 nm and the fraction of condensed counterions can be calculated from

$$\theta = 1 - 1/\xi/z .\qquad\qquad (3-3)$$

DNA in B conformation has 2 charges per .34 nm; hence d = 0.17 nm, ξ = 4.2 and θ = 0.76 which means that 76% of the counterions form an ionic cloud in the case of a univalent counterion. Furthermore, the net charge, 1–θ, equals d/7.14 indicating that there is one net charge per 0.714 nm. We can substitute this net charge with e in the Poisson–Boltz-mann equation and calculate electrostatic free energy and use it for further evaluation of the solution behavior of DNA. This is the so-called weakly charged polyion approach and Debye-Huckel approximation can be used because $|\Psi(r)| \ll 1$ (in kT units). Potential at a distance r from the polyion with radius can be calculated from

$$\Psi''(r) + (1/r)\,\Psi'(r) = \kappa^2\,\Psi(r) \tag{3-4}$$

where κ^{-1} is Debye length, r_D, which can be expressed by Bjerrum length $1_B = e^2/\varepsilon kT$ as

$$\kappa^{-1} = r_D = \left(8\pi 1_B c_o\right)^{-1/2} = \left(\varepsilon kT/e^2\; 8\pi\; c_o\right)^{-1/2} \tag{3-5}$$

and the boundary conditions are

$$\Psi'(a) = 2\xi/a \;\text{ and }\; \Psi(R) = 0. \tag{3-6}$$

The solution of the equation is

$$\Psi(r) = -2\,\xi\,\left(K_0(\kappa r)/K_1(\xi a)\right) \tag{3-7}$$

where $K_m(x)$ is a modified Bessel function (Frank-Kamenitskii et al., 1987).

From the known potential we can calculate electrostatic free energy and a relatively simple result can be obtained (Manning, 1978):

$$G_{el} = -R_g T/\xi \cdot \ln\left[1 - \exp(-\kappa d)\right] \tag{3-8}$$

and for diluted solutions, assuming that $\kappa d \ll 1$

$$G_{el} = -R_g T/\xi \cdot \ln(-\kappa d) \tag{3-9}$$

Debye length is defined in univalent electrolyte solution as

$$\kappa^2 = 8\pi 10^{-3} L_A \left(e^2/\varepsilon\; kT\right) I \tag{3-10}$$

where I is ionic strength and L Avogadro's number and can be approximated by

$$\kappa = 3.3(I)^{1/2}\; \text{nm}^{-1} \tag{3-11}$$

which gives 0.95 nm in biological fluids and $\kappa d = 0.88$.

This model assumes only atmospheric binding of counterions. Site specific binding is not taken into account. Electrostatic free energy would try to compensate all the charges and that would lead to complete neutralization which would cause spontaneous bending, folding and condensation (self-collapse, "collapsing upon itself") of DNA. That would be the hypothetical case at absolute zero temperature. A term which opposes this is entropy and free energy of such system is described as a sum of electrostatic and mixing entropy terms, which describes counterions and water. The first term therefore drives to complete binding and the last one to complete dissociation; the balance between the two determines the actual fraction of counterion condensation. Entropic contributions to free energy include mixing of free cations, bound cations, and solvent molecules and can be expressed as

$$G_{mix} = \theta \ln \left(1000\theta/cV\right) \qquad (3\text{-}12)$$

where θ is a fraction of ions associated with each charge, c concentration of counterions, and V the volume of the region surrounding the DNA within which cations are bound (Manning, 1978).

According to the condensation model, the driving force for DNA behavior in solution is the counterion diffusion potential which, due to electrostatic attraction, cannot diffuse freely. DNA tends to relieve its stress originating in the repulsion of phosphate groups and this is accomplished by the counterion atmosphere. From Equation 3-3 we can see that higher valence ions are much more effective in relieving this stress, due to stronger interaction and smaller loss in entropy upon neutralizing equal charge. When more than 90% of the negative charge is compensated, DNA can spontaneously condense. This model therefore does not distinguish between various polyvalent cations, polycations or positively charged polyelectrolytes. It does not assume dehydration upon binding and therefore DNA condensates produced upon any of the above agents should be similar and redissociable upon increasing salt concentration above 1.2 M NaCl what was indeed observed experimentally (Leung and Lasic, unpublished).

Using this theory, we can get more insight in the local geometry, melting and other properties of DNA. Recent developments in the theoretical treatments of electrostatic interactions in macromolecular solutions added to charge–charge interactions also terms due to charge–solvent interactions. However, due to complexity and nonuniversality of such models, it seems that there is not much interest in their development.

This theory, however, cannot account for the differential effects of counterions. For instance, the affinity of DNA for divalent cations decreases in the order Ca > Mg > Co > Mn and obviously other effects are important. These include geometric terms in the Poisson–Boltzmann equation as well as non-electrostatic effects, including steric interactions, hydrophobic effect and other entropic contributions.

It was shown however, that Debye-Huckel approximation is not good enough for DNA and that better agreement with experiments and numerical solutions can be obtained by using more rigorous electrostatic approach (Frank-Kamenitskii et al., 1987).

A more sophisticated theory for the description of polyelectrolyte behavior was described by the cell model (Katchalsky, 1976). However, it was found to be applicable mostly in dilute solutions of rigid polymers and not for the solutions of DNA. However, we can use the electrostatic potential around the rigid rod to describe electrostatic behavior of short rodlike segments of DNA, by using the Poisson–Boltzmann equation, which describes electric potential around charge(s) at a distance r

$$\Delta\Psi = -\left(4\,\pi\,e_o/\varepsilon\right)\Sigma\,n\,z\,\exp\left(-z\,e_o\,\Psi\left(r\right)/kT\right) \qquad (3\text{-}13)$$

where Δ is Laplace operator. While for flat surfaces one can use $\Delta\Psi = \partial^2\Psi/\partial x^2$ and for spherical symmetry one can express the Laplace operator in spherical coordinates, for rodlike symmetry the introduction of cylindrical coordinates yields

$$\left(1/r\right)d/dr\left(r\,d\Psi/dr\right) = -\left(4\,\pi\,e_o/\varepsilon\right)\Sigma\,n\,z\,\exp\left(-z\,e_o\,\Psi\left(r\right)/kT\right) \quad (3\text{-}14)$$

and using boundary conditions (potential is zero at r = ∞ and equals surface charge at r = a, where a is the radius of the polymer rod) one gets the following solution (Fuoss et al., 1951; Dolar, 1972)

$$\Psi = -kT/e_o\ \ln\left\{2\beta^2/\kappa\ \cos^2\left(\beta\ln\left(r/a\right)-C\right)\right\} \qquad (3\text{-}15)$$

where the integration constants β and C are given as

$$\xi = z^2 e^2/\varepsilon\,kTd = 1+\beta^2/\left(1+\beta\ ctg\ \beta\,\gamma\right) \qquad (3\text{-}16)$$

$$C = arctg\ \left(\xi-1\right)/\beta\ ,\ ar \qquad (3\text{-}17)$$

$$\gamma = \ln\left(R/a\right) \qquad (3\text{-}18)$$

where R is the distance where the potential from the polyion fades away. This boundary condition is not well defined at higher concentrations (neighboring molecule is closer than R) and therefore the deviations of experimental data and theoretical predictions may be above 20 to 30% at higher concentrations and at lower ionic strengths.

For low ionic strengths Poisson–Boltzmann equation can be written as:

$$\Psi''\left(r\right)+\left(1/r\right)\Psi'\left(r\right) = \kappa^2\ sh\,\Psi\left(r\right) \qquad (3\text{-}19)$$

and the boundary conditions are $\Psi'(a) = 2\xi/a$ and $\Psi(R) = 0$. The solution can be approximated for low ionic strengths as

$$\Psi(a) = 2\xi \ln(\xi a), \qquad\qquad \xi < 1 \qquad\qquad (3\text{-}20)$$

$$\Psi(a) = 2\ln(\xi a) - \ln\left[4(\xi - 1)^2\right], \quad \xi > 1 \qquad (3\text{-}21)$$

and it was shown that at $c_0 = 0.1$ M the potential is correct within 5% as compared to the numerical calculation of Equation 3-16.

A geometric parameter appears in these equations through the parameter ξ which is the dimensionless charge per unit length. Note that $\xi = 1_B/d$, where d is the separation between charges and that Debye length contains L_B. For instance, in studies of B-Z configuration transition one has 2d = 0.34 nm and correspondingly at room temperature $\xi = 4.2$ for the B conformation and 2d = 0.37 nm and $\xi = 3.9$ for the Z form.

For the absence of salt Katchalsky et al. (1976) derived equation

$$\Psi''(r) + (1/r)\Psi'(r) = \left((1/r)d/dr\left(r\, d\Psi/dr\right)\right) = -0.5\,p^2\,e^{-\Psi(r)} \qquad (3\text{-}22)$$

where parameter p is proportional to the outer radius R_o of the cell where the potential is zero (Frank-Kamenetskii et al., 1987). This equation can be solved analytically and potential decays as a logarithm of distance

$$\Psi(r) = \ln\left[C'\left(1_B c^+\right)^2 r^2 \cos^2\left(C'' \ln r\right)\right] \qquad (3\text{-}23)$$

where C' and C'' are integration constants which can be obtained from the boundary conditions (Frank-Kamenetskii et al., 1987).

Currently it is accepted that Debye Huckel approximation, despite its attractive simplification, is too simplified and that the distinction between condensed and noncondensed counterions does not reflect physical reality. Because Poisson–Boltzmann equation also contains ad hoc assumptions, a more rigorous theory was developed, which showed that Poisson–Boltzmann equation is a much more accurate approach than Debye Huckel approximation and condensation approach used by Manning. While estimates can still be made by using the condensation theory, Poisson Boltzmann formalism is recommended for better precision. Detailed analysis of more delicate processes, such as helix-coil or B-Z transition show that the condensation theory yields even erroneous predictions (Frank-Kamenitskii et al., 1987). In conclusion, we can use condensation model for rough estimates while for more detailed analyses more rigorous treatments are required.

Empirical mechanical models would, in contrast to statistical mechanical models, define certain deformations, such as bending and torsion and define measurable constants, such as bending, elasticity, and torsion modulus to characterize minimal energy states of DNA in diluted solution. Experimentally, the elasticity of a single DNA molecule was measured in molecules attached with one end onto a cover slip by photodigoxigenin bond and at the other end had attached a magnetic bead via biotin streptavidin bond. A magnetic field was used to rotate and pull the beads and forces around piconewtons were used. It was shown that the elastic behavior is important in transcription and replication as well as in theoretical description of twisting and bending contributions which may not be harmonic and isotropic (Strick et al., 1996). Similarly, nowadays DNA is being manipulated with optical tweezers, lasers, attached to optical fibers and its mechanical properties, such as bending, stretching or unwinding can be studied.

■ DNA CONDENSATION

Bearing in mind the large size of DNA makes it apparent that special packing must occur in order to fit these long molecules into a relatively small nucleus of a cell or into a core of a virus. Typically, the diameter of the cell nucleus is around 5 to 8 μm and chromosomes contain about 50% of proteinaceous material. Figure 3-9 shows a bacteriophage T2 which released its DNA after osmotic shock. Contour length of the DNA is around 0.17 mm.

In eukaryotic cells high concentrations of DNA-binding proteins are present and complex DNA into chromatin. The most abundant are histones, which can be classified in five different groups and which contain large fractions of the basic amino acids lysine, arginine, and histidine.

Histones are small positively charged proteins (around 5000 Da) around which DNA is wound. These particles are called nucleosomes and contain octamers of histones which form a short cylinder-like particle around which DNA is wound twice (at 147 bp/nucleosome). They are connected by a linker DNA and form chromatin which in electron micrographs resembles a "bead-on-a-string" structure after higher-order packing is unfolded. Nucleosomes pack into 30-nm-thick fibers which have to be further packed because this condensation decreases the size of a human gene to 1 mm and therefore has to be condensed approximately 100-fold more to fit into the cell nucleus. This allows approximately a centimeter-long molecule to be packed into a relatively small cell nucleus. Nucleosomes can also be used in the preparation of very monodisperse short DNA molecules. Linker DNA can be enzymatically cut, and after separation around 50-nm-long DNA is obtained. Milder lysis followed by separation on a gel chromatographic column can lead to dinucleosomal DNA. Condensation of DNA with histones and its packaging into a chromosome are shown in the scheme which shows the preparation of short fragment DNA (see Figure 3-10).

Bending of DNA, which is a necessary condition for its tight packing, can also be increased by specific sequences, such as the AA dinucleotide

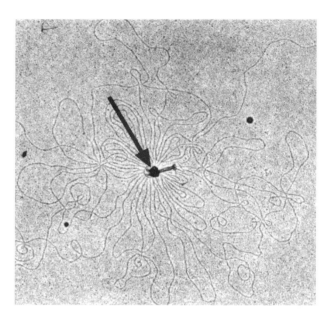

Figure 3-9 Bacteriophage T2 with released DNA upon osmotic shock. The density of DNA in the viral head (arrow) is approximately 500 mg/mL and upon placing the virus in distilled water osmotic pressure of 100 atm (1500 psi) bursts the virus. (From Kleinschmidt et al., *Biochim. Biophys. Acta,* 61, 252, 1961.)

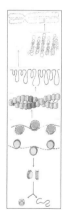

metaphase chromosome (1400 nm)

condensed section of chromosome (700 nm)

extended section of chromosome (300 nm)

chromatin fibers of packed nucleosomes (30 nm)

"beads-on-a-string" form of chromatin, linker DNA and core histones (11 nm)

nuclease digests linker DNA. released nucleosome bead (11 nm)

dissociation in high salt concentration, histone core + 146 bp DNA fragment

DNA fragment of 146 bp = 49.6 nm

Figure 3-10 Packaging of DNA in a chromosome. Reverse process is partial and sequential dissolution of the supramolecular structure which is used to produce very homogeneous DNA. At the last step, when DNA stretches between histone octamers are lysed, uniform 146-bp-long DNA is prepared. (Courtesy of R. Podgornik.)

that can become an AATT stack that acts as a wedge in the DNA. Such wedge elements introduce bending anisotropy. Highly repeated sequences may induce turns; inverted repeats (also known as palindromes) may form hairpins, while moderately repetitive DNA may be responsible for winding around histones or protamines. Additionally, bending can be enhanced if only one side of DNA has its charges neutralized (Strauss and Maher, 1995). In addition to natural DNA condensation into nucleosomes, DNA can also be condensed artificially.

A random coil of DNA occupies between 10^3 and 10^6 times the physical volume of the condensed polymer. DNA molecules can be effectively condensed (random coil–compacted particle transition) with up to a millionfold reduction in the volume occupied by a variety of cationic agents. Polyvalent positively charged species not only condense electrostatically on DNA, similarly to the monovalent ones, but also cause the collapse of the tertiary structure of DNA when more than approximately 90% of the charge is neutralized. According to the polyelectrolyte theory, monovalent ions can neutralize only about 76% of the charge and therefore cannot condense DNA (Equation 3-3). Multivalent cations (hexamine Co^{3+}, La^{3+}, etc.), polycations (spermidine^{3+}, spermine^{4+}), as well as positively charged polyelectrolytes (polylysine, polyhistidine, polyarginine, polyethyleneimine, etc.) have been found to condense DNA molecules (from 400 to 40,000 bp and longer) into either a doughnut-shaped toroid or rod. Interestingly, most condensation methods give rather similar shapes and dimensions of particles, a torus of 40 to 60 nm outer and 15 to 25 nm inner diameter and rods of 30 nm diameter and length of 200 to 300 nm for DNA molecules of very different lengths (Lerman, 1971; Laemmli, 1975; Eickbush and Moudrianakis, 1978; Bloomfield, 1991). It seems that longer DNA favors torus formation. The length of the rod resembles the circumference of the torus and the widths are also similar. Condensate contains many DNA molecules. In the case of DNA length of 1.35 kb there are approximately 25 molecules in a torus or rod; doubling the DNA size halves this number and very long DNA molecules (>30 kb) can form monomolecular condensates. Figure 3-11 shows this process and two typical structures formed. The fact that condensation of DNA is size independent probably indicates the predominance of enthalpic rather than entropic contributions to free energy. DNA can condense also in disordered particles and the structure of the condensates can change in time. Shorter segments cannot condense into toroidal or rodlike particles but form ordered liquid crystalline precipitates.

Although the main interaction is electrostatic, hydrogen bonding, hydration repulsion, and steric and hydrophobic forces also contribute to the condensation as different binding sites of different agents demonstrate. Also, the structure of the condensate depends on the nature of the condensing agent. Aliphatic diamines ($NH_3^+-(CH_2)_n-NH_3^+$) with different spacers were shown to condense DNA differently: molecules with an odd number of n were much more effective while the even ones for n = 2, 4, and 6 were not effective. Furthermore, DNA can be condensed by neutral polymers, such as polyethylene glycol, in the presence of high salt (NaCl), which form morphologically more compact aggregates. Such condensed DNA is called Ψ-DNA to indicate polymer salt induction. The mechanism of their condensation is not electrostatic but is due to phase

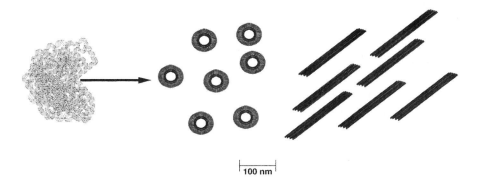

| 100 nm |

Figure 3-11   Condensation of DNA. Typical condensed structures are rodlike and toroidal particles. They are formed upon the action of various different condensing agents, such as Co^{3+} ions, spermine, spermidine, and others. In some other cases, DNA may not form regular condensates. Such condensates may structurally change in time while toroids and rods can precipitate. (Drawing courtesy of Stan Hansen.)

TABLE 3-1

BINDING ENTHALPY (CAL/MOL DNA$_P$) OF VARIOUS AGENTS TO SALMON SPERM DNA			
Agent	**Spermine**	**Poly-L-lysine**	**Mg**
ΔH	0	–300	+350

Adapted from Manning, G.S., *Q. Rev. Biophys.,* 11, 179–246, 1978.

separation. Also, the condensation can be driven by repulsive interactions of negatively charged polymers, such as polyglutamic acid.

Condensation is in general entropically driven. Very small enthalpies of the binding of various ligands to the DNA were reported (Table 3-1). The entropical contribution can be assessed also by the influence of anions. Chaotropic counterions, such as perchlorate can enhance condensation if the cation binds site specifically. The amount of (poly)cation cross-bridging is at present still not well understood. It seems that it can vary from agent to agent. Typically, binding to the minor groove releases water and the gain in binding enthalpy is balanced by the loss of dehydration energy, resulting in an entropically driven reaction. The binding into major groove, however, is normally enthalpically controlled, as is intercalation.

In addition to the above-described thermodynamic factors, kinetic factors are also very important in the condensation process. The reaction itself may take hours, and condensates can restructure after formation.

Packaging agents modulate the secondary structure of DNA into a highly ordered conformation which can exhibit special binding sites. Therefore, structural polymorphism, from specific exposure of specific sequences at specific writhe or twist sites to short segments of a non-B conformation, introduces many possibilities for the action of gene regulatory proteins.

The best-known example is RNA polymerase which has to attach to a specific site on DNA and then temporarily unzip the supercoiled DNA in which the double-stranded helix is twisted around itself. In addition to a special recognition site this also requires energy to forcefully untwist DNA and unzip the base pairs. RNA polymerase can therefore also be viewed as a molecular motor. In contrast to better-known kinesin and myosin which generate movements up to 10 nm, it generates movement of only few tenths of nanometers, but at slower motion generates much more force, about 14 pN, as measured by optical tweezers experiments. Chemical energy, derived from ATP–ADP conversion, is transformed into mechanical energy at around 10 to 20% efficiency.

▄ RECOMBINANT DNA TECHNOLOGY

Perhaps the greatest progress was achieved in recombinant DNA technology and genetic engineering which involve cutting and splicing of genes, cloning DNA segments into plasmids, and the introduction of plasmids into certain organisms, which can change their genetic basis and, in principle, that of their progeny.

It was discovered that various bacteria, as part of their defense against viruses, contain many different enzymes which can cut DNA only at specific points determined by the local sequence of nucleotides. They are called restriction enzymes and they normally recognize from four to eight nucleotides (minimally two). The DNA cuts produced by these enzymes may be flush (blunt) or staggered (sticky), as schematically indicated in Figure 3-12.

At present, a whole library of these enzymes exists. This field is constantly evolving, particularly to meet the needs of genome mapping. Therefore, in order to isolate larger genomic DNA fragments, restriction

flush ends   *sticky ends*

GATACGT   **CTGAT   ACGTAAGT**
CTATGCA   **GACTATGCA   TTCA**

Figure 3-12 Flush and sticky ends. Flush ends can be enzymatically converted into sticky ones. The sticky end shown above can ligate with another end with a sequence TGCA at the end of the double helix.

enzymes that recognize longer DNA sequence stretches continue to be discovered and made available commercially (currently an enzyme which recognizes a 39-nucleotide-long sequence is available). Restriction enzyme digestion, combined with ligation and purification, can be used to join various genes together as well as to determine the sequence of genes. Figure 3-13 shows schematically the formation of a plasmid. This creates a recombinant plasmid. Such a plasmid normally also contains a gene for resistance against a particular antibiotic which simplifies identification of transfected bacteria. Briefly, these plasmids are introduced into host cells, mostly *E. coli* bacteria which can replicate it several hundredfold. Bacteria transfected with the correct plasmids are selected upon treatment with a selective agent, such as an antibiotic. Bacteria transfected with the correct plasmids will survive, and after their growth in a bioreactor they are lysed and plasmids are purified. In large-scale preparation large batches of bacteria are used (1 to 100 L) which yield cake (a couple hundred grams per liter broth) which contains 1 to 10 mg of plasmid per liter of bacterial broth. Yields, of course, depend on the size and nature of the plasmid and the strain and harvesting time of the bacteria.

In recombinant DNA technology these bacteria are grown in fermentors and the expressed proteins are harvested, while gene therapy requires harvesting of transfected and multiplied plasmids.

DNA Plasmid Preparation and Purification

With current developments larger and larger quantities of plasmids are required. Several purification recipes have been improved and allow large-scale preparation. The purity of the plasmid is very important not only for transfection but also for complexation with cationic species. Very often contamination with RNA, proteins, short fragments of degraded DNA and chromosomal DNA occurs which adversely (and irreproducibly) affects the properties of DNA, and complexes as well as transfection experiments. Some researchers have told me that none of the commercially available DNA preparation kits can purify DNA adequately and that they do additional extractions and precipitations. For *in vivo* applications special care must be taken to ensure minimal levels of endotoxins. Their role in transfection is not known while in the *in vitro* experiments it was shown that increasing levels decreased gene expression (Weber et al., 1995). Briefly, gene expression decreases rapidly with increasing endotoxin. At 100 units of lipopolysaccharide per microgram of plasmid, DNA gene expression halves lipofection while Ca phosphate transfection is ten times more sensitive. Endotoxin-contaminated preparations cause death in laboratory animals which can be observed by the pathology of the digestive tract and swollen spleen and liver.

Definitively, a thorough evaluation of DNA concentration (adsorbance at 260 and 280 nm) and purity, including agarose gel electrophoresis, lipopolysaccharide analysis (chromogenic limulus amebocyte assay), analysis of RNA contamination (polyacrylamide gel electrophoresis followed by staining by silver nitrate), protein presence (protein kit assays or

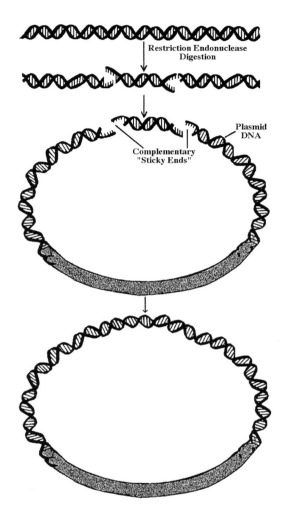

Figure 3-13 DNA can be cloned into plasmid. Normally, the correct gene is either synthesized or cut from the nonmutated gene with the aid of specific restriction nucleases. Blunt ends can be made into sticky ones enzymatically. Such a DNA sequence can be inserted into a particular location of plasmid which was opened with appropriate nuclease to create complementary cohesive ends. (Courtesy of Stan Hansen.)

electrophoresis in reducing 10% sodium lauryl sulfate–polyacrylamide gels and AgNO$_3$ staining), and presence of genomic DNA (1% agarose gels and Southern blotting) must accompany each batch of DNA. High pressure liquid chromatography (HPLC) and capillary electrophoresis should also accompany each DNA preparation. However, because of retention of genomic DNA in the guard columns a precise recovery has to parallel the determination. I urge scientists to thoroughly characterize DNA because many irreproducible results probably originate in DNA variability which is, in general, much larger than variability in the liposome preparations.

Traditionally, methods of DNA plasmid manufacturing include growth of transfected bacteria, their lysis (base and detergent), and purification of DNA by precipitation with polyethylene glycol (PEG), ultracentrifugation in CsCl–ethidium bromide system, or anion exchange chromatography. We shall briefly discuss three preparation schemes.

The most widely used is the commercially available Qiagen method. Custom preparation and purification of desired plasmids are also offered. Briefly, the method involves a modified lysis procedure followed by binding of plasmid DNA to a special anion-exchange resin at low-salt conditions. RNA, proteins, and low-molecular-weight impurities are removed by a medium-salt wash. Plasmid DNA is eluted by a high-salt buffer wash and concentrated and desalted by isopropanol precipitation. If done properly, the manufacturer claims, plasmids are pure, as determined by a 1% agarose analytical gel. Yields for a high-copy plasmids, such as pBS, pUC, pT2, or pGEM, are up to 3 to 5 mg of plasmid per liter of the culture, while for low-copy plasmids (pBR322 and cosmids) the yield is 0.2 to 1 mg/L of the broth. Losses on the columns are rather large and for large scale preparations these methods are normally not practical. Possible presence of detergent Triton may also interfere with colloidal properties and interaction characteristics.

Most researchers use the so-called Maniatis procedure (Sambrook, J., Fritsch, E.R., Maniatis, T.) for purification of DNA. According to this method, the bacterial pellet is dissolved with NaOH and SDS in the presence of lysozyme. An ice cold solution of potassium acetate and glacial acetic acid precipitates the chromosomal DNA, RNA, and protein/SDS/lipid complexes. After spinning and filtration, nucleic acids are precipitated with isopropanol. After rinsing the pellet plasmid can be purified by equilibrium centrifugation in CsCl–ethidium bromide gradients or by precipitation with PEG. Different variations of this procedure, such as a proteinase K digestion step after RNase digestion, can improve purity and yield and currently seem to be the preferable method for large-scale preparation of ultrapure DNA (Templeton et al., 1996).

A good manufacturing practice (GMP) protocol for the preparation of >100 mg of pure plasmid was recently published. In GMP settings for injectable drug substances special care has to be taken to remove all endotoxins and traces of host RNA and DNA. Briefly, after cell growth, alkaline-mediated cell lysis, 2-propanol extraction, ammonium acetate precipitation, PEG-8000 precipitation, and column chromatography are employed before final aseptic processing. No toxic extractions and animal-derived enzymes are used (Horn et al., 1995).

A laboratory procedure with enhanced separation of supercoiled and nicked DNA was recently published. It allows up to 10 mg protein and RNA-free plasmid DNA to be extracted from 500 mL of bacterial culture (Baumann and Bloomfield, 1995). Major steps of the procedure are listed below:

- Grow bacteria transfected with plasmid for approximately 1 day at 37°C

- Harvest bacteria and spin them down at 5000 rpm

- Resuspend the pellet in the lysis buffer

- Lyse with alkali and detergent (0.2 M NaOH, 1% SDS)

- Precipitate cellular debris with ammonium acetate and spin down

- After separation precipitate plasmid with isopropanol and spin down

- Resuspend pellets in Tris (10 mM) EDTA buffer (1 mM, pH = 8) (TE)

- Spin down undissolved material

- Add RNase and incubate 1 h at 37°C

- Extract with TE buffer-phenol

- Dialyze aqueous fraction

- Precipitate DNA with 5 M NaCl and ethanol

- Wash twice with cold 70% ethanol

- Measure concentration by 260/280 nm adsorption.

According to original reports, all these and many other protocols yield high-purity DNA plasmids. When speaking with various scientists, however, one gets the idea that each prefers his or her own method and does not trust other protocols. Large variations in plasmid properties can be traced to contamination with either chromosomal DNA, fragments of DNA, nucleosides, proteins, or RNA, which may not be detected by agarose gel chromatography, absorbance measurements (260/280 nm ratio), capillary electrophoresis, and HPLC. Before the preparation procedure is firmly established, a thorough characterization by the above-mentioned methods is recommended because DNA plasmids are often the least-defined reactant in gene delivery.

Genetic Engineering

Genetic engineering is a technology for constructing novel genetic elements from pieces of naturally occurring genes and regulatory sequences. These are then inserted into cells (bacteria, yeast, insect, plant, and mammalian cells) and various organisms produce molecules whose codes were inserted into them. By far the most frequently used are bacteria, especially *E. coli*. This technology allows production of relatively large amounts of engineered proteins, including various therapeutic proteins, cytokines (granulocyte macrophage-colony-stimulating factor, interleukins, interferons, etc.), various growth factors, and others. Additionally, genetically engineered microbes, plants, and animals can do many other beneficial tasks, as will be briefly described below. Also, methods of recombinant DNA technology have a potential to revolutionize human identification and offer invaluable, but unfortunately not yet appreciated, evidence in various criminal proceedings. In another example, the remnants of Czar Nicholas II and his family can finally rest in peace because of DNA analysis. Another application which caught general interest is recovery of old DNA from fossils. After initial optimism and some successful extractions and sequence determinations, it seems now that really old DNA can be preserved only in amber-embedded insects and that some other results were simply contaminants (Service, 1996).

Improved understanding of evolution can be obtained by comparing DNA from various species. Along these lines is also the controversial Human Genome Diversity Project in which researchers would compare genes from approximately 500 different ethnic groups in order to map relationships, track prehistoric human migration, and find family ties among the groups. Such genealogic study would improve the knowledge of human population history and perhaps answer some biomedical questions, such as some aspects of immunity. However, due to the resistance of some groups it is not clear if the project will ever be concluded in the original sample size.

Production of Materials and Goods

Here we shall only very briefly mention a few better-known examples. For instance, some anaerobic bacteria which ferment sugar-rich sap into alcohol can be genetically engineered to produce ethanol from xylose from woody biomass. Some other genetically engineered bacteria can synthesize biodegradable plastics. Such protocols are being studied more and more, and it is hoped that they may solve some local ecological as well as energetic problems.

From the daily press we are well aware of the genetically engineered "flavr-savr" tomato, which can be harvested when completely grown. Scientists have identified a gene that causes the tomato to rot. The gene codes for an enzyme (polygalacturonase) that breaks down cell walls during ripening. They cloned the gene and inserted back a nonactive form. The shelf life of tomatos is extended to 10 days, and it allows growers to pick tomatoes at the blush stage, i.e., the fruits ripen on a vine and retain much flavor, instead of when they are still green and to forward them to the markets before they get mushy. Other plant engineering includes plants with higher yields and products of quality, such as larger fractions of unsaturated oils in seeds. Cotton plants can grow better fibers, rapeseed plants lauric acid for the soap industry, while some other plants can produce vaccines and antibodies.

The world crop (>$1 trillion), which spends over a billion dollars annually on pesticides (which in addition to the toxicity to the environment can damage the ozone layer), loses more than 10% of the crop to various pests. There is an effort to generate transgenic plants which would be resistant to pests due to systemic acquired resistance genes which code for various proteins, such as peroxidases, chitinases, glucanases, ribosome-inactivating proteins, defensins (antimicrobial peptides), lysozymes, and so on. Currently, more than 50 different transgenic maize variations are in field trials. Other crops include rice (inclusion of insecticidal protein against leaf-folder and stem-borer insects), other cereals, and potato in which the production of larger quantities of more-valuable starch is also being engineered.

Prudent and honest work is required because recently it was reported that, against all the expectations, transgenic plants can cross-pollinate with wild types. This is one of the biggest worries about genetically engineered plants because it can make new generations of weeds. Oilseed rape, engineered in such a way that it can survive specific herbicides, was found to cross-pollinate with its weedy relative and both crop and weed produced, unexpectedly, nonsterile hybrid seeds; in many cases herbicide resistance was passed on.

Transgenic Animals

Direct injection of foreign genes into the pronucleus of the fertilized mouse egg with subsequent oviductal implantation of the surviving zygotes results in the integration and retention of the exogenous genes in the newborn animal and is also transmitted into progeny.

Transgenic animals are laboratory animals which have overexpressed certain genes or can carry genes for various human diseases. Alternatively, they can lack some genes or have a target gene inactivated. These are the so-called knock-out animals and are useful models for the studies of atherosclerosis, hypercholesterolemia, osteoporosis, spontaneous tumors (lack of p53 protein), cystic fibrosis, thalassemia, Duchenne muscular dystrophy, sickle cell anemia, and other diseases. Severe combined immunodeficient (SCID) mice can grow various human tumor xenographs and are used in investigations of human cancers.

Mice are especially useful because their genetics, biochemistry, and physiology are well understood and rather similar to humans. They reach sexual maturity in 6 weeks and during the reproductive life have around eight litters with an average size of six to eight. Genetically standardized inbred lines permit studies where the only difference between test and control animals is the mutation in question. In addition to being invaluable models in efficacy studies of many drugs, such animals are useful also for the investigations of gene functionality.

Other examples of transgenic animals are cows which synthesize various proteins in their milk and pigs with human genes growing humanized organs, which we hope can be used as implants into humans that are less likely to be rejected. In the times when xenotransplantation is perceived as a real possibility because of the lack of human donors and the inapplicability of mechanical devices, pigs and baboons are bred as organ donors. However, the interior of blood vessels is covered with molecules which human antibodies immediately recognize as foreign and subsequent immune attack of the system kills the implanted organ. In contrast, human blood vessels bear various molecules that prevent this process. Now, researchers have produced pigs which bear these molecules and it is hoped that these organs (such as heart, liver, kidneys) will be much more compatible with the human immune system and will eventually allow transplantation of the organs from these animals into humans. Pigs are also used to produce human hemoglobin and in the future undoubtedly many new applications will follow in this fast-growing scientific branch.

■ SUMMARY

In this chapter DNA was introduced from physical, chemical, biological, and synthetic points of view. DNA structure in solution is determined by its concentration and the presence of solutes, while in living organisms complex compaction processes condense DNA into small, dense structures. DNA molecules can be cut and pasted into new molecules. These can be amplified in bacteria and plasmids can be isolated and used in various applications.

■ ADDITIONAL READING

Arms, K., Camp, P. S., *Biology,* 2nd ed., CBS College Publ., 1982.

Bloomfield, V. A., Crothers, R. M., Tinoco, I., *Physical Chemistry of Nucleic Acids,* Harper and Row, New York, 1974.

Boulikas, T., Nuclear envelope and chromatin; functions of chromatin and the expression of genes, *Int. Rev. Cytol.,* Suppl. 17, 493–571; 599–684, 1987.

Davidson, F., *The Biochemistry of the Nucleic Acids,* rev. 8th ed., Academic Press, New York, 1976.

Lehninger, A. L., *Principles of Biochemistry,* Worth Publ., New York, 1982.

Sambrook, J., Fritsch, E.R., Maniatis, T., *Molecular Cloning,* 2nd ed., Cold Spring Harbor Press, pp. 1.38–1.39, 1989.

4 GENE EXPRESSION

Genes can be delivered into cells *in vivo* primarily by two methods: as a part of the viral (or retroviral) genome or as a bacterial plasmid. Viral vectors with reconstituted gene and depleted viral proteins use viral transfection pathways, while bacterial plasmids are not infectious per se and must be inserted into cells by appropriate gene delivery systems. We shall briefly discuss viral vectors in the next chapter and will mostly concentrate on the design of plasmids.

We shall distinguish between gene transfection and gene expression. The former describes delivery of genes into cells, while gene expression indicates that the protein, encoded in the delivered DNA, was synthesized. Obviously, successful gene transfection is a necessary but not sufficient condition for gene expression.

Prokaryotic cells, such as *Escherichia coli,* contain genetic material in the form of the single DNA molecule. The length of DNA exceeds cell dimensions almost a thousandfold, and the molecule is condensed into a small chromosome. Genetic information, however, is also contained in small episomal plasmids, such as the ones which can confer antibiotic resistance to bacteria. These plasmids contain codes for enzymes which can deactivate drugs. In contrast, in eukaryotic cells, the genetic material is separated from the cytoplasm by the nuclear membrane.

Eukaryotic genes contain several coding regions, the so-called exons, which lead via mRNA to protein synthesis. These stretches are separated by introns whose function is still not well understood. They probably stabilize RNA and regulate gene expression. Genes contain several other stretches of DNA whose specific properties help to regulate gene expression and will be mentioned below. Recombinant DNA technology allows the construction of new genes by cutting genes and after separation of the fragments splicing them with new ones into novel sequences.

For effective plasmid replication and gene expression, either *in vitro* or *in vivo,* DNA vectors have to be very carefully constructed. The DNA vector is a construct which, in addition to the cDNA of interest, contains sequences that can enhance gene expression by appropriate binding specificity, stabilization of RNA, and catalysis. Such sequences can provide autonomous replication and nuclear retention; can have a potential to induce homologous and site-specific recombination; and can contain tissue-specific promoters, enhancers (because in synthetic plasmids they are normally adjacent they are usually referred to as the pro-moter+enhancer region), introns, translation enhancer region, and a 3' untranslated terminal repeat unit (UTR) that includes the polyadenylation (polyA) signal. The function of these will be discussed below, while for a comprehensive review the reader is referred to Kriegler (1990).

In addition to the above, standard sequences which are required for effective growth, selection, and purification of plasmids are required. They include an origin of replication (ORI), an antibiotic resistance gene, and possibly another marker.

When cDNA is flanked with appropriate sequences the whole con-struct can be inserted in a commercially available plasmid, such as pBR322.

These reconstituted plasmids are inserted into bacteria. The trans-fected bacteria can be easily selected by incubating the medium with an antibiotic because the transfected gene also contains the antibiotic resis-tance gene. These bacteria are grown in fermentors, and at appropriate times the growth is stopped, cells are lysed, and plasmid purified as discussed in the previous chapter. These plasmids, normally complexed with a carrier system, are used for transfection.

The gene expression region of the plasmid can contain, in general, the following blocks going downstream, i.e., from the 5' to the 3' end. A block for nuclear retention can be followed by a sequence for homol-ogous recombination, which is followed by a tissue-specific promoter. Downstream follows the promoter+enhancer region, intron, translation enhancer, and cDNA, i.e., the gene of interest. The construct ends with 3' UTR which includes sequences for the polyA signal. Various response elements can be also included between the promoter and the 3' end. Some of the most important blocks will be discussed below and are schematically shown in Figure 4-1.

The nuclear retention block may simply consist of an appropriate sequence which enhances via induced DNA conformation adhesion to chromosomes via electrostatic, electrodynamic, and/or hydrophobic forces.

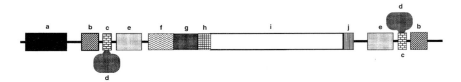

Figure 4-1 A segment of a plasmid which is responsible for gene expression. Various stretches with specific functions are schematically shown. a. Autonomous replication/nu-clear retention sequences; b. Sequences for homologous recombination; c. Sequences for site-specific integration; d. Site-specific recombinage; e.Tissue-specific promoter; f. Promoter + enhancer region; g. Hybrid or synthetic introns; h. Translation-enhancing sequences DNA; i. cDNA; j. 3' Untranslated Region Including the Polyadenylation Signal. (Drawing courtesy of Stan Hansen.)

Each chromosome or plasmid must also contain an ORI. This is the site where the replication fork begins. This is a sequence of between 100 to 200 bp which is recognized by a replication enzyme. Replication is bidirectional and, as an example, the rate in *E. coli* is 45,000 bp/min. In other words, the rate of DNA unwinding is 4500 turns per minute!

■ PROMOTERS AND ENHANCERS

These are DNA stretches, normally up to several hundred (50 to 500 bp) base pairs long, with specific functions. Promoter contains an mRNA cap site and acts as a binding site for RNA polymerase, an enzyme that initiates mRNA transcription, while enhancers increase the initiation rate of transcription. They modulate gene expression in a time- and tissue-specific manner by forming part of a specific structural assembly for DNA–protein interactions. While enhancers can enhance gene expression a few thousand base pairs up- or downstream, promoter sequences, such as TATA box (highly repetitive sequence of thymines and adenines, which is normally located just 25 bp upstream of the mRNA cap site), actually position the start of transcription. Promoter sequences contain a lot of homology between various species. For instance, herpes simplex thymidine kinase and human β-globin promoter are rather similar (Kriegler, 1990). Such homology indicates an important function which was preserved in the development of species. Promoters and enhancers are recognition sequences for transcription factors. A compilation of such regulatory sequences has revealed distinctive classes of AT-, GC-, TG-rich sequences (Boulikas, 1995). Because there may be several thousand different transcription factors in a single cell and only a few hundred have been identified, it is likely that improved understanding of the structures and mechanisms involved will further increase the efficiency of expression.

Viral, cellular, and inducible promoter+enhancer regions exist. The most widely used is viral promoter+enhancer region from the human cytomegalovirus (CMV) region. This regulatory sequence produces the highest levels of gene expression in practically all tissues of most species. Other promoter+enhancer regions include simian virus (SV40), which gives significantly lower gene expression, and enhancers from polyoma virus, HIV, gibbon ape leukemia virus, hepatitis B, and some others.

Cellular enhancers can be used to increase expression in appropriate cell types. For instance, albumin gene enhancer and the apolipoprotein A-1 enhancer can be incorporated to increase gene expression in the liver. Some other cell- or tissue-specific promoters are α-fetoprotein for expression in fetal liver, surfactant protein B&C promoter for expression in respiratory endothelium, immunoglobulin heavy-chain enhancer for B-cell specific expression, β-globin enhancer for expression in erythroid cells, the insulin gene enhancer for expression in pancreatic islet cells, and many others. Constitutive promoters bring persistent gene expression in a wide variety of cells and include the phosphoglycerate kinase and *Pol* II promoters.

Gene expression by some promoters and enhancers can be induced or repressed. The best-known examples are mouse mammary tumor virus promoter and metallothionein promoter which can be induced by gluco-corticosteroids (dexamethasone) and heavy metal ions (zinc, cadmium, copper), respectively. On the other side, tetracycline-responsive promoters (Gossen and Bujard, 1992) can be in the presence of low concentrations of tetracyclines completely turned off. Such enhancers+promoters can be used as gene switches. For instance, radiation-sensitive promoters (Egr-1) can induce, after introduction into the patient, expression of tumor necrosis factor-α only in tumor tissue after irradiation and thus prevent expression of this potent agent in other tissues where it may have arrived after administration via a systemic route.

Five- to tenfold greater gene expression was achieved when CMV immediate early promoter in plasmid was exchanged for tetracycline regulated chimeric transactivator (Liang et al., 1996). Furthermore, by positioning of the tetracycline control element the expression of the reporter gene could be either repressed or activated by the transacting proteins whose binding is regulated by a tetracycline.

■ INTRONS AND polyA TAILS

Functional introns can increase the mRNA production up to two orders of magnitude. They are placed immediately downstream from the promoter+enhancer region and can significantly increase gene expression. The mechanism of their action remains unknown although it is likely that they facilitate transcription. Their function can be sensitive to *in vivo* vs. *in vitro* conditions. cDNA, being a marker or therapeutic gene, is followed by 3′UTR which provides for mRNA stability, its efficient transport to the cytoplasm, and can increase the efficiency of mRNA translation. The stability of mRNA varies from minutes to hours and therefore rates of mRNA decay regulate gene expression. Stability is a function of structure and it is likely that the polyA tract protects RNA against rapid degradation. The polyA signal is a sequence which specifies to the cell to add about 300 A bases to the 3′ end of RNA transcript. Transcription is terminated at highly curved, AT-rich motifs.

The efficiency of mRNA translation can be increased by adding sequences for an internal ribosome entry site (IRES), which are placed next to the 5′ end of the cDNA coding region.

■ COMPLEMENTARY DNA

These are genes (exons) which code for the protein whose expression in a particular cell type is desired. For optimization of DNA plasmids and gene delivery systems normally reporter genes are used while the ultimate goal is, obviously, to deliver therapeutic genes into appropriate cells. Therapeutic genes include genes for cystic fibrosis regulatory protein (CFTR), factors VIII and IX, cytokines, apolipoproteins, HS-tk, tumor suppresor genes, and multidrug-resistance genes whose expression yields glycoprotein P which effluxes many antineoplastic drugs (anthracyclines, taxol, vincristine) from the cells. Systems, however, are normally optimized by the use of various reporter genes and the detection of their expression will be described below.

cDNAs are the reverse transcriptase products for mRNA representing appropriately spliced coding regions of the gene lacking the introns. These are used frequently in gene therapy because they are the shortest pieces of DNA specifying the protein; however, introns may contain enhancer elements and future gene therapy studies may include genomic copies of the gene much larger than the cDNA (Boulikas, private communication).

■ CYTOPLASMIC GENE EXPRESSION

Some results with nonviral lipid delivery systems show that only a small fraction (~1%) of DNA introduced into the cell cytoplasm actually reaches the nucleus. There, DNA must be transcribed into mRNA which, upon further changes, migrates into cytoplasm to ribosomes where protein synthesis commences (Chen et al., 1993). It may be advantageous if gene expression would begin in the cytoplasm. Indeed, some vectors, such as bacteriophage T7 which encodes for an enzyme T7 RNA polymerase which can transcribe DNA into RNA in the cytosol of mammalian cells with high transcriptional activity, can express cDNA in the cytoplasm. For such a system to work, a T7 RNA polymerase protein must be present in the cytoplasm along with the cDNA of interest. It can be introduced together with DNA, encoded in the DNA, or both. Expression of both genes is induced by T7 RNA polymerase promoters and rapid cytoplasmic gene expression independent of nuclear transcription factors was observed. Transcripts are not capped and an IRES sequence is inserted into the 5′UTR for efficient translation of transcripts. Although high levels of expression can be achieved, it is only transient because polymerase is degraded. By using a T7 autogene, however, a continuous synthesis of T7 RNA polymerase can be achieved, and expression for a week was reported (Gao and Huang, 1993). Such an approach may be useful when a fast, transient, and high level of transgene expression is preferred.

■ REPORTER GENES

A variety of reporter genes can be used. The synthesized proteins must be easily detectable and should not occur in mammalian cells. Detection includes enzyme-linked immunoassays (ELISA) for specific proteins, fluorescence (luciferase, green fluorescent protein), immune staining (β galactosidase), or protein activity (chloramphenicol acetyltransferase, CAT). The quantitative detection of these marker genes is often not trivial and careful and artifact-free analytical assays are needed for reliable optimizations.

Some of the reporter genes are additionally labeled in order to allow follow up of the biological fate of DNA, including its possible integration into chromosomes. These markers include thymidine kinase, neomycin phosphotransferase II, multiple drug resistance, and similar genes which give cells resistance against particular drugs. Cells can be then grown under positive or negative selection conditions and the frequency of integration assessed.

■ VECTORS

Many different gene transfer vectors are commercially available. They include pBR322 and derivatives, pUC, pBluescript, pGEM vectors, and many others. Another vector, pSPORT 1, contains a cloning site with recognition for 19 restriction nucleases which increases the potential of cloning strategies. The expression of cloned genes can be controlled by *lac* promoter and repressor genes which are contained in the plasmid. Such plasmids are also availble in a precut form. Typically they are between 3 and 5 kb long. Researchers can insert the gene or cDNA of interest into these vectors for transient or stable gene transfection. Complete reporter genes containing plasmids are also available and some researchers use them to study the influence of different introns and other sequences on gene expression. Transient transfection is less time-consuming and less labor-intensive, but it yields gene expression in a single burst. Stable transfection yields continuous expression, normally at moderate levels, or, if combined with selective gene amplification, at high levels in a continuous culture.

Most vectors are based on animal virus genomes. Parts of viral genomes are inserted into bacterial plasmids, such as pBR322, containing ampicillin resistance to facilitate propagation in bacterial cells and their manipulation. The chimeric molecules formed could be propagated in *E. coli* and the isolated plasmid concomitantly transferred to tissue culture cells where they could express either viral, bacterial, avian, mammalian, or any conceivable gene and could replicate in either bacterial or animal cells. They contain the SV40 ORI to be capable of replicating in a cell permissive for its replication. The most frequently used ORI is from SV40. Other vectors use EBV-ORI, HSV 1 or 2 ORI, polyoma and bovine papilloma virus ORI, and some others.

Plasmids constructed following some of the above guidelines are multiplied, purified, and used in gene delivery with an appropriate transfection carrier.

■ SUMMARY

In this chapter we introduced DNA plasmids and their sequential construction. Various active functions in appropriate elements (sequences) must be present to optimize gene expression. Typically, the coded gene must be flanked by a promoter, enhancer, intron, and some other sequences which are then introduced into a plasmid containing a sequence for multiplication in bacteria. Selection of transfected bacteria is eased by introducing a gene for an antibiotic resistance. The composition of optimal plasmid is therefore a process of cutting and pasting together appropriate stretches and requires good knowledge of molecular biology.

■ ADDITIONAL READING

Kriegler, M., Gene transfer, in *Gene Transfer and Expression: A Laboratory Manual*, W. H. Freeman, New York, 1990, 3–81.

Lasic, D. D., Templeton, N.S., Liposomes in gene therapy, *Adv. Drug Del. Rev.*, 20, 221–266, 1996.

5

GENE DELIVERY

In order for genes to be expressed they must be in the cell nucleus. Plasmids are very large molecules. Typically, they contain between 3 and 15 kb which equals, at approximately 660 Da and two negative charges per base pair, a molecular weight of 2 to 10 million Da and 6000 to 30,000 negative charges per molecule. Knowing that cell membranes are effective permeability barriers to even small molecules, one can appreciate the problem of intracellular delivery of plasmids. The problem is even more pronounced in *in vivo* transfection because free DNA is quickly degraded by extracellular DNA nucleases, which protect the body against exogenous genes. This is especially true for systemic administration. The only exception seems to be intramuscular injection, where upon local injection of naked DNA some activity was observed. However, the entry of DNA molecules into intact cells still presents an enigma, and we shall discuss some possibilities of DNA internalization in Chapter 10. It could be a consequence of mechanical rupture, osmotic imbalance, or hydro-dynamic or local pressure (upon bolus injection) effects.

Numerous DNA delivery systems exist (Table 5-1). Mechanical methods include direct microinjection into the cell nucleus, ballistic methods, in which plasmid-coated gold particles are shot into the tissue, and laser methods, which burn transient pores. In agriculture, seeds are mixed with sharp crystalline (silicon carbide) needles coated with DNA. Physical transfection techniques involve osmotic shocks, freeze-thawing, ultrason-ication, and electroporation which became a very popular transfection method in *in vitro* work. Chemical methods rely on DNA precipitation or complexation by using Ca phosphate; cationic polyelectrolytes such as DEAE dextran, polybrene, or polyethylenemide; cationic micelles or liposomes; polycations; basic polypeptides or proteins; or any combination of these agents. Plasmids can be also encapsulated in conventional liposomes (negatively charged, pH sensitive, fusogenic) or sterically sta-bilized liposomes, virosomes, or some other microparticles. Biological methods use viral constructs for DNA delivery.

Most of these techniques cannot be applied *in vivo*. We will not discuss mechanical and physical methods. After briefly mentioning viral systems, we shall concentrate on chemical and colloidal systems for DNA transfection into cells. cDNA reconstituted into genetically modified viruses and plasmids complexed with various agents into colloidal DNA represent two major and fundamentally different transfection pathways.

TABLE 5-1

VARIOUS GENE DELIVERY METHODS

Mechanical	Microinjection, gene gun, sharp needles
Physical	Electroporation, sonication, osmotic shock, freeze-thawing
Chemical	Complexation with multivalent cations, polycations, polyelectrolytes, micelles, lipids/liposomes
Biological	Viral or bacterial transfection

Physical and mechanical methods normally deliver naked DNA plasmids into cells. Viral systems integrate a gene into a viral genome which is depleted of replication-competent sequences. Viral vectors are reconstructed from packaging cells which are transfected with plasmids expressing deleted genes and vector plasmid. These particles resemble viruses and use viral pathways to deliver genes. Bacterial plasmids are not infectious and have to be delivered through a cell membrane by a special carrier system, as will be shown below. As discussed in a previous chapter, plasmids should have at least five major components: (1) a multicloning site for insertion of gene, (2) a strong promoter sequence, (3) a polyadenylation signal, (4) an antibiotic resistance stretch for positive selection, and (5) an *Escherichia coli* origin of replication for the generation of multiple copies in bacteria.

■ NAKED DNA

During studies of the transfection of muscle cells *in vivo,* it was surprisingly discovered that "negative" controls — naked DNA — resulted in gene expression when injected in the muscle. When 100 μg of DNA coding for influenza A nucleoprotein was injected into the hind leg of mice, the expressed antigen stimulated an immune response, and cytotoxic T lymphocytes specific for conserved viral antigens were shown to respond to different strains of virus (Ulmer et al., 1993). This may allow us to bypass the perennial problem of developing vaccines in response to ever-changing viral surface proteins. Genetic vaccination is now being studied for other diseases, such as hepatitis C, tuberculosis, malaria, HIV, and other viral infections.

Later, naked DNA was also injected in cardiac muscle and in tumors. It was shown that upon direct injection of 30 μg of DNA about 2 ng of reporter protein was synthesized (Yang and Huang, 1996) while the presence of cationic liposomes inhibited gene expression in a dose-dependent manner. At constant DNA concentration gene expression linearly increased with the volume of DNA solution. Glucose (5%) was the best diluent, especially if 0.01% Triton X-100 was added. Hypertonic solutions did not improve expression while the expression was reduced to about one half when distilled water was used as diluent.

▬ VIRAL SYSTEMS

The most frequently used delivery systems *ex vivo* and in *in vivo* applications in current human therapy are viral constructs, i.e., genes inserted into viral DNA with some sequences deleted and reconstituted into noninfective viruses. In addition to intravenous administration, these gene carriers can be delivered by direct intramuscular, subcutaneous, localized, and intraperitoneal injection, as well as by inhalation of an aerosol.

Various viruses have been used as DNA delivery vehicles. They differ mostly with respect to safety, plasmid-loading capacity, immunogenicity, and the nature of their interactions with cells and chromosomes. Ideally, one can develop viral carrier on the basis of viruses that transfect the type of cells which are targeted in a particular disease.

The most widely used viruses are *retroviruses*. They are single-strand RNA viruses which after entering the cell nucleus incorporate the gene directly into the chromosome. This presents a safety concern because of a potential carcinogenicity and infectivity despite the fact that several viral protein codes are deleted. Also, contamination with intact retroviruses during the preparation, which can be highly oncogenic, cannot be ruled out. These vectors include the retroviral long terminal repeats that are necessary for the production of viral RNA and for integration in the host genome. *Gag, pol,* and *env* genes are deleted and replaced with gene(s) of interest. Mostly murine retroviruses are used which are unable to replicate on their own and require a packaging cell line, i.e., cells carrying (the deleted) retroviral genes encoding proteins essential for packaging. *Adenoviruses* are less hazardous (an example is a common cold virus). They are double-stranded DNA viruses (36 kb) which can incorporate larger genes than retroviruses. They are much more efficient in transfection, especially the cells of the airways because of their tropism for this tissue. Compared with retroviruses where 5 to 10% transfection efficiency is considered high, they can be tenfold more effective. They do not incorporate into the genome and thus reduce the risk of malignant transformations but also the persistence of expression. Additionally, an immune response may develop, besides the fact that many people already possess immunity against these viruses. It is a common experience that typically a second injection is ineffective due to the development of the immune response. The appearance of neutralizing antibodies and cytotoxic T lymphocytes is also a possibility. Other viruses, such as adeno-associated viruses or herpes simplex virus have been also employed. Therefore, it is not surprising that some scientists envisage the creation of several different viral systems for consecutive administrations and/or use of immune system–suppressing drugs such as cyclosporin. *Adeno-associated viruses* seem to be free of safety issues, such as insertional mutagenesis and immunogenicity. They cannot replicate without adenoviruses or herpes viruses. They insert into a specific location on chromosome 19 and do not require dividing cells for expression. Efficiency of transfection is moderate and their DNA-carrying capacity is low, below 4 kb. Production of these viruses is also complicated because they require helper viruses.

Such viral systems are being constantly improved. Recently, Kovesdi's group reported on a modified adenovirus with increased host range. Its fiber was modified with a lysine-rich sequence in order to improve binding to heparin sulfate which is present on a variety of cell types and is also used by herpes simplex virus to bind and enter the cell. Other functions, such as targeting Fab fragments and retrovirus *env*-ligand fusion proteins, can be also added to adenoviruses.

At present, it is still not clear which viruses will be the mainstream in the development. It is possible that it will be none of the above-mentioned viruses but a novel viral construct with more deletions and some additional sequences.

Sometimes inactivated viruses are combined with liposomes or other DNA condensates to improve the transfection yield, as will be shown in Chapter 11.

Genetic alteration of plants is also very important. In addition to permanently altered plant DNA, transient gene expression systems may offer many advantages without breeding true lines. Tobacco mosaic virus is an RNA virus (6.4 kb, capped at the 5′ end, and not polyadenylated). The viral coat protein gene can reach 10% of the leaf dry weight, and genetically engineered virus was found to be able to express foreign protein to a high concentration of at least 2% of soluble proteins (Grill, 1993).

Because of the above mentioned inherent problems associated with viral vectors, such as potential carcinogenicity, infectivity, and development of an immune response and inflammation, many researchers believe that liposome- or lipid-based transfection systems will become the mainstream of gene therapy. Ultimately, I believe that stronger synergy between viral components and synthetic particles will have to be employed to achieve effective, durable, and safe transfection.

■ NONVIRAL DELIVERY SYSTEMS

As already mentioned, injections of high doses of DNA result in only minimal transfection, with a possible exception of intramuscular injection (where expression of 1 ng of gene product from 10 to 100 μg of plasmid DNA was observed) (Wolff et al., 1990). Some transfection can also be observed in thyroid glands, tumors, and lymph nodes, as well as in airway cells upon intratracheal or pulmonary delivery. Other cells, with a possible exception of mucosal cells in the digestive tract, are more resistant to transfection. This is due to the chemical instability of the plasmid in extracellular fluids and in circulation, to its inability to enter into the cells, and to the fact that not many cells *in vivo* are phagocytic in general. A possible solution is to complex and/or condense DNA plasmid. This can protect it against nucleases in the extracellular milieu and can substantially alter its surface properties and hydrophobicity and, most importantly, reduce its size, which may be a necessary condition for the entry into the cell.

Several different complexing and condensing agents can be used. They include polyvalent cations (Ca^{2+}, Mn^{2+}, $Co(NH_3)^{3+}$, La^{3+}), polycations (spermine, spermidine, polyamines, histones, and other basic proteins), cationic polyelectrolytes including polypeptides and dendrimers, and cationic colloidal particles.

Such DNA condensates can be further coated with biocompatible coatings or encapsulated into conventional liposomes. An example is a cationic complex coated with neutral/anionic lipids or condensed DNA encapsulated into conventional liposomes. Although encapsulation of supercoiled DNA (noncondensed) into conventional liposomes did not have much impact yet, I believe that with improved methods for DNA encapsulation and vastly improved control of the behavior of such vehicles over cationic complexes the situation may change.

Polycations, Polypeptides, and Polymers

Since 1961 it has been known that cellular uptake of polynucleotides can be enhanced by complexing them with protamine (Amos, 1961), while spermine and spermidine did not increase the uptake but did protect them against enzymatic degradation.

Later, other complexing agents were tried. Since the late 1960s, the most widely used continues to be $Ca_3(PO_4)_2$ precipitation. Because of the formation of precipitates, these systems are not effective for *in vivo* applications. Other polyvalent ions are rarely used for DNA transfection. Encapsulation of such condensates, such as $Metal_n$-DNA_m, into nonpermeable liposomes has not been reported yet.

DNA can be condensed also by high salt and addition of polypeptides or poly(ethylene) glycol, a neutral polymer. The latter does not interact with DNA via electrostatic forces but mostly via a phase separation mechanism. Obviously, rather high concentrations are required and the technique can be used mostly for DNA separation and purification. Some polymers, such as polyvinylpyrrolidone, can interact with DNA via H bonding.

The same is true for polypeptides (polylysine, polyarginine, and polyhistidine). Polypeptides are in general toxic and several authors report that polylysine is toxic. Poly(L-lysine) is, in contrast to poly(D-lysine) and polybrene, biodegradable and is less toxic. Many new and shorter polypeptides are being synthesized and studied but the information on their *in vivo* activity and toxicity has not been reported yet.

Some transfection efficacy was observed for $M_w > 20,000$ Da polylysine–DNA complexes. *In vivo* some activity was observed for anionic polylysine and polyhistidine complexes while cationic ones were not effective (Lasic et al., unpublished). Several groups are trying to synthesize less-toxic natural polypeptides to condense DNA. For instance, scientists from GeneMedicine reported that 10-mers were very effective in DNA

Putrescine	$NH_2 - (CH_2)_4 - NH_2$
Spermidine	$NH_2 - (CH_3)_3 - NH - (CH_2)_4 - NH_2$
Spermine	$NH_2 - (CH_3)_3 - NH - (CH_2)_4 - NH - (CH_2)_3 - NH_2$

Figure 5-1 Chemical formulae of various polycations: putrescine spermidine and spermine. These are written in the form of free bases, while in biological conditions they are normally phosphate salts. All primary and secondary amines can be protonated at physiological values of pH and putrescine, spermidine, and spermine can bear 2, 3, or 4 positive charges, respectively.

condensation with a greatly increased safety profile. For efficient transfection they use condensing and fusogenic peptide. The former can be galactosylated to target hepatocytes (Tomlinson, 1995).

Polycations, such as spermidine or spermine are not very effective gene transfection agents for systemic applications as studied by tail vein injection of a complex of the agent with DNA (CAT marker) in mouse lungs a day after injection. Both anionic and cationic complexes were prepared. Colloidally soluble complexes at 0.3 to 0.5 mg DNA/mL can be prepared at a ratio of $\rho = 2$ and 0.5, respectively (Lasic et al., unpublished).

Recently, polyamine transfection reagent TransIT™ (1.33 mg/mL in 80 to 90% ethanol solution, PanVera Corp., WI) became available. The prospectus claims that at high transfection activity *in vitro* the reagent reduces cellular damage.

Polyelectrolytes

Polyelectrolytes are charged polymers. Cationic polymers include weak bases such as poly(vinylamine) and poly(vinylpyridine) which become charged in acidic solutions. When weakly basic poly(vinylpyridine) is quaternized with an alkyl halide, such as butyl bromide, the highly ionized poly(4-vinyl-N-butylpyridinium bromide) results. The properties of this polyelectrolyte can be greatly controlled by N-alkyl substituent. Even nucleic acids can become positively charged at low pH due to the protonation of amino groups in heterocyclic bases. Some examples of polybases are shown in Figure 5-2.

In principle, it is possible to complex/condense DNA at low pH, and when pH increases polyelectrolyte molecules deprotonate and DNA decondenses. This property may also be exploited in gene delivery for effective DNA decondensation upon entry in the cytoplasm.

In light of the importance of DNA condensation and following the recent burst of cationic lipid synthesis it is surprising how little has been done in polymer chemistry to complex and/or condense DNA. Some nonionic polymers can interact with DNA and perhaps they can find some utilization in localized DNA delivery instead of naked DNA. Indeed, GeneMedicine scientists reported that polyvinylpyrrolidone polymer increases DNA transfection upon intramuscular injection (Tomlinson,

poly(vinylamine): $(- CH_2 - CH)_n-$
                                    |
                                   NH_2

polyethylemeimine: $(- CH_2 - CH_2)_n-$
                                    |
                                   NH

poly(4-vinylpyridine) $(- CH_2 - CH)_n-$
                                    |
                                   C_5H_5N

poly(4-vinyl-N-alkylpyridinium halides): $(- CH_2 - CH)_n-$
                                                      |
                                                     $C_5H_5N^+RX^-$

Figure 5-2 Chemical formulae of monomers of various positively charged polymers.

1995). Results are much more reproducible and gene expression shows more uniform and diffuse distribution as opposed to the focal localization of naked DNA. It is possible that complexation via hydrogen bonds may decrease polymer size and improve intracellular delivery in the environments which do not have many DNA digestive enzymes present.

Mostly, however, cationic polymers are used. DEAE-dextran polymer is used in transfection, but so far it was not found efficient for *in vivo* applications. While branched copolymers have not been used yet, starburst polymers (dendrimers) have shown activity *in vitro*. To date, despite some chemical modifications, such as reducing the number of branches, they have not been found efficient for *in vivo* applications. These polymers are spherical polymers which grow from one molecule in successive layers of branching as shown in Figure 5-3. Their size can be similar to histones, but it seems that they cannot encapsulate DNA and protect it. Topologically, this is not surprising; as they have around 60 to 110 charges each, it is obvious that many of them have to interact with plasmid, which may result in large, noncompact aggregates (repulsion between nonneutralized charges) which still may have exposed DNA on the surface and therefore compromised stability in biological environments. Although tightly wound DNA seems to be resistant to dye intercalation and DNase degradation, it is not clear if adsorption of plasma factors does not change that.

While a look into a textbook shows many different cationic polymers, not many of them were used in DNA transfection. Polyethyleneimide was shown to be as effective as cationic liposomes in *in vitro* tests, as will be described in Chapter 11. Undoubtedly, synthetic chemists will be able to synthesize improved polymers but their systemic applicability will depend on their ability to protect or coat complexed/condensed DNA, which may be more difficult to achieve in polymer systems than in self-aggregating bilayers. On the other hand, polymers can achieve the highest charge per molecular mass density (Table 5-2).

Polymer chemistry has introduced a variety of special polymers recently for drug delivery and I am sure that new, rationally designed

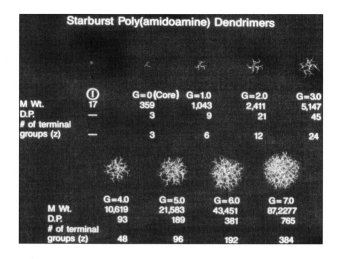

Figure 5-3   First seven generations of dendrimers. (Courtesy of D. Tomalia.)

TABLE 5-2

CHARGE PER MASS RATIO OF VARIOUS CATIONIC SYSTEMS

System	+Charge/Molecular Weight (Cb/Da)	Ratio
Poly(ethyleneimine)	1/44	44
Poly(4-vinyl-N-alkylpyridinium halides)	1/158	158
Spermidine	3/145	48
Spermine	4/202	50
Calcium phosphate	6/310	52
Cobalt(hexamine)	2/155	77
Polylysine	1/142	142
CTAB	1/378	378
DODAB	1/631	631
DOTAP	1/732	732
DOTMA	1/700	700
DOGS	4/902	225
Lipofectin	1/1374	1374
Lipofectace	1/2124	2124
Lipofectamine	3/908	302
DOSPER	4/1089	272
DC-Chol	1/504	504

Note: See Appendix E for explanation of abbreviations. Molecular weight may vary due to different counterions.

(polyethylene glycol) and cationic segments as well as comblike copolymers may yield effective gene carrier systems, especially perhaps for localized injections due to the fact that at those sites the concentration of degradative enzymes is smaller. Topological problems, such as exposed DNA, may be shielded by a steric shield provided by a neutral component.

Cationic Liposomes and Other Colloidal Particles

Cationic detergents has been used in DNA purification since the 1950s. Early experiments with cationic liposomes for DNA transfection were less effective than with negative liposomes, and as a result of the toxicity of stearylamine-containing liposomes, these studies were not continued (Fraley and Papahadjopoulos, 1982).

In parallel, physicists and colloid scientists studied DNA in the presence of oppositely charged colloidal particles and polymers. These studies revealed some basic properties of solubility and interaction but never had any input into transfection protocols. We can use these results, however, to improve our understanding of DNA interactions on the colloidal level. Briefly, solubility gaps at specific charge ratios were found, and the precipitates and soluble complexes were studied by a variety of physicochemical methods (Li et al., 1994).

In the late 1980s, however, the cationic liposome-based *in vitro* transfection systems renewed interest in liposomal delivery of DNA (Felgner et al., 1987). Micelles, based on alkyl trimethylammonium surfactants, were also tried for DNA complexation. Low transfection efficiencies were found and they were shown to be toxic. When mixed with diacyl lipids or cholesterol they formed bilayered liposomes which were characterized by increased transfection efficacy. However, single-chain cationic amphiphiles are in general toxic and interest in these systems decreased (Pinnadewuge et al., 1989).

Many different cationic liposomes were prepared and tested in transfection. Not many structure–activity or even structure–toxicity relationships were published. Basically, scientists mostly mix components and apply them into cell cultures or inject them into animals and follow transfection efficiency and/or gene expression. In general, many systems were found to be effective for *in vitro* administration, but only a few systems were found to transfect also *in vivo*, as will be described in Chapter 8. While several cytotoxicity studies were published, practically all the researchers claim that they observed no apparent toxicity in *in vivo* applications and that laboratory animals tolerated treatments well. In most cases, however, mice were injected with less than 0.5 μM cationic lipid per mouse which may explain the good tolerance. No necroscopies were reported which would describe the appearance of liver, spleen, lungs, and other organs. Typically, animals are sacrificed after 1 day, which may be too soon for some toxic effects to show up. No blood chemistry studies are reported which would show liver damage. Studies in humans used minute concentrations of these agents. Obviously, rigorous safety experiments remain to be done. The same is true for the immunogenicity of the formulations or apparent lack of it.

To increase biocompatibility these particles can be coated with negatively charged bilayers and perhaps a sterically stabilized coating and other condensing, fusogenic, or targeting agents can be included. At the end, we shall discuss some novel lipid-based carriers.

In addition, hydrophobic DNA–lipid complexes were prepared in organic solvents (Bally et al., 1995) and these can be formulated into emulsions (Huang, 1996).

Conventional Liposomes

Classic liposomes did not contribute significantly to gene delivery. Neither did pH-sensitive and fusogenic liposomes. This does not mean, however, that with improved understanding of DNA condensation and/or encapsulation they may not reemerge as a potent gene delivery system. Their disadvantages are nonqualitative DNA encapsulation and more-demanding preparation of formulations, but the ease of tailoring their surface characteristics as well as their biocompatibility and safety may outweigh the manufacturing disadvantages. While there is practically no control over very reactive cationic complexes and their biodistribution after systemic application, such complexes may have controllable surface characteristics and therefore their *in vivo* fate (see Chapters 11 and 13).

It is possible that current cationic liposome–DNA complexes will be replaced, at least in many current applications, by more-advanced delivery systems. In the case of liposomes one can think of employing neutral or anionic liposomes, possibly sterically stabilized ones (with targeting ligands) which are biocompatible and nontoxic as compared with cationic lipids. These liposomes will be targetable and will be able to deliver DNA into cytoplasm. One possibility is fusogenic liposomes which will fuse with target cells because of the presence of fusogenic lipids, polymers, proteins, or peptides. Another possibility is disruption of endosomes before lysosomal degradation by a similar fusogenic mechanism or by addition of lytic agents, such as polypeptides, or by buffering the endosomal interior. It is also possible that coated pit entry via some receptors results in the direct transfer of encapsulated plasmid into the cytoplasm. Liposomal particles that will fuse with the plasma membrane directly because of a lipid-mediated membrane destabilization are another possibility.

Apart from these surface ligands or (co)-encapsulated agents, the encapsulation of large DNA plasmids remains the largest obstacle. Two possibilities arise. To minimize liposome size and improve encapsulation, large plasmids may be precondensed or supercoiled plasmid may be encapsulated. At present, the optimal conditions of DNA precondensation and its encapsulation are not known yet.

DNA can be precondensed by polypeptides, high salt, high salt and polypeptides, cationic lipids, polymers and dendrimers, or histones. Liposomes can be prepared by hydrating lipids with such a solution and subsequent size reduction. It is known that condensed DNA can be stable against some mechanical treatments, including a few minutes of sonication (Wasan et al., 1996; Bennet et al., 1996). As we shall see in the liposome chapter, high encapsulation efficiency of these large particles may be a problem. Simple treatment includes brief sonication, extrusion, or homogenization at very high lipid concentrations to ensure large encapsulated volumes, i.e., fractions of medium inside the liposomes. Special lipid ligands including PEGylated lipids can be incorporated by incubation of liposomes with appropriate micelles or by detergent dialysis techniques. Reverse phase methods are known for high entrapment efficiencies of hydrophilic substances, and the presence of organic phase may help with DNA condensation. Most of these methods, however, have not been tried yet.

After the liposome formation the damage to DNA will have to be assessed. Also, in some cases condensed DNA is stable only in a high-salt or high-multivalent-cation solution. The stability of liposomes formed in such conditions, such as 1 M NaCl upon dilution with physiological medium, will have to be assessed.

Properties of liposomes may be further improved by designing pH-sensitive or fusogenic liposomes as well as targeted liposomes. Their characteristics will be presented in the next chapter.

Similar systems were already used for the delivery of antisense oligonucleotides, including pH-sensitive and folate-PEG-lipid containing liposomes. Other possible delivery systems for specific applications, such as controlled-release systems, can be lipid foam, liposome paste, biogel, all of which can release DNA complexes slowly.

Targeted Systems

In addition to the possibilities discussed above, some systems were already tested *in vivo*. Conjugates of cationic polymer and targeting ligand may act as an efficient delivery vehicle for systemic application. Targeting of liver hepatocytes via internalizing an asialoglycoprotein receptor by covalent conjugates of polylysine and targeting molecule (asialorosomucoid) demonstrated therapeutic activity (see Chapter 13). Polylysine conjugated to transferrin was used to target neoplastic cells which exhibit this receptor because rapidly dividing cells require a high level of iron. Similarly, insulin conjugated to positively charged N-acylurea albumin was also used as a receptor-specific carrier to cells expressing insulin receptor. Macrophages can be targeted by macrophage-expressed lectins which bind mannose, glycans, galactose, or fucosyl-glycoconjugates (Monsigny et al., 1994).

These conjugates are taken up by endocytosis. While this ensures internalization it also degrades DNA. *In vitro,* chloroquin can be used to inhibit lysosomal degradation, while, *in vivo,* different strategies will have to be thought of. One strategy is direct cell entry via fusion, fusion with endosomal membrane, such as conveyed by the influenza virus fusogenic protein or a part of it, or inclusion of endosome disruption or buffering components. *In vitro* ionophores were also used.

The hybrids between such structures and adenoviruses have been also tried. The function of the former was to enhance the escape rate from the endosomes. Also, alternatively, some more components of the viruses can be included in the plasmid itself to improve transfection without adding the virus with its possible safety concerns.

Targeted Liposomes

Typical ligands that are attached to liposomes can be antibodies or parts of thereof, lectins, oligosaccharides, or simple molecules such as folic acid. Tumor cells require larger quantities of folate, an essential cofactor in the synthesis of purines and pyrimidines, and therefore overexpress the folate receptor due to their increased metabolic rates. These cells may have over 20-fold higher concentration of folate-binding protein (over half a million receptor molecules in some cell lines), and it is believed that they can transcytose the material engulfed in caveolae which are rich in glycosylphosphatidylinositol without exposing the contents to lysozymes.

Epithelial growth factor is also overexpressed in many tumor cells and can present a suitable target. Hepatocytes may be targeted via asialoglycoprotein receptor and simple lipids, such as lactosylceramide, may improve delivery if particles are smaller than ~100 nm. Macrophages can be targeted by including lipids such as phosphatidylserine in the bilayer as well as via incorporation of mannose-containing glycolipids in the bilayer.

The main concern with these ligand-bearing and target-searching particles is accessibility of the target. Mostly, these applications are limited to the vascular system and perhaps the peritoneal cavity and some other body cavities containing nonviscous fluids. Also, we must keep in mind that targeted sterically stabilized liposomes have not performed according to the expectations of many scientists. Further, their immunogenicity has not been critically assessed yet. I doubt that repeated administrations of antibody-bearing liposomes are feasible at present. Even the solution of shorter fragments and/or humanized antibodies may not bypass the clearance by the immune system upon repeated administrations. The same may be true for peptide ligands.

Minichromosomes

This approach consists of adding an independent chromosome by electroporation or microinjection, which becomes maintained throughout the division process. The minichromosome contains DNA elements for the human centromere, mouse telomeres, phage insertion sequences, and the antibiotic-resistance gene. Promoters and regulatory genes are also included and can respond to normal physiological triggers in the host organism.

Minichromosomes segregate normally during mitosis and are a stable part of the cell genome. They operate in all animal cells and have a potential for the transformation of plant cells as well.

Transkaryotic Therapy

This is an alternative to *in vivo* and *ex vivo* procedures using viral vectors. It can be used for secretion of soluble proteins. The concept resembles the *ex vivo* approach. A small number of cells are obtained from the patient and they are genetically engineered in the test tube. After propagation and control of their activity, they are administered back to the patient. Typically, this is a skin biopsy and cells are injected subcutaneously.

In addition to the above-discussed optimization of the carrier system, plasmid itself will be very likely improved by adding specific sequences, such as nuclear targeting, nuclear retention, self-replication, chromosome integration, and, ultimately, homologous recombination. Perhaps more information from the virus genome can be incorporated into plasmid without any safety concerns. It is likely that additional karyotypic DNA stretches will be found and included on the plasmid to improve their nuclear localization. Therefore, carrier would maximize cytoplasmic delivery while DNA intranuclear. New sequences that can improve stability, delivery, and binding and processing of RNA intermediates will be also used. Such a synergistic approach may lead to gene therapy pharmaceutical products.

RNA Delivery

Due to its stability and ability to integrate into the host genome DNA was predominantly used in gene transfection. However, since large quantities of RNA can be synthesized *in vitro* via bacteriophage RNA polymerases and because the target is cytoplasm and not cell nucleus, RNA transfection may offer some advantages. By using Lipofectin, similar results as with DNA transfer were obtained: transfection efficacy varied with respect to the RNA/lipid ratio (optimal at 1:3 to 4 ratio) and with the cell type (Malone et al., 1989). Additionally, these systems can be also used to deliver some proteins.

In conclusion, in this chapter we introduced several delivery systems and speculated on some future developments. The same, or similar, systems can also be used to deliver antisense nucleotides and ribozymes where scientists are only now realizing that the synthesis of stable compounds may be a lesser challenge than their delivery into cells.

Finally, none of the currently existing gene delivery systems seems to be efficacious and safe enough for commercialization. It is very likely that significant improvements mostly in safety, inflammatory response reduction, and efficacy and duration of expression will have to be made before the first formulations will be on the market. Table 5-3 summarizes the most-studied gene delivery systems.

■ SUMMARY

One of the major problems in gene expression is effective delivery of plasmids into appropriate cells, especially *in vivo*. For applications in

TABLE 5-3

COMPARISON OF DIFFERENT GENE DELIVERY SYSTEMS FOR *IN VIVO* APPLICATION

Vehicle Vector	Safety Efficiency	Capacity Persistence	Loading Capacity	Insertion	Dividing Cells	Targeting
Retrovirus	High	High	Moderate	Yes	Yes	No
Adenovirus	Very high	Low	High	No	No	No
AAV[a]	Moderate	Moderate	Low	Yes	No	No
Herpes	Unknown	High	High	No	No	Nerve cells
EF[b]	Low	Moderate	High	No	No	No
Naked DNA	Low	Low		No	No	Muscle only
Liposomes+	Low	Low	High	No	No	Potentially
Liposomes−	Low	Low	Moderate	No	No	Potentially
PL-receptor	Low	Low	Low	No	No	Liver
Polymers	Low	Low	High	No	No	No
Artificial virus	High?	High?	High?	Yes?	No	Yes

Note: +,− cationic and anionic liposomes; PL, polylysine.

[a] Adeno-associated virus.

[b] Electroporated fibroblasts (implant).

genetic therapy practically only viral and colloidal gene carriers can be employed. The plasmid of interest is either reconstructed in a virus with deleted sequences or complexed with a carrier for intracellular delivery. Viral vehicles have problems with safety, low titers, and in some cases with efficiency, while colloidal carriers have problems with efficiency and duration of expression, and possibly with potential adverse effects of cationic species. Among many colloidal systems, lipid- and liposome–based delivery systems seem to be the most widely studied and used.

◼ ADDITIONAL READING

Kriegler, M., Gene transfer, in *Gene Transfer and Expression: A Laboratory Manual*, W. H. Freeman, New York, 1990, 3–81.

Lasic, D. D., Templeton, N. S., Liposomes in gene therapy, *Adv. Drug Del. Rev.*, 20, 221, 1996.

LIPOSOMES

6

Liposomes are vesicular colloidal particles composed of self-assembled amphiphilic molecules. Amphiphiles are molecules that contain two groups with different solubility. The hydrophilic group, often referred to as the polar head, is "water loving," while the hydrophobic part, the so-called nonpolar tail, is "water hating." Therefore, these molecules self-assemble and form ordered structures in aqueous solutions. Single-chain amphiphiles, such as soaps and detergents, form micelles. These are small spherical structures in which surface polar heads shield the nonpolar interior against water. Many natural amphiphiles, such as lecithin (diacyl phosphatidylcholine), have two nonpolar tails and due to a bulky non-polar part cannot be packed into micelles. These molecules normally self-assemble into lipid bilayers in which two polar surfaces shield the nonpolar interior. Bilayered lamellae have their edges exposed to water, therefore, at lower concentrations they self-close into spherical structures to eliminate this unfavorable exposure, and lipid vesicles or liposomes are formed. Figure 6-1 shows the structure of micelles and lipid bilayers schematically.

In general, however, aqueous systems of amphiphiles exhibit a very rich phase behavior and some of the structures formed are shown in Figure 6-2. While in drug delivery basically only the dispersed self-closed lamellar phase — the liposome — is important, in gene transfer several other structures and phases, including the open lipid bilayer fragment, the inverse hexagonal phase, and the micelle, may be also important.

The structure of lipid systems can be approximated by taking into account the geometric properties of these amphiphiles. In the case when the polar part is larger than the nonpolar tail, the molecules tend to pack into structures with high radii of curvature. For similar areas of polar heads and cross sections of nonpolar tails, molecules pack into bilayers while lipids with a relatively small polar head pack into inverse structures, as shown schematically in Figure 6-3. A structural parameter P is defined as

$$P = v/(a * l) \tag{6-1}$$

where v is the volume of the lipid molecule, a the area of the polar head, and l the length of the hydrocarbon chain. For values of P below 1/3, micelles are favored structures; for values between 0.8 and 1.1,

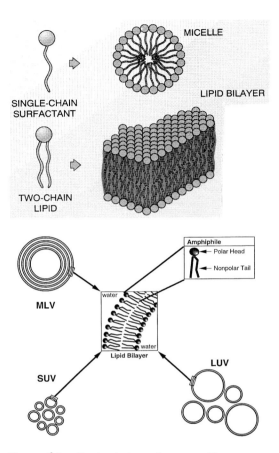

Figure 6-1   Single-chain surfactants self-aggregate into micelles (top) while double-chain surfactants form bilayers. Because bilayers have exposed edges they self-close in aqueous suspensions into spherical structures called lipid vesicles or liposomes.

preferably around 1, bilayers are the most stable structure, while for values P > 1 to 1.1 inverse structures form. I did not follow exact numbers from the literature (Israelachvili, 1985) mainly because this is only an approximation which only takes into account molecular geometry and does not consider entropy and other interactions. Furthermore, it is based on the assumption that all the structures are at thermodynamic equilibrium which in the case of liposomes is normally not true. In any case, however, it offers good estimates about the structure of particular lipid mixtures, especially because we can define an average P as the sum of mole fractions of individual values of P of individual lipids:

$$\langle P \rangle = \Sigma_i x_i P_i \tag{6-2}$$

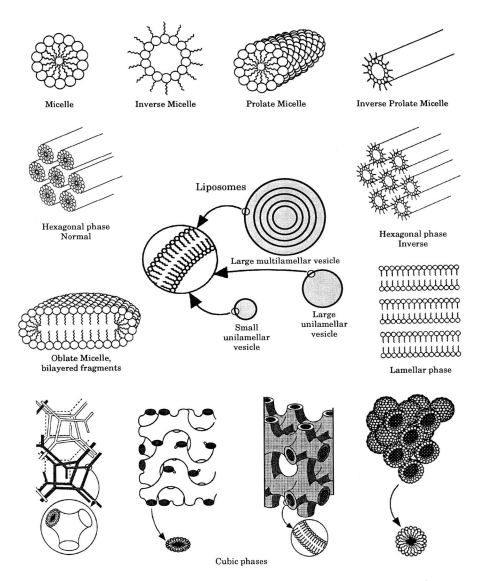

Figure 6-2 Several structures formed by lipids in aqueous solutions. In mixed systems phase behavior is even richer. Liquid crystalline phases and micellar solutions are stable thermodynamic phases while lamellar colloidal suspension — liposomes — is a kinetically trapped state. Despite the excess energy due to the bilayer curvature, these systems can be stable for prolonged periods of time, from years to possibly decades.

where fractions are taken for lipid i. We shall use this concept later to explain liposomes with built-in instability.

Liposomes can be defined as self-closed spherical particles where one or several lipid membranes encapsulate(s) part of the solvent in

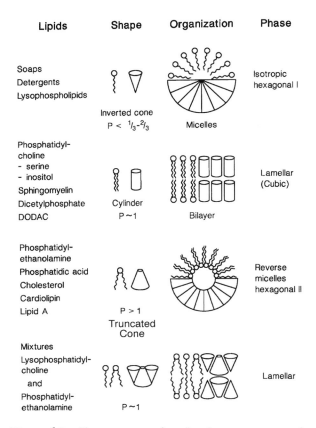

| Lipids | Shape | Organization | Phase |

Figure 6-3   The concept of molecular geometry and structure of the amphiphilic phases as deter mined by packing of surfactant molecules (steric effects) as developed by Israelachvili and collaborators (1985).

which they freely float into their interior. With respect to the size and number of membranes we distinguish large multilamellar vesicles (LMV or MLV) and unilamellar vesicles which can be small (SUV), large (LUV), or giant (GUV), as shown in Figures 6-1 and 6-2. Small liposomes are normally defined as the ones where curvature effects are important for their properties. This curvature depends on the lipid composition and can vary from 50 nm for soft bilayers to 80 to 100 nm for bilayers composed of mechanically very cohesive bilayers. Giant vesicles are normally those with diameters above 1 μm. The thickness of the bilayer is around 4 nm while they can contain surface grafted polymers which can extend up to 5 to 10 nm above the surface.

Another important liposome characteristic is composition which determines surface and membrane properties, including surface charge, steric

Figure 6-4 Phase transitions in a lipid bilayer. Crystalline phase transforms into a gel phase at T_c', and when hydrocarbon chains melt the liquid crystalline phase occurs above T_c.

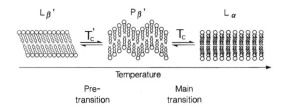

interactions, and membrane rigidity. This is another important property of bilayers which is characterized by a phase transition from ordered solid to disordered fluid membrane at the temperature T_c as shown in Figure 6-4. This temperature depends on the length and degree of saturation of hydrocarbon chains. For phosphatidylcholine polar heads it varies from approximately –15°C for dioleoyl chains to 24, 42, and 55°C for dimyristoyl, dipalmitoyl, and distearoyl chains, respectively. Fatty acid chains and phospholipids will be introduced in the next section (see Figure 6-5). Phosphatidylethanolamine polar heads attached to the same fatty acid chains have slightly higher values of T_c, while charged groups in general reduce this temperature a few degrees. With increasing concentration of cholesterol the ordered phase becomes more disordered and the disordered more ordered. This eventually results in an ordered fluid phase which has no phase transition for cholesterol-saturated bilayers (50 mol% in the case of phospholipids). These are also mechanically the most cohesive bilayers, while liposome stability against proteins and membrane permeability is saturated at the lipid to cholesterol ratio of 2:1. Saturated C_{18} chains interact with cholesterol more strongly than any other and therefore form mechanically the strongest membrane (Lasic and Needham, 1995).

■ LIPIDS AND LIPOSOME COMPOSITION

Typically, liposomes are composed of neutral or anionic lipids, which can be extracted from natural sources or prepared synthetically. The most-used natural lipids are lecithins (phosphatidylcholines), sphingomyelins, and phosphatidylethanolamines (PE) (kephalins) which are normally extracted from natural substances, such as egg yolks, soya beans, and (ox) brains. These lipids are at physiological values of pH zwitterionic (neutral). Negatively charged lipids are phosphatidylserines, phosphatidylglycerols (PG), and phosphatidylinositols (PI). Natural lipids contain various mixtures of lipid chains. In contrast, synthetic lipids can have well-defined acyl chains attached to the same polar heads. The most used are dimyristoyl, dipalmitoyl, distearoyl, dioleoyl, and palmitoyl–oleoyl chains. The structure of these lipids is shown in Figure 6-5. Cholesterol is often added to improve mechanical stability of the bilayer and decrease leakage of the encapsulated material.

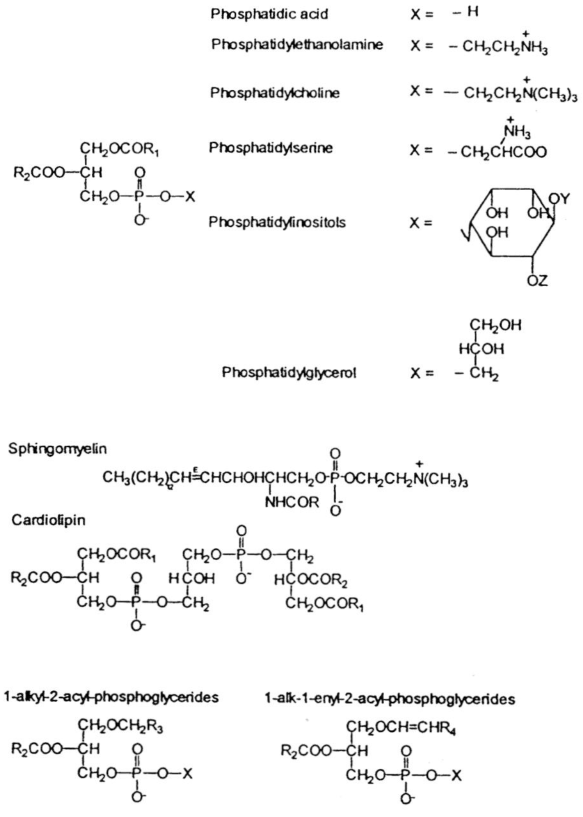

Figure 6-5 Typical phospholipids and fatty acid chains encountered in liposome work.

Fatty Acid Chains

Saturated	Unsaturated
$CH_3-(CH_2)_n-COO-$	$CH_3-(CH_2)_7-CH=CH-(CH_2)_7-COO-oleoyl$
n = 10 = lauryl	$(CC_7C=CC_7COO-oleoyl)$
n = 12 = myristoyl	$CC_5C=CC_7COO-palmitoleoyl$
n = 14 = palmitoyl	$CC_4C=CCC=CC_7COO-linoleyl$
n = 16 = stearoyl	$CCC=CCC=CCC=CC_7COO-linolenyl$
n = 20 = arachidyl	$CC_4C=CCC=CCC=CCC=CC_3COO-arachidonyl$

In addition to these liposomes which are characterized by nonspecific interactions with the environment, and are normally referred to as conventional, three other liposome groups can be defined with respect to their functionality (Lasic and Papahadjopoulos, 1995), as schematically

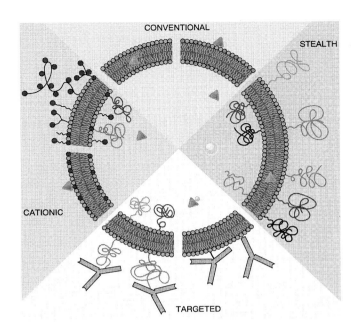

Figure 6-6 Four different classes of liposomes as defined according to their functionality. Conventional liposomes interact with the milieu nonspecifically. Sterically stabilized liposomes do not interact while targeted (ligand-bearing) liposomes react specifically. Polymorphic liposomes change their phase upon interaction with a specific agent or medium.

shown in Figure 6-6. Inert liposomes which have pronounced stability in the biological milieu are referred to as sterically stabilized liposomes due to surface coating with inert hydrophilic polymer, such as polyethylene glycol (PEG). Typically, 5 mol% of lipid with covalently bound polymer with the degree of polymerization around 50 (range 30 to 120) are incorporated in the membrane. Liposomes with attached targeting ligands, such as monoclonal antibodies, lectins, or oligosaccharides can also be targeted to specific targets. Conventional targeted liposomes are normally used for *in vitro* experiments and tests while sterically stabilized liposomes with attached ligands are used for systemic targeting of specific cells. The fourth group consists of very reactive liposomes which change their phase and structure upon a particular interaction and are called polymorphic liposomes. Because these are rather important in gene delivery we shall describe their properties. These include liposomes sensitive to ions, heat, light, target, or degree of degradation/dissociation. Ion-sensitive liposomes can change their structure upon change of concentration of a particular ion. For instance, pH-sensitive liposomes undergo phase transition lamellar–hexagonal phase upon acidification and release their contents. If pH-sensitive polymers are bound to the liposome surface or coexist as free in solution this can induce increased membrane permeability, liposome disintegration, or fusion. Liposomes can be sensitive to other ions, such as Ca^{2+} or polyions. An example is cationic liposomes which can change their structure upon interaction with the negatively charged polymers.

Although pH-sensitive liposomes can be made from mixtures of lecithins and fatty acids, by far the most common lipid is dioleoyl phosphatidylethanolamine (DOPE). These molecules can form lamellar phases only at higher values of pH when the amine group is charged. By lowering pH it deprotonates; this decreases its polar head area (a) as a result of reduced hydration, and packing parameter P increases from around 1 to a higher value which prefers packing into a hexagonal array. As a consequence, DOPE liposomes become unstable at pH values below 8. Because this pH range is normally not suitable for *in vivo* applications it is usually used in mixtures with hemisuccinate lipids. In this composition negatively charged cholesterol hemisuccinate protonates at lower pH values and decreases polar head group area. Reduced packing parameter P causes liposome destabilization at pH values below 5.5. As a consequence, liposomes can fuse with nearby membranes or disintegrate and flocculate. Similar release of entrapped material can be achieved if DOPE is packed with lipids with P ~0.5, such as polymer-bearing lipids, and polymer either slowly breaks away by hydrolysis or thiolysis (Kirpotin et al., 1996) or these lipids dissociate from the bilayer due to higher aqueous solubility. The mean value of packing parameter ⟨P⟩ increases, and above critical value liposome disintegrates (see Figure 6-7). If the mean value of ⟨P⟩ decreases, such as upon cleavage of double-chain surfactant into two single chain amphiphiles, liposome disintegration follows as well, as schematically shown in Figure 6-7.

Additionally, if liposome contains other active groups hidden in the polymer coat, they can become exposed and change liposome interaction characteristics. Similarly, in another example of liposome with a built-in structural instability, asymmetric membrane composition can be held by a pH gradient across the vesicle membrane which dissipates in time and which results in liposome destabilization.

lamellar - micellar phase transition

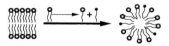

lamellar - hexagonal II phase transition

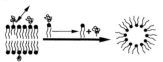

Figure 6-7 Schematic presentation of liposome disintegration. Lamellar–micellar phase transition occurs upon hydrolysis of lipids and lamellar–hexagonal II phase transition in the mixed lipid bilayer is caused by PEG–lipid dissociation from the bilayer or cleavage of PEG from PE or lipid hydrolysis. (Courtesy of Stan Hansen.)

Surface-attached pH-sensitive proteins or peptides can be used to induce liposome fusion upon a trigger, such as pH drop. Some viruses employ this mechanism to fuse with cells or endosomes after endocytosis. Most frequently used is influenza fusion protein (Wilschut and Dijkstra, 1991) while many laboratories have problems with reproducibility of Sendai virus–triggered fusion. This virus, however, is attractive because it can facilitate DNA entry directly into the cell cytoplasm, bypassing the endocytotic pathway and possible lysosomal degradation, because it can neutralize pH.

Another example of polymorphic liposomes is cationic liposomes. They avidly interact with anions and anionic polyelectrolytes. Simple anions decrease liposome stability because of the reduction of electrostatic shielding of the surface charge by anions in the solution. This interaction in general obeys the Derjaguin–Landau–Verwey–Overbeek (DLVO) model while anionic polyelectrolytes, like polyglutamic acids, polystyrene sulfonate, and most notably DNA, adsorb and can induce bridging and/or possibly lipid phase change. Analogously to the anionic liposomes, cationic pH-sensitive liposomes can be prepared. In this case, however, by lowering pH the basic groups become more charged and bind DNA tighter and the benefit for transfection is not obvious.

Cationic liposomes are currently the most widely used lipid transfection system, and below we shall introduce some cationic lipids and liposomes.

■ CATIONIC LIPIDS

Positively charged lipids, with the exceptions of sphingosine and some lipids in primitive life forms, practically do not exist in nature. Before the explosion in lipid synthesis in the early 1990s several cationic detergents were used for preparation of liposomes with positive charge. The most popular single-chain amphiphiles are chloride and bromide salts of the alkyl trimethyl ammonium surfactants. The most widely used have either a dodecyl (C_{12}) or a hexadecyl (cetyl, C_{16}) chain, and the abbreviations DDAC/B or CTAB/C are normally used. To impose positive charge on liposomes, such detergents were incorporated in the lipid bilayer. Mostly stearylamine was used because it has lower aqueous solubility and is less toxic. In the beginning, basically only two families of two-chained amphiphiles were in use: dioctadecyl dimethyl ammonium bromide/chloride (DODAB/C)* and DOTAP family (dioleoyloxy-3-(trimethylammonio) propane). These liposomes were mostly used to study theories of colloid stability as a counterpart to anionic ones.

There are several very important parameters describing properties of detergents and lipids. These are their molecular geometry which influences

---

* In biological literature these abbreviations are often used incorrectly with respect to previously established trends and DDAB is actually DODAB.

the structures they form, hydrophilic–hydrophobic balance, detergent power, and critical micelle concentration (cmc). The latter one is simply the ratio between free molecules in solution (as monomers) and molecules in aggregates. Because lipid exchange between the two states is a highly dynamic process we must be aware that the systems, which are stable in the test tube, can practically immediately change their structure and properties (for instance, surface charge) upon dilution if the cmc values are high (approximately $>10^{-3,-5}$ M). Phospholipids have cmc values below $10^{-8,-9}$ M and this is not an important instability problem. However, charged single-chain detergents, such as stearylamine, can pop out from the liposome membrane in milliseconds upon dilution or intravenous administration and this has resulted in many artifactual studies where the real surface charge was much less than expected from the bulk concentrations.

Since it was realized that cationic liposomes can complex DNA (Behr, 1986) and that these complexes can transfect DNA, as was shown by Felgner et al. (1987) for liposomes containing DOTMA (dioleoxy propyl trimethyl ammonium chloride), numerous new lipids were synthesized to improve gene transfer efficiency and to decrease their toxicity. DOTMA is in fact DOTAP with a sole difference that acyl chains are linked to the propyl backbone via ether and not ester bonds. Transfection efficacy studies of this structural family have led to another efficacious lipid DMRIE (dimyristooxypropyl dimethyl hydroxyethyl ammonium bromide) (Felgner et al., 1994). Polyelectrolytes, such as polylysine were also attached to acyl chains (Zhou and Huang, 1989). This, however, increases aqueous solubility of these compounds. Natural cations, such as spermine^{4+} and spermidine^{3+}, can be also coupled to fatty acids. These lipids form micellar rather than vesicular structures. The best-known examples are DOSPA and DOGS (see Figure 6-8) (Behr et al., 1989). Positive charge can be associated also on the sterol backbone, with DC-Chol (Figure 6-8) being the best-known example (Leventis and Silvius, 1990; Gao and Huang, 1991). Many other (poly)cationic groups such as spermine and spermidine were linked to cholesterol as well. I am not aware of any other sterols being used for linkage of (poly)cations.

The chemical structures of lipids most frequently used in gene complexation are shown in Figure 6-8. The three most common neutral lipids are also shown. Numerous other lipids exist but mostly they are variations of ammonium salt or polyamine with respect to group stereochemistry, number of positive charges, branching and separations between them, spacer groups, backbone molecules, hydrophobic anchors, and so on. Practically all naturally occurring cations and polycations have been attached to fatty acid chains or sterols.

While detailed studies of the chemical stability of cationic lipids have not been performed yet, experiences show similar stability profiles to neutral and anionic lipids. The major degradation reactions are hydrolysis and oxidation.

Neutral Lipids

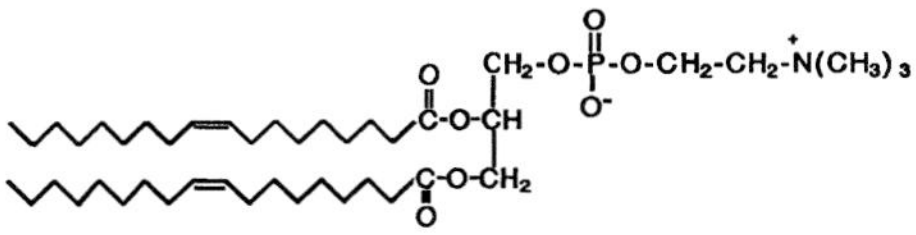

DOPC

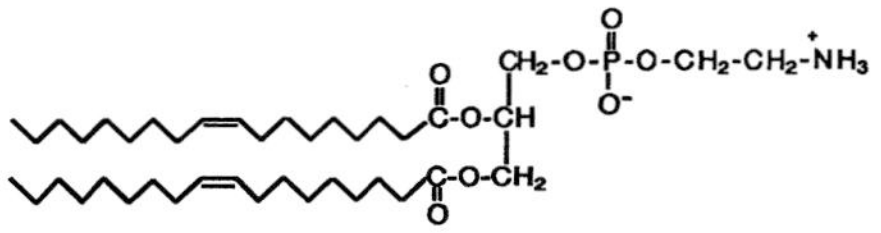

DOPE

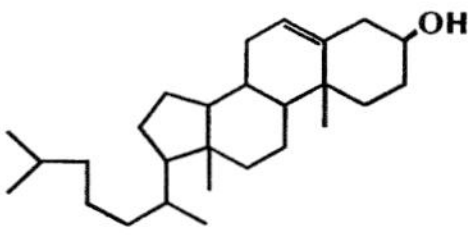

CHOL

Figure 6-8 Some neutral and cationic lipids used in gene transfection. Chemical names are described in the text and Appendix E. (Courtesy of Stan Hansen.)

■ ELECTROSTATIC PROPERTIES OF CHARGED LIPIDS AND LIPOSOMES

Polar lipids can have various degrees of charges in aqueous solutions at various pH ranges. Primary phosphate (phosphatydic acid) has two values of pK, at 3.5 and 8.5. Secondary phosphates, such as are present in PG, PI, and cardiolipin (DPG), have pK (PI, DPG) = 2.0 and pK = 3.0 for PG. If quaternary ammonium is bound to the phosphate, such as on phosphatidylcholine or sphingomyelins, the pK of phosphate becomes 2.5 and the pK of quaternary amine is around 13. Adding amine to the secondary phosphate, such as in the case of phosphatidylethanolamine, leaves pK of phosphate around 2.5 and pK of the amino group around 9. Cholines are isoelectric in pH range 3 to 10, while ethanolamines are negatively charged above pH > 8. Negatively charged phosphatidylserine, which has a carboxyl group attached to a secondary phosphate, has three pK values. The phosphate group has pK of 2.5, the carboxyl has pK = 4.5, and the amino group is characterized by pK = 10.3.

pK values of cationic lipids have not been reported yet. From ammonia and amines one can expect them in a range from 8 to 11, typically above 10, depending on the side groups, which means that at normal values of pH they are almost completely charged. Accordingly, DOTAP and DOTMA have pK values around 12. If the charge is delocalized on a heterocycle ring, the pK can be lower.

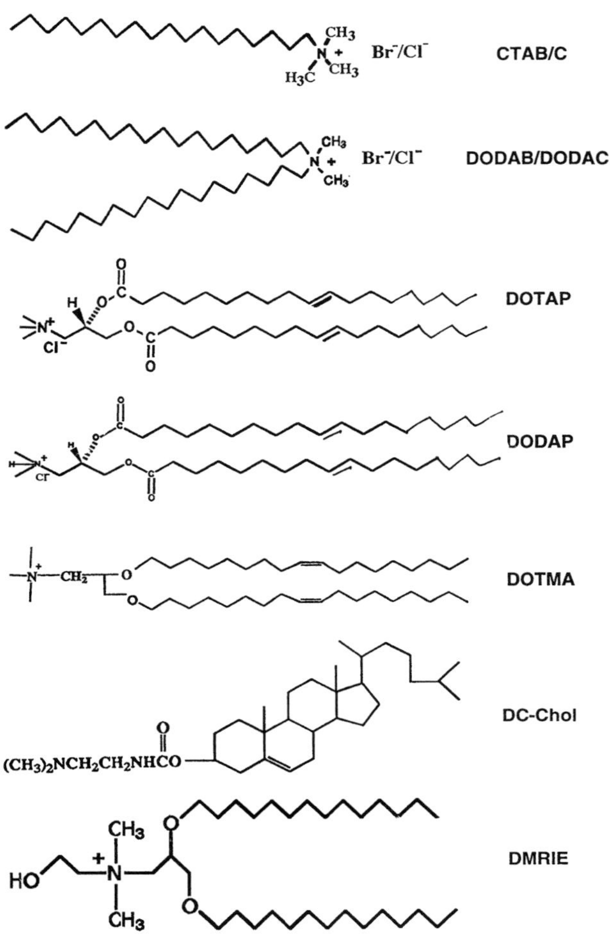

Figure 6-8 (continued)

The majority of positive charges of cationic lipids are based on (poly)amines and quaternary ammonium salts. Not many specific details are known about the pK values of these cationic lipids and counterion associations with the bilayers. Amines are weak bases and upon interaction with acids yield aminium salts. When the central nitrogen atom is charged but is not attached to a hydrogen atom, the compound is called a quaternary ammonium salt. Quaternary ammonium salts and guanidine-based compounds are very strong bases and pK_a values are above 12. Tertiary amines (RR'R"N, where R is an alkyl group) are less basic than secondary (RR'NH) and primary (RNH₂) amines. For simple alkyl amines pK_a values are typically above 10 for primary and secondary amines and

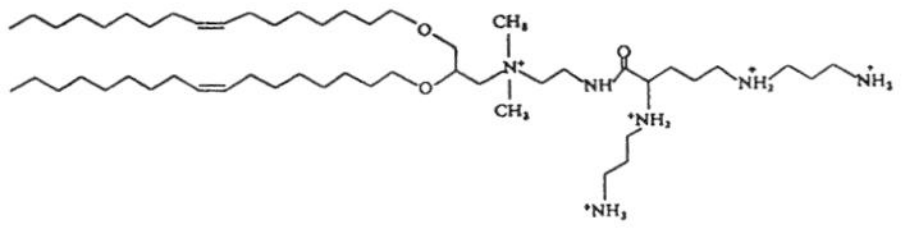

DOSPA

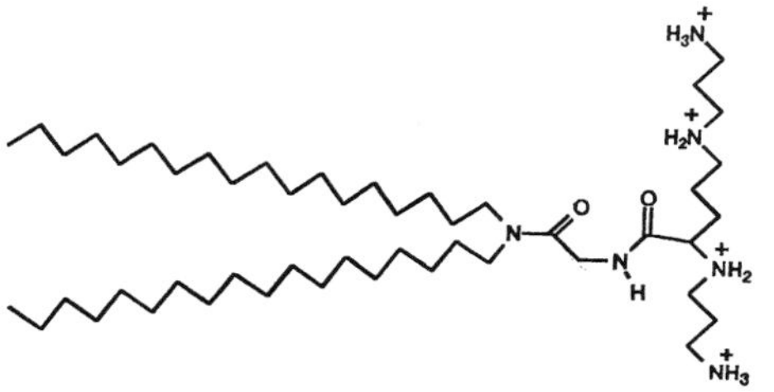

DOGS

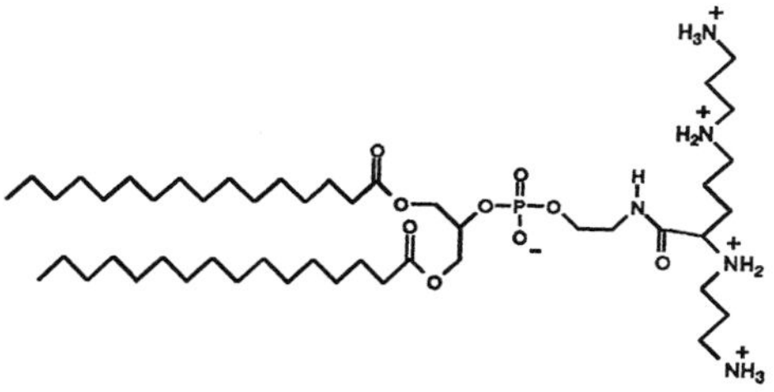

DPPES

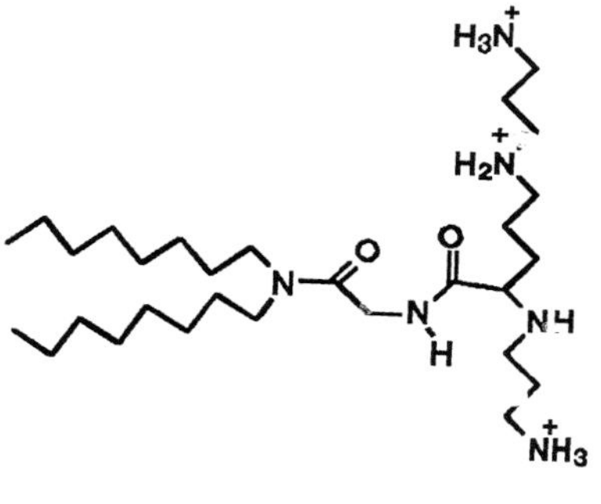

C_8Gly Sper $^{3+}$

Figure 6-8 (continued)

above 9 for tertiary. Arylamines are weaker bases and aromatic amines are very weak bases. The presence of double bonds and nearby charges, however, can reduce the pK_a values and in dense networks, such as in dendrimers the pK_a values may be below 6. Amides (one R is oxygen) are very weak bases. In addition to unknowns about the pK values of various polyamines conjugated to hydrophobic parts also the surface pH is not well defined. Positively charged surface attracts hydroxyl ions and surface pH increases. If one performs simple electrostatic evaluation this increase can be up to 3 pH units in low salt conditions. However, this crowding of hydroxyls also drastically reduces their activity which may

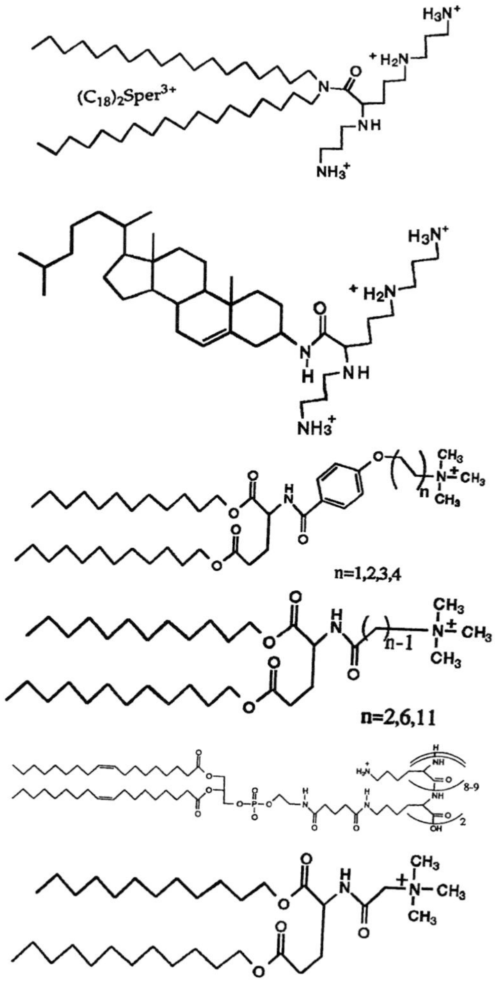

$(C_{18})_2$ Sper $^{3+}$

Sper-Chol

$C_{12}GluPhC_nN^+$

$C_{14}GluC_nN^+$

LPL

TMAG

Figure 6-8 (continued)

compensate for the increased concentration and the real surface pH has not been yet precisely determined.

The surface of charged liposomes is characterized by a surface potential which decays into the bulk solution proportionally to the Debye length κ^{-1}. Counterions are smeared in the vicinal double layer because of thermal energy. The electrostatic potential of a plane with surface charge σ in z,z valent electrolyte with concentration c is given at temperature T by Gouy–Chapman approximation (Cevc, 1993) of the Poisson–Boltzmann equation:

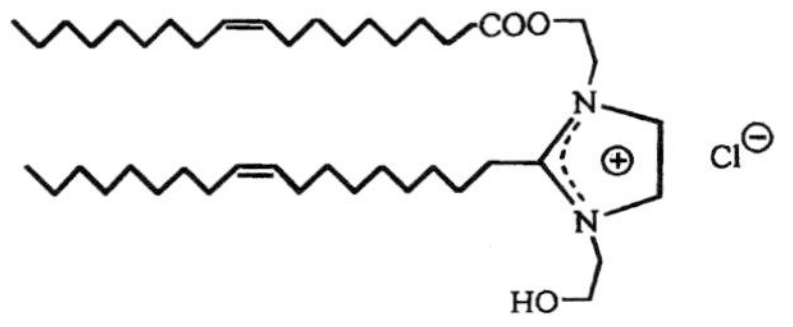

DOIC

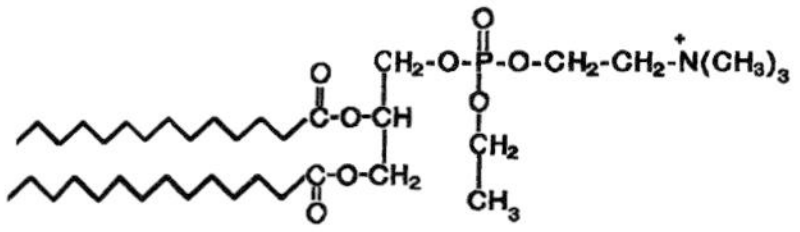

DMEPC

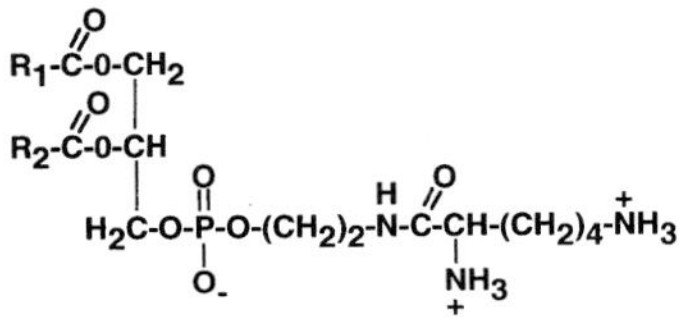

Lysinyl PE

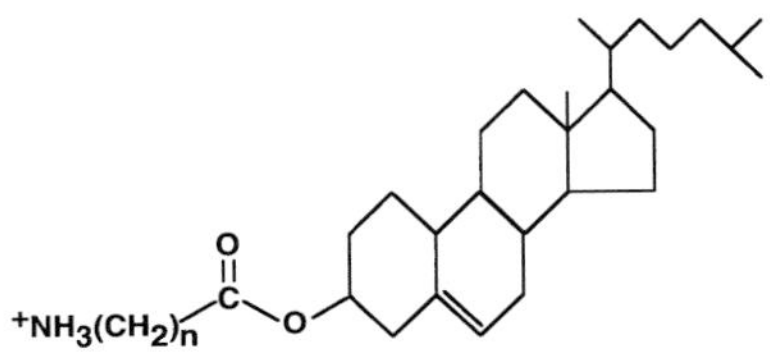

AE Chol

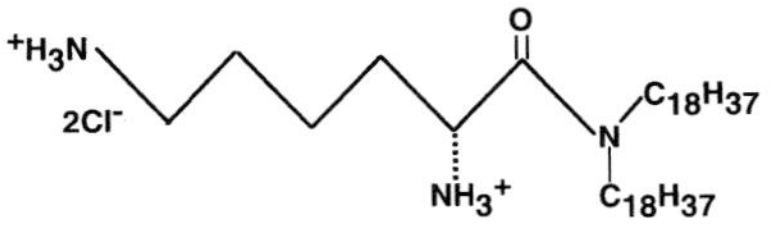

GENZYME #47

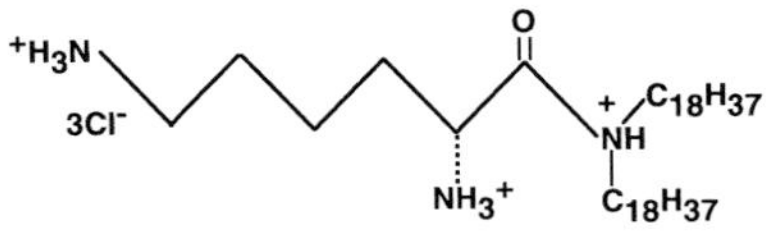

GENZYME

Figure 6-8 (continued)

$$\Psi = \left(2kT/Ze_o\right)\sinh^{-1}\left(ze_o\sigma\kappa/2\epsilon\epsilon_o kT\right) \quad \text{for} \quad \Psi > 50\,\text{mV} \qquad (6\text{-}3)$$

and by

$$\Psi = \sigma\kappa/2\epsilon\epsilon_o \quad \text{for} \quad \Psi \ll 20\,\text{mV} \qquad (6\text{-}4)$$

The net surface charge is defined as

$$\sigma = \alpha z'e_o/a \qquad (6\text{-}5)$$

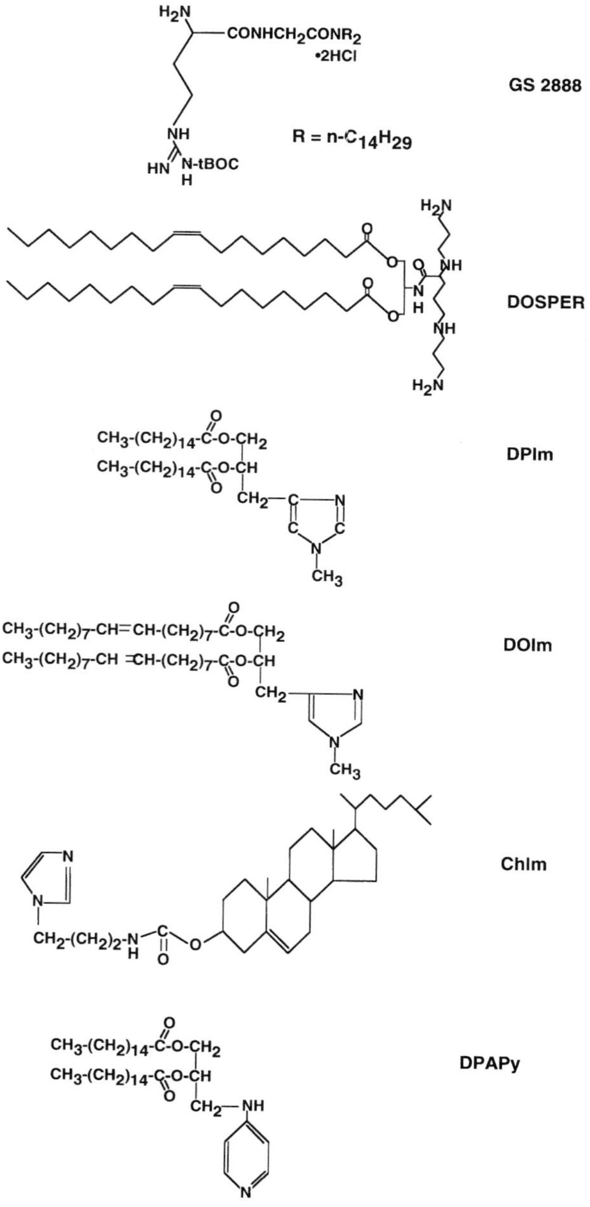

Figure 6-8 (continued)

where z' is the valency of charged lipid and α the degree of ionization, which may be, especially in the case of strongly charged cationic lipids, small. Lipid area a takes into account the density of charges (i.e., membrane composition). The potential decays in the bulk medium as

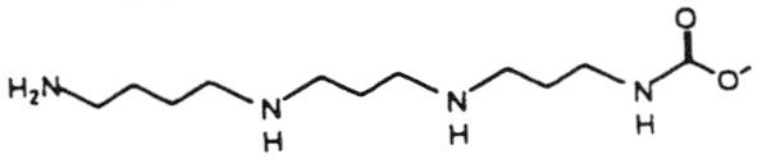

No 32 Genzyme

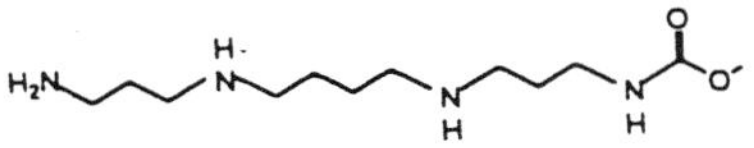

No 37 Genzyme

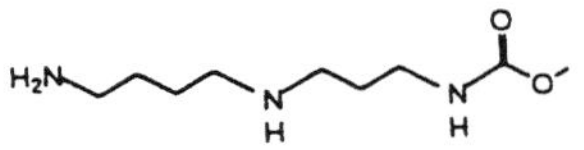

No 48 Genzyme

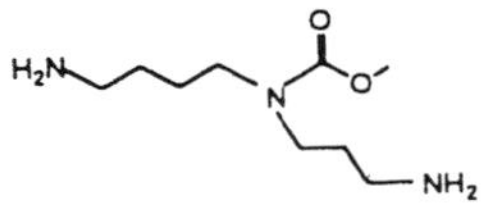

No 53 Genzyme

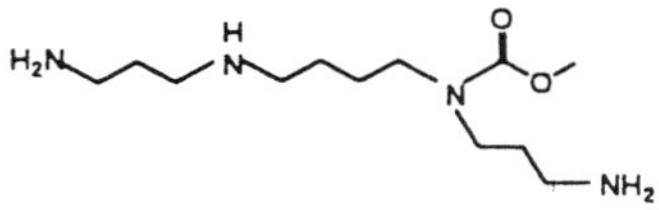

No 67 Genzyme

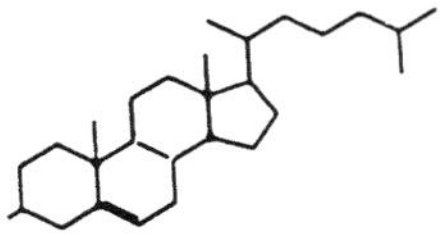

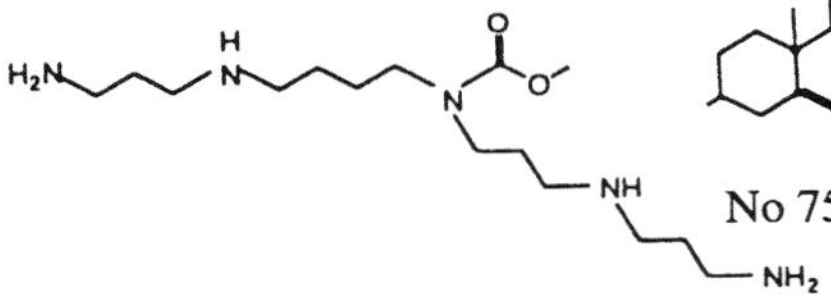

No 75 Genzyme

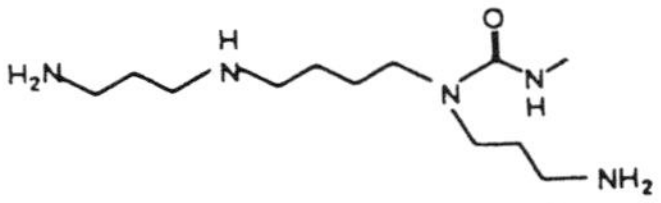

No 86 Genzyme

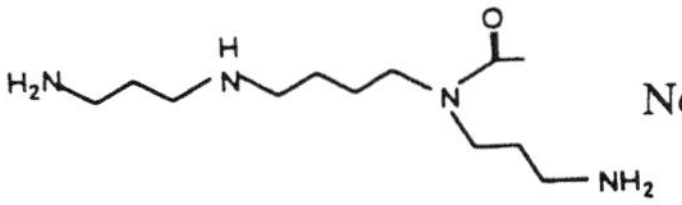

No 101 Genzyme

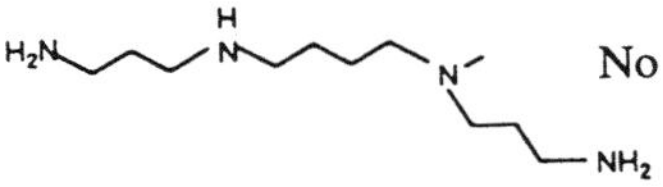

No 106 Genzyme

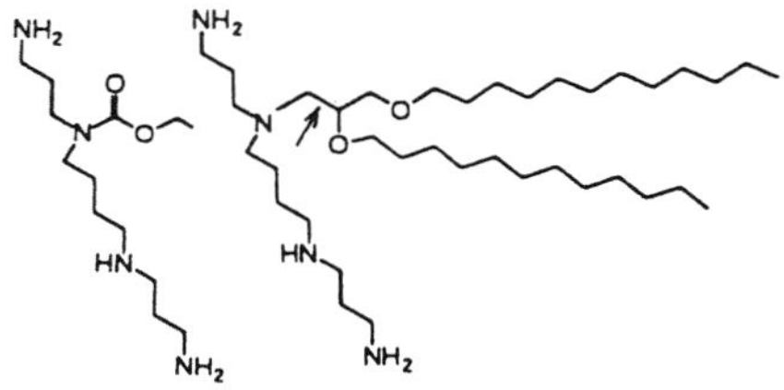

Diacyl anchor
No 89 No 102 Genzyme

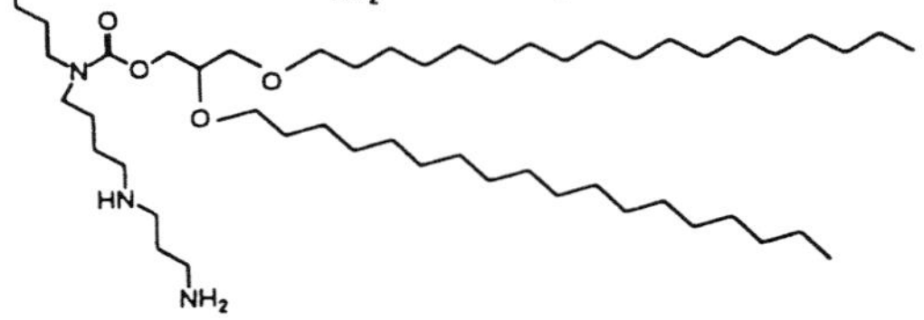

No 111 Genzyme

Figure 6-8 (continued)

$$\Psi(x) = (4\,kT/ze_o)\tanh^{-1}\left[\exp(-x/\kappa)\tanh(ze_o\Psi/4\,kT)\right] \qquad (6\text{-}6)$$

which can be approximated for low surface potential to

$$\Psi(x) = \Psi\exp(-x/\kappa) \qquad (6\text{-}7)$$

Surface charge can be measured by binding of various fluorophors or spin probes and by measuring ζ potential. The latter method measures surface potential at an imaginary slip plane (approximately two to three water molecules away from the surface) via measurement of mobility μ of particles in the medium with viscosity η. According to the Smoluchowsky equation the ζ potential can be calculated from

$$\zeta = \eta\mu/\epsilon\epsilon_o \qquad (6\text{-}8)$$

These equations are valid for low surface charges while the situation at high surface charges may deviate from these approximations.

◼ CATIONIC LIPOSOMES

In the first 20 years of liposome research cationic liposomes were not studied extensively, especially not in medical applications, due to their toxicity. Scientists used stearylamine to impose a positive charge on neutral liposomes and study their properties. Colloidal studies have shown that the DLVO theory can be applied to explain their stability although in the case of sonicated DODAC liposomes their stability was found to be lower than expected and observed with anionic liposomes (Carmona-Ribeiro, 1989; 1992). In general, pK values of cationic groups are closer to the physiological pH values and anions may be associated with bilayers to a larger extent than cations in the case of anionic liposomes. In addition, entropy effects of anions are rather different from those of normally well-hydrated cations. Many anions are also rather hydrophobic. As an example, we can state that in many cases the same cationic amphiphile may form different structures depending on the nature of the anion: for instance, chloride, bromide, or hydroxide salts form bilayers and liposomes whereas tosylate and acetate salts form micelles. Such counterion dependence is not characteristic for anionic liposomes and may influence their interaction properties. The lower than theoretically predicted stability of sonicated DODAB liposomes was explained by the presence of hydrophobic defects on the membranes of these liposomes (Carmona-Ribeiro, 1992).

The molecular geometry of these surfactants is often less ideal to form bilayers (very low values of P of highly charged lipids, such as DOSPA or DOGS and P > 1 for lipids with small polar heads and no molecular backbone, such as DODAB) as compared with phospholipids, and therefore liposomes may be less stable. Also DOTAP and DOTMA have a smaller backbone with no phosphate group. Especially in the case of high surface charges in low-ionic-strength media, where Debye length (distance where the influence of surface potential fades into thermal noise) can exceed the dimensions of the liposome, the optimal shape of a self-closed liposome may not be well defined (Helfrich, 1994, private communication). In general, higher charges and lower ionic strengths make bilayers more rigid. Furthermore, high charges may stabilize some bilayer defects. Indeed, in pure DODAB solutions, many lenslike structures (a = 30 to 50 nm, b = 10 to 15 nm) and micellar structures (open fragments) were observed by cryoelectron microscopy (Frederik et al., in preparation).

Cationic liposomes used in gene delivery are normally mixed with neutral lipids, such as DOPE. Normally, small unilamellar liposomes are prepared by sonication, extrusion, or homogenization (microfluidization) of LMVs which are prepared by hydration of thin lipid films. Cholesterol is often used as a neutral lipid, especially for *in vivo* applications while in some cases pure cationic lipids yield the highest transfection.

Numerous cationic liposome transfection kits for use in gene transfer are commercially available. Probably due to economic and marketing reasons the concentrations of these liposome solutions are rather low and they cannot suspend DNA at concentrations sufficient for effective *in vivo* transfection. Table 6-1 shows some of those kits and some useful data.

Cryoelectron microscopy has revealed a variety of shapes of different cationic liposomes. Surprisingly, even SUV are often not spherical, but show dumbbell or oval structures. While small sonicated liposomes are mostly spherical, DOIC/Chol and DMEPC/Chol SUV were often observed to contain two lamellar, pear-like liposomes of about 130 nm (5 to 10% of particles) in equilibrium with small dumbbells (60 × 40 nm), some disklike micelles and SUV (50% of particles, diameters around 60 in DOIC and 80 in DMEPC system). DODAB liposomes show lenslike particles (50 × 25 nm) and flat fragments, while unsized formulations often contain large invaginated liposomes. Extruded vesicles do not look spherical. Small vesicles (80 nm) resemble elongated ovals and pearlike particles, while larger extruded liposomes (200 to 250 nm) show many tubular structures and predominantly completely invaginated liposomes which appear like two lamellar vesicles with an opening. DOTAP/Chol and DOTAP:DOPE systems look rather similar. Figure 6-9 shows cryoelectron micrographs of several cationic liposome samples.

The origin of these shapes is not known, but it is possible that at these very high surface charges and counterion interactions, where sizes of particles approach the Debye length, spherical shapes may not have the lowest energy. Actually, similar deviations from sphericity and large invaginations were also shown in anionic liposomes (Schmutz and Brisson, 1994), and it is possible that only the advent of cryoelectron microscopy made these observations really possible. If the images are real, theoretical

TABLE 6-1

COMMERCIALLY AVAILABLE CATIONIC LIPOSOME KITS

Name	Composition (w/w)	Concentration mg/mL	mM	Producer	Price[a]	M_w[b] (Da)	+ch/mol[c]	Cell Types[d]
Lipofectin	DOTMA:DOPE (1:1)	1	1.45	LTI[e]	133	687	0.53	HeLa, BHK-21, CHO-K1
Lipofectamine	DOSPA:DOPE (3:1)	2	2.04	LTI	172	977	3.36	BHK-21, HeLa, CHO-K1
Lipofectace	DODAB:DOPE (1:2.5)	1	1.41	LTI	99	708	0.32	HeLa, BHK, CHO-K1
DOTAP	DOTAP	1	1.36	B-M[f]	130	732	1.00	BHK-21, HeLa, COS7
CellFectin	TMTPSp:DOPE (1:1.5)[g]	1	1.12	LTI	149	891	1.12	CHO-K1, COS, BHK-21
Transfectam	DOGS	1	1.11	PM[h]	295	902	4.00	HeLa, HepG2, PC12
TFX-50	TDA:DOPE (1:1)[i]	—	2.1	PM	175	891	1.0	HepG2, 293, COS-7, HeLa
DC-Chol	DC-Chol:DOPE (3:2)	—	2.0	—	—	606	0.62	A431, A459, 1B, HeLa, L929
DOSPER	DOSPER[k]	1	0.92	B-M	—	1089	4.0	CHO-K1, HeLa, HepG2

Note: Pan Vera Corp. is selling three different polyamine transfection reagents under the name TransIT™.

Abbreviations: See Appendix E.

[a] In approximate price in $/mg in liposome solution.

[b] Calculated from composition. Some numbers are estimates because exact structures and counterions were not reported.

[c] Positive charge per mole of formulation [e+/M].

[d] Many other cell lines, over one hundred, were transfected with these cationic liposome kits. The efficiencies between various cell types, however, can vary by a factor of 1000.

[e] Life Technologies, Inc. (Gibco).

[f] Boehringer-Mannheim.

[g] Tetramethyl tetra palmityl spermine.

[h] ProMega™

[i] *N,N,N*-Tetramethyl-*N,N*-bis(2-hydroxyethyl)-2,3-dioleoyloxy-1,4-butanediammonium iodide. This formulation is sold as a dry lipid film and the experimenter has to hydrate it and use MLV produced (150 to 350 nm, recommended 2.1 mM. The ratio is mol/mol).

[j] Used by R-Gene, University of Pittsburgh, etc. (now, available from Sigma).

[k] 1,3-Di-oleoyloxy-2-(6-carboxy-spermyl)-propyl-amide.

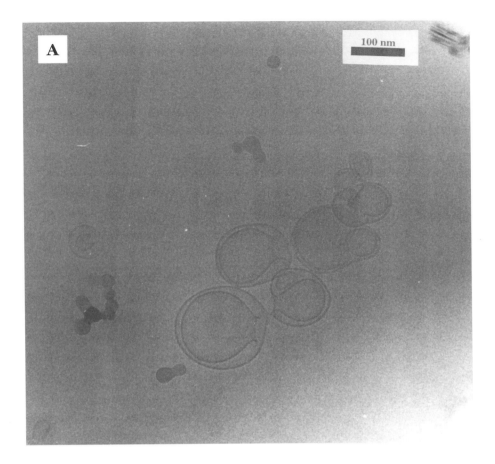

Figure 6-9 Cryoelectron microscopy of cationic liposomes. Unusual shapes may either be an artifact of impurities or, perhaps, may require reevaluation of theories of vesicle shapes. (A) sonicated DOTAP (commercial product 6 months old. Freshly sonicated DOTAP suspensions contain small and spherical liposomes.) (B) extruded DOTAP:Chol. Arrows indicate openings of invaginated liposomes. (Courtesy of P. Frederik.)

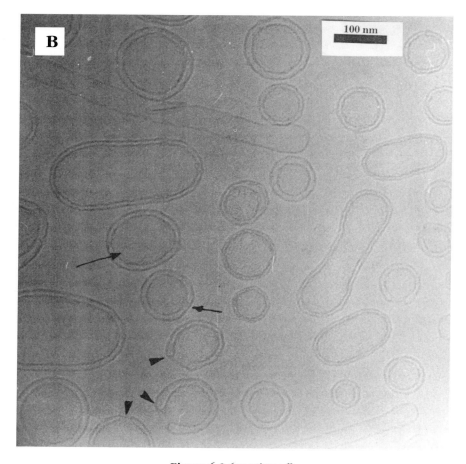

Figure 6-9 (continued)

studies of vesicle shapes will have to be refined, possibly by including Gaussian curvature in the transformation open fragment–vesicle. Alternatively, shape changes may be due to lipid phase segregation due to chemical degradation and/or multicomponent composition.

LIPOSOME PREPARATION METHODS

The same preparation methods that are used for the preparation of anionic and neutral liposomes can be used for the preparation of cationic liposomes. Before we explain details below, we shall very briefly characterize a typical procedure: lipids are mixed in an organic phase, dried, hydrated during agitation, and sized down to ensure a homogeneous population of vesicles, as shown schematically in Figure 6-10. Dry crystalline lamellae swell upon addition of water and agitation breaks the growing tubules (the so-called myelin figures); MLV are formed.

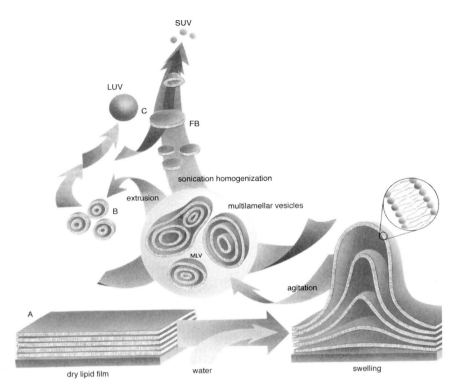

Figure 6-10 Growth of myelin figures upon hydration of dry lipid film. Agitation detaches hydrating lipid mass and particles self-close into large multilamellar vesicles. These can be sonicated, extruded, or homogenized to prepare a uniform population of smaller vesicles. (From Lasic, D.D., Rècherche 20, 904, 1989.)

Hydration of Lipids

Typically, lipid concentrations between 5 and 50 mM are employed. For the preparation of liposomes with mixed lipid composition, lipid components must be mixed in an organic solvent in order to assure optimal mixing of lipids. Organic solvent is then evaporated and dry lipid hydrated with an appropriate buffer. Most frequently, chloroform or a chloroform/methanol mixture (3/1 vol/vol) is used and thin lipid film is prepared in a round-bottomed glass flask upon rotary evaporation. To increase surface area rather large flasks are recommended (for instance, for the preparation of 10 mL of 20 mM liposomes containing equimolar lipid with molecular weight 1000 Da and DOPE, 100 mg of lipid and 79 mg of DOPE are weighed in a 1-L round-bottomed flask and dissolved with 10 to 20 mL of organic solvent). After removal of organic solvent, traces of organic solvents are removed by a vacuum pump, normally overnight at pressures below milli Torr (~0.1 Pa). For preparations which will be used in humans the use of chloroform is not advised despite the fact that it can be pumped off below 1 ppm relatively quickly. In such cases one can use tertiary butanol. Lipids are weighed into a container, dissolved in this solvent at 30 to 50°C and quickly frozen, most frequently in a dry ice–ethanol or acetone mixture. The frozen lipid cake is then lyophilized for at least 1 day. The thickness of the cake should not exceed its diameter. Another way to mix and dry lipids is spray drying. Despite the fact that liposomes containing high mole percents of cholesterol abolish phase transition and can swell below T_c of lipid, it is still recommended that the mixture swells at temperatures above the T_c.

This dry lipid film, cake, or powder is hydrated during vigorous mixing at temperatures above the gel–liquid crystal transition temperature (T_c) of the lipid with highest T_c. Typically, most of the cationic lipids contain dioleoyl or dimyristoyl chains and work at room temperature suffices. Charged analogues have lower values of T_c than their phospholipid counterparts. Transition temperature of DODAB is 37°C. As a hydration medium one can use distilled water, buffer solution, saline, or nonelectrolytes such as sugar solution. For *in vivo* use physiological osmolality (290 mOsm/kg) is recommended and can be achieved by using 0.9% saline, 5% dextrose, or 10% sucrose solution. Hydration should be performed at temperatures above T_c of the most rigid lipid during vigorous mixing, shaking, or stirring, and it is recommended that it lasts at least 1 h. Often aging (standing overnight) of MLV eases downsizing.

Highly charged lipids may swell into a very viscous gel, especially when hydrated with low-ionic strength solutions. Viscosity is due to electrostatic repulsion between charged lipid bilayers and can have already occured at very low concentrations (< 1 wt%). The gel can be broken by addition of salt or by downsizing the sample. For this case, only sonication can practically be used for liposome preparation because it is nearly impossible to quantitatively empty the hydration vessel. In such a case one dries lipid(s) in the sonication test tube. For liposomes that contain more than 20 to 40% of neutral lipid, gel normally does not occur.

A slightly more cumbersome hydration method is by dissolving the lipids in ethanol (or iso-propyl alcohol or propylene glycol) and injecting this solution directly into the aqueous phase during vigorous stirring. This step requires additional dialysis or diafiltration to remove organic solvent. For topical applications these solvents are normally not removed because they provide sterile protection. Water-immiscible solvents like ether or petrol ether are rarely used. In the case of ethanol injection appropriate conditions, mostly low lipid concentration and quick mixing, may result in the direct formation of SUVs.

LMVs are formed during the hydration procedure. In the case of charged bilayers the lamellarity is low and birefringence in the polarizing microscope is rarely observed. In some cases, especially at lower lipid concentrations, these liposomes may be used directly for genosome formation. The majority of applications, however, requires smaller and better-defined liposomes. For DNA complexing SUVs are normally preferred. This is due to the fact that during genosome formation lipid restructuring occurs and these liposomes are the most amenable to such transformations. Downsizing can be performed by sonication, extrusion, or homogenization.

Sonication

LMV dispersion is placed in test tubes which are either sonicated in a bath sonicator or by tip sonication. Normally, 5 to 10 min sonication above T_c suffices for the preparation of SUVs with radii below 50 nm. With some lipids, radii below 20 nm can be obtained while some diacyl cationic lipids (including DOIC and DOGS) can even form micelles. DODAB/neutral lipid liposomes cannot be sized below 130 nm. Bath sonication is preferred because temperature can be better controlled and the sonicator tip can shed titanium particles during direct sonication, which must be centrifuged away (typically 5 to 10 min on the bench top centrifuge suffices). Bath sonication requires small sample volumes, typically about 1 mL/tube. Thick glass tubes are less likely to break during sonication and an argon blanket to reduce lipid oxidation is recommended. This method is the most suitable for samples which did not swell well (some neutral lipids often remain sticking on the surface of hydration vessel) or are gelly. Obviously, in these cases lipids have to be weighed directly in the test tube in which sonication will be performed. Tip sonication, which dissipates more energy into the sample, can contain, depending on the tip and container size, from 1 to 5 mL of sample. Besides the lipid composition and concentration, the size of vesicles produced depends on temperature, sonication time and power, volume of samples, as well as tuning; i.e., by carefully adjusting the position of the tip (level of water and tube position in a bath sonication experiment), one can achieve much better energy dissipation.

Extrusion

In this technique the lipid dispersion is forced through filters with different pore sizes. Typically, LMV solution is prefiltered through a filter with pores around 1 μm and then 5 times through 0.4- and 0.2-μm pores. This is followed by 5 to 10 extrusions through a filter with a pore size of 100 nm. This forms large unilamellar vesicles (LUVs) with diameters slightly above pore sizes, around 110 to 120 nm. If smaller vesicles are desired, one can continue filtering through 80- and 50-nm pores. Smaller pores (30 nm and in the case of some more-rigid bilayers also 50 nm) do not reduce the size further down but rather increase it. This is due to the imposition of a too high curvature to vesicles which are therefore unstable and fuse. The extrusion method yields the best vesicles with respect to the homogeneity of size distribution and is the best one to control the size distribution of vesicles, especially for larger (100 to 500 nm) diameters. Typical cells have volumes from 10 to 100 mL, can hold polycarbonate membranes of 25 or 47 mm diameter and can sustain pressures up to 1000 psi. For lipids with higher values of T_c, temperature jackets are available (or one can perform extrusion in a water bath). A

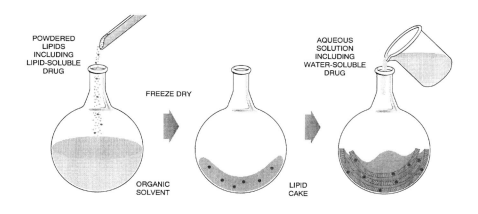

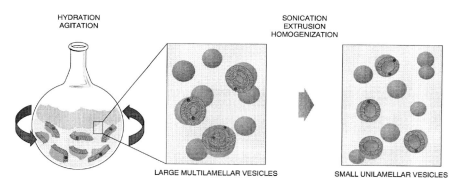

Figure 6-11   Schematic presentation of liposome preparation. Dry (or organic solutions of) lipids are dissolved (mixed) in an organic solvent. Following rotary evaporation and vacuum the thin lipid film is suspended in aqueous solution during shaking. LMVs are formed which can be sized down into SUVs by sonication or homogenization. (From Lasic, D. D., *Sci. Am. Sci. Med.*, 3, 34–43, 1996.)

very convenient and quick extrusion can be performed in a 1-ml syringe kit shown in Figure 6-11.

Homogenization

Homogenization is the easiest method for the scaleup. Liposome dispersion is forced at high pressures through a small hole and is collided into a wall, small ball, or tip of the pyramide. Microfluidization devices split the beam into two parts, which are collided head on at pressures up to 20,000 psi. The pros of the method are its simplicity, large capacity (depending on the size of the homogenizer one can prepare from 10 mL to hundreds of liters in 1 h), and speed. The cons are minimal volumes of around 10 mL (dead volume in small homogenizers is around 5 to 8 mL and this can result in substantial sample dilution), possible sample degradation, and contamination of the sample with very small lipid particles and some large ones. Samples can be run continuously or in batches. Typically, 3 to 5 passages through the interaction chamber are enough to achieve minimal size. Further treatment results in size growth due to too high curvatures. It is a common mistake that people overdo homogenization and do not control temperature well. Lipids can oxidize (especially unsaturated dioleoyl chains) and hydrolize, and liposome samples must be tested for lipid degradation products. It is my experience that careful tinkering with the valve tubes, turbulences in the connectors, and reduction of possible noncirculating volume spots can significantly improve the homogeneity of the vesicle preparation. Terminal filtration to remove large liposomes is in any case highly recommended.

Figure 6-12 shows a commercially available extrusion device and a homogenizer. High hydraulic pressure pumps liposomes at high pressure and it can also push them through a filter of an attached extrusion unit.

High entrapment efficiencies of water-soluble substances in liposomes were achieved by preparing liposomes from reverse phases. The substance to be encapsulated is dissolved in an aqueous phase and dispersed into the excess organic solvent containing lipids and forming water-in-oil emulsion. Upon removal of organic phase systems gels and gel is broken by addition of aqueous phase which will subsequently form exterior solution while the primary polar solution containing drug or nucleic acids becomes mostly entrapped into liposomes. This method was used in the first studies of DNA entrapment into conventional liposomes.

Other methods for liposome preparation are detergent depletion, ether injection, and ethanol injection. They are more cumbersome and are practically never used for the preparation of cationic liposomes. We shall mention only the detergent depletion methods which may be useful if some ligand-bearing lipids or proteins are to be included or embedded in the membrane. The lipid mixture is solubilized by a detergent with high aqueous solubility (critical micelle concentration). The components which are to be included are also dissolved in the detergent solution. Detergent is then removed by dialysis, gel chromatography, or by using detergent-adsorbing beads. This results in the formation of unilamellar vesicles. If octyl glucoside is used liposomes are above 100 nm while the use of sodium cholate results in the formation of SUVs. While this method doesn't seem promising for large-scale liposome preparation, it can be used in conjunction with DNA to coat DNA–lipid particles with appropriate bilayers. Virosomes, vesicles containing viral lipids and some viral proteins, are typically produced by such a method also.

Typically, viruses are dissolved with detergent, normally $C_{12}E_8$ (dodecyl octaoxyethylene) and capsid material is removed by centrifugation. The system is reconstituted into vesicles by detergent removal by using detergent-adsorbing beads. In contrast to reconstituted virosomes, synthetic virosomes can be made from appropriate lipids and proteins (or their fragments) by using pure compounds and possible contamination with viral constituents is eliminated.

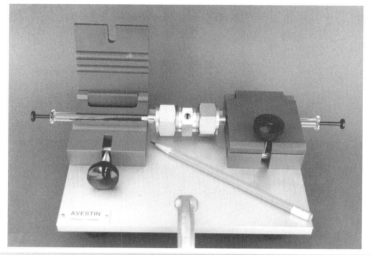

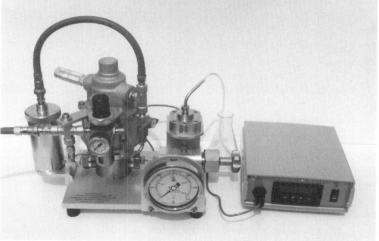

Figure 6-12 Extrusion of liposomes through a membrane placed between two syringes is a simple and quick method for producing milliliter quantities of liposomes. Homogenization is a simple and scalable method for preparation of larger volumes of liposomes. (Courtesy of Avestin, Ottawa, where the two devices are produced.)

We have already mentioned that lipids can be hydrated by injection into an aqueous phase. Mostly ethanol lipid solutions are used. In the case of quick injection of low concentrations, SUVs are formed while the use of experimentally useful concentrations results in heterogeneous mixtures of MLV, which have to be dialyzed to remove organic solvent.

Single-component cationic liposomes can be prepared by weighing the appropriate amount of lipid into a tube and hydrating directly, without preparing thin film, cake, or powder. In such a case, the hydration step should be performed more extensively, especially if liposomes are not intended for downsizing. As mentioned before they may swell into a gel, and sonication in the same tube is recommended to reduce lipid losses in the formulation.

Table 6-2 shows the most popular liposome preparation methods.

TABLE 6-2

PROS AND CONS OF LIPOSOME PREPARATION METHODS

Method	Advantage	Disadvantage
Sonication	Easy	Not scalable, contamination with small/large liposomes
Extrusion	The most homogeneous liposomes, scalable	Labor intensive
Homogenization	Easy, scalable	Contamination with too small/large liposomes

Spontaneous vesicles were prepared by mixing cationic and anionic single-chain surfactants at nonequilibrium ratios (Kaler et al., 1989). The size of the vesicles produced is rather heterogeneous and therefore their interaction with DNA resulted in a significantly larger amount of precipitation.

■■ MECHANISM OF VESICLE FORMATION

Liposomes are formed upon hydration of lipid molecules or their mixtures. Normally, lipids are hydrated from a dry state (thin or thick lipid film, lyophilized cake, or spray-dried powder), and stacks of crystalline bilayers become fluid and swell. Myelin figures — long, thin cylinders — grow and upon agitation detach and self-close into large, multilamellar liposomes because this eliminates unfavorable interaction at the edges (see Figure 6-9). Once these large particles are formed they can be either broken by mechanical treatments into smaller bilayered fragments which close into smaller liposomes. An alternative pathway makes use of asymmetric membrane expansion or compression, upon asymmetric pH change, interaction with particular ions or molecules, and causes budding off of smaller unilamellar liposomes. The two mechanisms are schematically shown in Figure 6-13A.

While the size of liposomes in the budding-off mechanism is very difficult to calculate, in the "self-closing" bilayer mechanism the liposome size depends, in the first approximation, on the dissipated energy into the system, the bending elasticity of the bilayer, and the edge interactions of open fragments. The balance between edge interaction and bending elasticity of the membrane determines final vesicle size. Over quite a range the two contributions are comparable, which can explain the rather

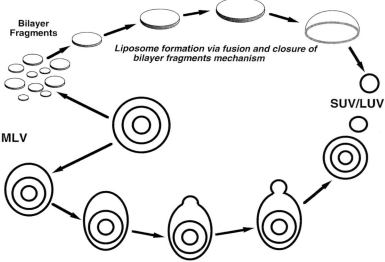

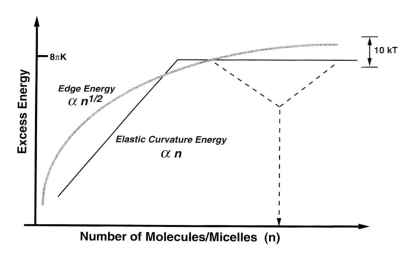

Figure 6-13 A, Liposomes can be produced either by fragmentation, aggregation, and self-closure of preexisting bilayers or by budding due to the asymmetric changes in the area of opposing monolayers. Preparation of liposomes from reverse phases probably follows the second mechanism because changes of solubility conditions induce curvature. B, Energy changes during the closing of a lipid fragment. Bending energy is increasing proportionally to the number of molecules until a constant value is achieved, while the edge interaction, which is proportional to the square root of the number of molecules at that point, vanishes (broken line). (Courtesy of Stan Hansen.)

heterogeneous vesicle preparations. Both interactions are unfavorable, as shown in Figure 6-13B (Lasic, 1993a). As a result, liposomes are in general not in a thermodynamically stable state (Lasic, 1993a). This fact can explain the heterogeneity of liposomal preparations, if they are not processed by an established preparation procedure. When a membrane closes it has finite, positive excess bending energy, as symmetric bilayers tend to be flat. However, it is just this property of liposomes which makes them useful drug and gene delivery vehicles. Systems at thermodynamic equilibrium change their phase upon application (dilution, temperature change, etc.), while kinetically trapped systems are rather stable against such perturbations and therefore hold their cargo better. For instance, micelles and microemulsions dissolve or aggregate upon dilution, while liposomes are invariant to the same procedure.

The excess bending energy associated with each liposome can be calculated from the general equation of bending energy, E

$$E/area = (1/2)K\left[C_1 + C_2 - C_0\right]^2 + kC_1C_2 \tag{6-9}$$

where K is the bending modulus, k is the Gaussian bending modulus, and the C terms are curvatures. In the case of a symmetric bilayer the spontaneous curvature C_0 is zero. By bending a plane into a sphere the two principal curvatures are equal ($C_1 = C_2 = C$) and neglecting the Gaussian term one gets

$$E = 2KC^2area \tag{6-10}$$

and expressing curvature with radius, $C = 1/R$, and using the area of a sphere of $4 \pi R^2$ one gets

$$E = 2Karea/R^2 = 8\pi K \tag{6-11}$$

This is the excess free energy associated with each vesicle. Typically, values of E are around 10 to 50kT, and because the energies to open the closed vesicles (creation of a hydrophobic boundary) are larger, liposomes are rather stable.

■ LIPOSOME STABILITY

Liposome stability is a complex issue which is composed from unrelated instabilities which on the other side synergistically cause the destabilization of the system. One can distinguish between physical (thermodynamic and colloidal), chemical, and biological stability of liposomes. In the pharmaceutical industry and in drug delivery, shelf-life stability, which is a cumulative property of physical and chemical stability, is also important.

Physical stability indicates mostly the constancy of the size distribution and the ratio of lipid to active agent of liposomes which indicates the stability of encapsulation or binding of the active agent. At high charges of cationic liposomes these vesicles can be stable at 4°C for years, if properly sterilized (however, in contrast to my experiences with anionic or neutral lecithin liposomes, I have never observed the growth of microorganisms in these samples).

Chemical stability primarily indicates hydrolysis and oxidation of lipids. Hydrolysis detaches hydrophobic chains, especially if they are attached via ester bonds (–CO–O–C–). Ether bonds (–C–O–C–) are rather stable. I have not seen a study of the stability of cationic lipids which would show optimal pH and degradation kinetics. We can assume, however, that they are similar to other lipids, meaning that careful work at optimal pH (normally between 5 and 6) and storage in liquid form at 4°C some 5 to 10% of the chains hydrolyzes in a year. Oxidation is more likely due to the presence of unsaturated chains. Again, careful work and the presence of antioxidants can reduce the degradation to similar levels as in hydrolysis. Some of the cationic lipids are synthesized by neutralizing negative groups on phosphate of phospholipids. These phosphotriesters are less stable with the attached group, such as ethyl, being the first one to leave. Phosphotriesters are in general toxic and the toxicity of such compounds should be carefully investigated (Eibl, private communication).

Biological stability of liposomes is rather limited. A simple test of plasma incubation often reveals extensive leakage and aggregation. This is especially true for cationic liposomes. *In vivo* stability is even more compromised. Again, cationic liposomes are because of negatively charged surfaces and colloidal particles in biological systems the least stable. Typically, these liposomes are adsorbed upon intravenous administration in seconds if they do not induce colloidal aggregation and blood clotting.

Industrial applications of liposomes require definition of shelf-life stability. As discussed above, highly charged cationic liposomes in low salt solutions, at optimal pH, and in the presence of antioxidants can be stable for years in liquid form. If prepared in the solutions of cryoprotectants these liposomes can be freeze-dried, which significantly increases their stability. For freeze-thawing, 5% dextrose is normally sufficient, while for freeze-drying and rehydration 10% sucrose seems to be the optimal cryoprotectant. Both are isotonic with physiological fluids.

Cationic liposomes have special interaction characteristics. In simple electrolyte solutions DLVO theory is qualitatively obeyed (an exception seems to be small vesicles which are less stable because of the presence of hydrophobic defects) and their interactions with DNA will be discussed in the next chapter.

Colloidal Stability of Liposomes: The DLVO Theory

The stability of colloidal systems is an important factor in their applications. Although no general model exists, the DLVO model can quantitatively explain stability of many charged systems. Briefly, it states that if electrostatic repulsion between two particles is larger than van der Waals attraction, the system is stable. With respect to the charge and ionic strength of the medium various force–distance profiles can be calculated and observed in many lyophobic colloids. We shall describe these forces for a homogeneous liposome or genosome suspension with diameter 2R, surface charge σ_o, at temperature T, and in z_i–z_j electrolyte solution at concentration (number density) ρ. The ubiquitous attractive force between liposomes is van der Waals attraction, while the long-range repulsive force is electrostatic repulsion. The balance between the two determines colloidal stability. Using the Poisson–Boltzmann equation to calculate electrostatic interaction potential and nonretarded van der Waals interaction by Hamaker summation method over atom–atom pair potential for spherical geometry, one determines the interaction energy between two particles at a separation D:

$$W(D) = \left(64\pi kTR\rho_\infty\, \gamma^2/\kappa^2\right)e^{-\kappa D} - AR/6/D \qquad (6\text{-}12)$$

where A is Hamaker constant, κ^{-1} Debye length,

$$\kappa = \left(\Sigma_i\rho_\infty\, e_2\, z_i^2/\epsilon\epsilon_o kT\right)^{1/2} \qquad (6\text{-}13)$$

and

$$\gamma = \tanh\left(ze\sigma_o/4kT\right) \qquad (6\text{-}14)$$

where k is Boltzmann constant and T is temperature.

As $D \rightarrow 0$, electrostatic repulsion increases more slowly (exponential) than the van der Waals attraction (power law), and the colloidal solution is inherently unstable. However, at larger separations, the electrostatic repulsion can exceed attraction, and with respect to surface potential and electrolyte concentrations, a series of DLVO interaction (distance) profiles can be obtained and are shown in Figure 6-14. In the case of a high barrier between the primary minimum and larger distances, the colloidal system is kinetically stabilized; therefore, it will not coagulate within reasonable time periods. With decreasing electrostatic repulsion, a secondary minimum appears. In such systems some flocculation or precipitation can be observed, but in the absence of other forces is easily redispersible. When the height of the barrier, b, becomes comparable with thermal energy kT (b < 5 to 10kT) the system is not stable and coagulation (precipitation) occurs. By titrating a stable system with electrolyte, one can define a critical coagulation concentration (CCC) at which W = 0 and dW/dD = 0. The coagulation behavior as a function of CCC often serves as a tool to study colloidal stability.

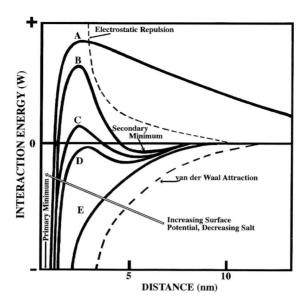

Figure 6-14 DLVO potential between colloidal particles. Depending on the system, various profiles between
exponential repulsion and power law attraction can be
calculated. The decreasing stability (curves from A to E)
can be a result of gradual addition of salt(s). (Courtesy
of Stan Hansen.)

A number of studies address the colloidal stability of charged liposomes. Similar behavior of anionic and cationic liposome stability was
observed. Later, other forces were introduced to explain instability of
small vesicles as compared with large ones. Namely, it was claimed that
small DODAC vesicles contain hydrophobic defects that could cause
precipitation. Although this explanation seems plausible, in line with
recent cryoelectron microscopy observations and previously reported
studies that claimed there is a coexistence of open fragments in DODAC
systems (Pansu et al., 1990), further work on better-defined systems will
be required to assess these issues. We shall use some of the above
concepts to explain the stability of genosomes.

It seems that in contrast to electrostatic stabilization, which was found
to be effective in many *in vitro* applications, steric stabilization is a
ubiquitous way to stabilize particles in biological systems and in media
with high or variable salinity. Addition of other interactions expands the
DLVO model to an extended DLVO interparticle potential. For the most
general case we propose that the total potential between the particles
should include all the above-mentioned forces, including hydrophobic
attraction and hydration, undulation, steric repulsion, repulsive protrusion
forces, and attractive ion correlation forces, and one can write

$$V_{tot} = -V_{vdW} - V_{hfo} - V_{icf} + V_{cst} + V_{hyd} + V_{und} + V_{st} + V_{pr} \qquad (6\text{-}15)$$

A treatment, analogous to the DLVO model for two potentials, should be performed to find the stability of the system. In a first approximation, potentials could be treated as additive. For rigorous treatment, however, one may expect dependence between various terms. It is reasonable to expect the interdependence of electrostatic, hydration, and steric interaction in the case of charged surface and covalently bound polymers due to different water structures at the surface.

When discussing the stability of the DNA–lipid complex we must distinguish two steps. During formation it is a colloidal interaction which results in the formation of complexes. The main interactions are electrostatic (attractive) with likely contributions from hydrophobic interaction and hydrogen bond formation. After their formation, however, a certain population of particles with a certain distribution of sizes and surface charges is formed and classic colloid stability can be applied to follow its stability as a function of ionic strength, pH, concentration, particle size, aqueous solubility of lipids (Ostwald ripening), and similar colloidal parameters. In this case interactive contributions originate in van der Waals forces, electrostatic repulsion, possible hydration and steric repulsion, and possible hydrophobic interaction (attractive). Entropy prefers smaller particles but because these contributions are in the order of thermal energy (kT), an order of magnitude below other interactions, they may not be too important. Qualitatively, DLVO is obeyed.

Ostwald ripening is another mechanism for the destabilization of colloidal systems. Colloidal particles are in equilibrium with their building blocks free in solution. Solubility of molecules or ions on surfaces with higher curvature is larger than on surfaces with lower radius of curvature. The reassociation of desorbed ions or molecules with colloidal particle scales with the surface area of the adsorbing particle and therefore it is normally said "the rich get richer and the poor get poorer." In conventional liposomes this is not a very important mechanism because of low lipid solubility. However, in systems with highly charged lipids this may be different (Lasic, 1993a).

■ CHARACTERIZATION AND QUALITY CONTROL

Liposomes prepared by one of the above methods must be characterized. Large-scale industrial applications rely on either large-scale extrusion or homogenization. While the former method yields better-defined product, the extra effort may not be needed in DNA delivery applications because liposomes are in the next step reacted and disintegrated anyway. Low-level contamination with large or small liposomes does not seem to matter because of the very large heterogeneity of genosomes produced. At high DNA and lipid concentrations, as needed for *in vivo* applications, however, the presence of large liposomes or long (chromosomal) DNA may catalyze precipitation via bridging interactions.

The most important parameters for liposome characterization are shown in Table 6-3. They include visual appearance, turbidity, size distribution, lamellarity, encapsulated volume, surface charge, osmolality, pH, conductivity, concentration, composition, presence of degradation products, and stability.

Simple naked-eye investigation of a liposome sample can tell a lot to an experienced researcher. Liposome suspensions can range, depending on concentration and especially particle size, from translucent to opaquely milky. One can see precipitation; if the turbidity shows a bluish shade this indicates that particles in the sample are homogeneous. A flat gray color may indicate that one has a nonliposomal dispersion, most likely a dispersed inverse hexagonal phase or dispersed microcrystallites. When aided by a (phase contrast) optical microscope one can see liposomes above 0.3 μm and contamination with larger particles. A polarizing microscope can tell us about lamellarity: LMVs are birefringent and display a Maltese cross. Also, waterlike surface tension and wetting of the glass, slight foaming, and quick rising of bubbles are characteristic for liposome solutions. If the "entrapped" bubbles rise slowly, get easily entrapped upon shaking, or if the glass does not de-wet quickly, all this may indicate nonliposomal lipid dispersions due to higher surface hydrophobicity. Most often these are dispersion of hexagonal II phases which can be frequently observed in samples containing nonionic neutral lipids or DOPE. Due to high surface charges, nonliposomal and nonbilayered lipid dispersions or suspensions can be very stable.

Size distribution is normally measured by dynamic light scattering. This method is reliable for liposomes with relatively homogeneous size distribution, while various bimodal size distributions may more reflect mathematical algorithms used in calculation to fit a multiexponential decay function than reflect the properties of the sample. A very simple but very powerful method is gel exclusion chromatography where truly hydrodynamic radius can be detected if the column is well calibrated. The line width of the peak indicates size distribution. For liposomes only Sephacryl S 1000 has pores large enough to separate liposomes. This column (typically 30 cm, diameter 1 cm, flow rate 5 to 8 mL/h, applied 1 to 5 μM of liposomes) can separate liposomes in the size range 30 to 300 nm. Sepharose 4B and 2B columns can separate SUV from micelles. All these columns are more difficult to operate with positively charged colloidal particles because of possible electrostatic interactions with gel medium, which can be slightly negatively charged, and because the addition of salt can cause the aggregation of the sample and clogging of the column. Many researchers use electron microscopy to measure liposome size. The most widely used negative staining and freeze-fracture methods are prone to artifacts due to the changes during sample preparation as well as to geometric reasons: it is difficult to estimate the size of collapsed dry vesicles in the negative stain procedure while in freeze-fracture or thin

TABLE 6-3

LIPOSOME CHARACTERISTICS AND QUALITY CONTROL PARAMETERS

General Characterization Studies

pH	pH meter
Conductivity	Conductivity meter
Osmolarity	Osmometer
Phospholipid concentration (PL)	Lipid phosphorus content (Bartlett method)
Phospholipid composition	TLC (combined with the Bartlett method), HPLC
Cholesterol concentration	Cholesterol oxidase assay, HPLC (normal and/or reverse phase)
Trapped volume	Measure of intraliposomal aqueous phase
Agent concentration	Spectrophotometry, HPLC, GC, spectrofluorimetry
Residual organic solvents and heavy metals	NMR, GC Standard protocols
Agent/phospholipid ratio	Determination of drug and phospholipid concentrations
$[H]^+$ or ion gradient for remote loading	Fluorescent indicators, ESR indicators, ^{31}P-NMR, ^{19}F-NMR

Physical Characterization and Stability Assays

Vesicle size distribution	
Submicron range	Dynamic light scattering (DLS), gel exclusion chromatography and specific turbidity, electron microscopy (various methods)
Micron range	Coulter counter, light microscopy, light diffraction, and specific turbidity
Electrical surface potential and surface pH	Use of membrane-bound electrical field probes and pH-sensitive probes
ζ Potential	Electrophoretic mobility
Thermotropic behavior, phase transition, phase separation	DSC, NMR, fluorescence methods, FTIR, Raman spectroscopy, ESR
Percentage of free drug	Gel exclusion chromatography, ion exchange chromatography, precipitation by polyelectrolyte
Liposome/aqueous phase partition coefficient (Kp) by dilution-dependent drug release assay	Dilution effect (up to 10,000-fold) on liposomal agent/PL ratio at equilibrium
k_{eff}^a	Effect of time on agent/liposome ratio
$[H]^+$ or ion gradient	Fluorescent pH indicators, ^{31}P-NMR, ^{19}F-NMR, intraliposomal ion concentration

Chemical Stability Assays

pH	pH Meter
Phospholipid acyl chain autoxidation	Conjugated dienes, lipid peroxides, TBARS and fatty acid composition (GC), UV/VIS
Phospholipid hydrolysis	TLC, HPLC, total PL and/or free fatty acid concentration

TABLE 6-3 (CONTINUED)

LIPOSOME CHARACTERISTICS AND QUALITY CONTROL PARAMETERS

Cholesterol autoxidation	TLC, HPLC
Antioxidant degradation	TLC, HPLC
Agent degradation	TLC, HPLC, spectrophotometry, spectrofluorimetry

Biological Assays

Sterility	Aerobic and anaerobic bottle cultures
Pyrogenicity and endotoxin	Rabbit and/or limulus amebocyte lysate (LAL) tests
Toxicity	Related to agent and use of liposomal product
Medium-induced leakage	Gel exclusion chromatography, ion exchange chromatography, precipitation by polyelectrolyte

From Barenholz, Y. and Lasic, D. D., in *Nonmedical Applications of Liposomes,* Vol. III, p. 23–41, CRC Press, Boca Raton, FL, 1996.

sectioning it is not known in which plane vesicles were fractured or cut. A novel development — cryoelectron microscopy — where a sample is frozen and directly observed in the electron beam, without any staining, shadowing, or replica preparation, is much more reliable (see Figure 6-9).

Lamellarity of liposomes is measured by electron microscopy or by spectroscopic techniques. Most frequently, NMR spectrum of liposomes is recorded without and with addition of a paramagnetic agent that shifts or bleaches the signal of the observed nuclei on the outer surface of liposomes. Comparing total signal with the signal of the nuclei protected in the vesicle interior allows calculation of the average lamellarity.

Encapsulation efficiency is measured by encapsulating a hydrophilic marker (radioactive sugar, ion, fluorescent label, dye), and after removing the outside label by gel chromatography (Sephadex G-25 or 50, or desalting column, 5 cm long, capacity 1 mL), one measures the marker in both samples after liposome lysis with detergent (typically, a nonionic detergent such as Triton is added at a detergent/lipid ratio of 10/1). Electron spin resonance methods allow determination of internal volume of preformed vesicles because some spin probes can freely diffuse through the bilayers while some interacting agents (polyvalent paramagnetic ions or reducing agents, such as ascorbic acid) cannot.

Surface potential is measured via ζ-potential. Particles migrate in an electric field, and their movement is detected either by the naked eye through a microscope or by laser (Doppler effect). Results are qualitatively very useful, but more for quality control than quantitative data on the structure of the complexes. Osmolality is normally checked by vapor pressure osmometer and pH with a standard pH meter.

Very important is lipid concentration determination. Phospholipids can be measured by quantitative phosphorus analysis in which lipids are digested and inorganic phosphorus is determined spectrophotometrically or by HPLC. For lipids either silica columns or reverse phase columns (C8 or C4) are used. Detection may present a problem. Evaporation laser light scattering detectors and refractive index detectors are normally much better than spectrophotometric detection. Cholesterol and its oxidation products can be detected on C18 reverse phase column with adsorption at 209 nm. HPLC also shows degradation products, such as fatty acids and lysocompounds in the case of hydrolysis or various oxidation products. Quicker, but less quantitive is TLC. Plates are sprayed by molybdenum dye or developed in iodine vapors for the detection of lipids.

With respect to physical and chemical stability, I am not aware of a single cationic liposome preparation that contains antioxidants, such as α-tocopherol (vitamin E), and chelators and is buffered. Obviously, the use of buffers will interfere with the DNA–liposome complexation reaction which strongly depends on ionic strength. Because pK of atmospheric CO_2 buffers the unbuffered systems, the pH actually remains in the range between 5 and 6, which seems to be optimal for minimization of hydrolysis. Oxidation is the other major degradation pathway of lipids. Knowing that these formulations normally contain up to 100% of oleoyl, chains we can understand the importance of the addition of antioxidants. Some of the liposomes also contain cholesterol which is, in contrast to common belief, quite prone to oxidation. In my experience cholesterol in liposomes was even more unstable than lipids with dioleoyl chains, with degradation rates in the range of 20 to 80%/year if liposomes were not manufactured properly. Oxidative products of cholesterol do not disrupt liposome structure but are toxic. Oleic acid is, contrary to common belief, rather stable. The stability problem present conjugated double bonds which this acid has none. At this point, however, I must mention that various data were presented in which the nonspecific antitumor activity of applied genosomes could be explained simply by the toxicity of lipid hydrolysis and oxidation products.

Not a single cationic lipid/liposome stability study has been reported. Some liposome kits are distributed as dry films which certainly improves their chemical stability while physical stability cannot be defined for such a preparation. In our hands cationic liposomes were physically and chemically stable for at least a year within 5% of required specifications. In some cases, however, the liposome size decreased in 12 h after formation for 5 to 15%. Ruling out chemical degradation I believe that in certain preparation methods surfactant-stabilized minibubbles of air are formed and their slow disappearance results in an apparent size decrease.

■ INTERACTIONS OF LIPOSOMES WITH CELLS AND *IN VIVO*

Because liposomes are extensively studied as a drug delivery system we shall very briefly describe their interactions with cells and in biological systems.

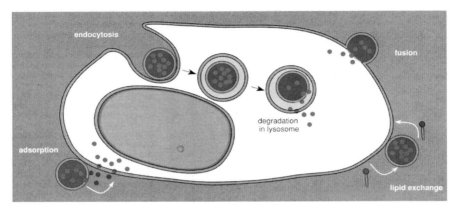

Figure 6-15   Four different interactions of liposomes and cells. It is likely that other interactions, such as direct membrane poration, or a novel internalization mechanism in some cell lines (fibroblasts, epithelial cells) may also exist. (From Lasic, D.D., *Am. Sci.* 80, 21, 1992.)

Figure 6-15 shows four different ways liposomes, possibly with encapsulated, attached, or associated molecules, can interact with cells. The first interaction is lipid exchange. Lipids themselves have small aqueous solubility and therefore liposome and cell membrane can exchange lipid molecules. In biological systems several proteins can increase this exchange significantly. Such exchange is higher for liposomes in liquid crystalline phase and for lipids with shorter hydrocarbon chains. The second interaction is adsorption. This is, in the case of smaller liposomes, largely independent of the fluidity of the membrane. If adsorbed liposomes leak, part of the encapsulated cargo can enter the cell by diffusion. The third interaction is fusion in which vesicle and cell membrane fuse via an intermediate, which can be an inverted micelle or, according to more-recent data, a short lipid stalk. This fusion process, however, is rather rare and later we shall discuss a few ways to increase its rate. The most important interaction is endocytosis in which the cell engulfs adsorbed or bound vesicle into vacuole (endosome) and after fusion with lysozymes, which deliver lytic agents (enzymes, protons -lower pH) which digest liposome and possibly its cargo. Throughout this book we discuss different ways to bypass this degradation.

A rather different interaction was observed between red blood cells and cationic liposomes. Erythrocytes are practically inert to any internalization and yet they engulfed cationic liposomes. Upon adsorption the membrane surrounds absorbed liposome which then becomes directly internalized. Increasing ionic strength reversibly decreases "zipping" of liposomes by erythrocyte lipids (Martin and MacDonald, 1978). Some detergents and ionophores can induce transient pores and some other interactions, still unknown, may exist, especially with some cells, as well.

In vivo interactions depend on the administration route. Orally administered liposomes in general are digested in the digestive tract by low values of pH, lipases, and detergent action of bile salts. With improved understanding of mechanical and colloidal stability of liposomes, more-robust liposomes can be prepared. For instance, small liposomes with composition DSPC/Chol (1/1) containing 5 mol% of PEG-DSPE are extremely stable in test tube experiments (leakage is induced only at high detergent concentrations and prolonged exposures at elevated temperatures). Their application for oral delivery, perhaps to the Payer's patch, however, has not been tried yet. Topically applied liposomes mostly dry on the surface and disintegrate. Some compositions, researchers claim, can penetrate a few micrometers into the skin. Liposomes injected in various body fluids interact with ions and molecules in the milieu. Additionally, thermodynamic factors, such as leakage upon dilution, can occur in the case of membrane-adsorbed or embedded molecules. Administration into the bloodstream typically results in fast liposome sequestration into the cells of the reticuloendothelial system, mostly fixed macrophages in liver and spleen. This is due to opsonization with plasma globulins and proteins of the complement cascade. Typically, the majority of liposomes ends up in the liver, depending on formulation, within 1 min to 1 h. Larger liposomes are retained by the spleen to a larger extent. The third organ where liposomes end up is bone marrow and circulating monocytes. Some are taken up also in the lymph nodes and deep skin macrophages. Only recently, it was shown that using sterically stabilized liposomes the phagocytosis can be reduced. Because surfaces and particles in living systems are negatively charged, cationic liposomes are much more reactive and immediately after administration they adsorb onto the nearest surface or become coated by plasma proteins (probably mostly albumin). They can also cause aggregation of negatively charged cells. Some of these aspects will be discussed in the next section.

■ TOXICITY AND SAFETY OF CATIONIC LIPOSOMES

Because biological systems are mostly negatively charged one can expect two different toxicities originating from cationic liposomes and lipids. Germicidal action of cationic surfactants against viruses, bacteria, fungi, spores, protozoa, and invertebrates is well known (Jungerman, 1970). On the colloidal level positively charged particles may induce aggregation, flocculation, thrombosis, or platelet aggregation. On the molecular level these lipids can act as surfactants, causing membrane solubilization, poration, hemolysis, as well as changing the properties of the membranes and membrane proteins, such as kinase C, in the membranes in which they insert. Protein kinase C inhibition by cationic lipids is the best-known example (Bottega and Epand, 1992). While colloidal toxicity seems unavoidable, biodegradation can mostly reduce the toxicity on the molecular level. Colloidal toxicity depends on the interactions of cationic particles in plasma which may differ for liposomes and genosomes containing different lipids. For instance, two liposomes (DOIC/Chol and

DMEPC/Chol 1/1), as well as genosomes prepared from them (charge ratio –/+, ρ = 0.5), differ significantly in *in vitro* plasma stability tests. While the former one flocculates in seconds, it takes hours before flocculation is observed with the latter ones (Lasic, 1994, unpublished). Liposomes show faster precipitation rates than genosomes which can be understood by their lower surface charge. The difference between various cationic lipids may be in the kinetics of adsorption vs. aggregation with oppositely charged particles. If upon systemic administration adsorption of albumin and some other macromolecules is quicker than colloidal aggregation, such systems may show prolonged stability and reduced colloidal toxicity.

Conventional liposomes are normally tested for toxicity by performing hemolysis, thrombosis, and cytotoxicity assays. Their effects on phagocytic activity of the reticuloendothelial system and pyrogenicity are tested as well. To date such studies have been performed with cationic liposomes.

The interaction of three different liposome systems with blood was tested and rather dissimilar behavior was observed. Liposomes containing stearylamine provoked a strong increase in plasma turbidity while DOTMA and BisHOP (2,3-dihexadecyloxy-propyl-*N,N,N*-trimethylammonium chloride) provoked a strong clotting response. BisHOP liposomes did not cause hemolysis while the other two did. Parameters measured, including turbidity, clot weight, and percent hemolysis, depended on the mole percent of cationic lipid in liposomes as well as on liposome concentration (Senior et al., 1991). Macroscopic effects were not observed below a threshold concentration of 0.25 μM/mL. It was speculated that increased uptake *in vivo* may be due to the high negative charge of these particles coated with negatively charged proteins. Interactions were reduced when more-rigid bilayers were used.

Despite the extensive safety studies that are undoubtedly performed in many organizations, no published study compares toxicity or cytotoxicity of different cationic liposomes. Scarce data exist on cytotoxicity of complexes. In general, it is believed that lowering the positive charge by adding larger quantities of DNA reduces the overall toxicity. DNA is a powerful activator of the complement system (Szebeni, Alving, & Lasic, unpublished, 1994), especially if it is not clean (some DNA samples contain bacterial endotoxins). Most liposomes were found to activate complement, and charge reduction by DNA complexation increased complement protein consumption.

Naked DNA is not toxic upon systemic administration. In complexes with cationic liposomes, however, cytotoxicity was observed. In general, toxicity is proportional to positive charge. Not many results have been published and in the next chapter we shall review a few studies of genosome toxicity. Even less is known about safety of cationic liposomes in *in vivo* applications. Despite the fact that most reports conclude that no adverse effects were observed and that animals tolerated treatments well, thorough evaluation of various tissues (lung, spleen, liver, and others) for pathology, swelling, bleeding, inflammation, and appearance should be performed.

After this short introduction of liposomes, we shall briefly describe some of their applications. Liposomes are also a very useful model, tool, and reagent to study biomembranes, as will be shown below.

■ LIPOSOMES AND CELL MEMBRANES

We shall very briefly show the similarities of liposomal bilayers and biomembranes. Cells as well some organelles in eukaryotic cells are separated from the medium by a cell membrane which represents a significant barrier for permeation of various species. Biological cells, in addition, contain membrane-spanning, embedded, inserted, and adsorbed proteins which regulate transport of various ions and molecules in either direction. Membrane proteins are anchored to the bilayer by a hydrophobic surface which may be long sequences of apolar amino acids, an apolar surface of an α-helix, or noncontinuous portions of the polypeptide chain brought together by the folding pattern of the protein. Polar surfaces of membrane proteins are exposed to water.

Permeability of water molecules is relatively high, while the low permeability of ions makes the lipid bilayer an excellent insulator, and there is normally a difference in electrical potential across the membrane. In living cells the nonequilibrium distribution of ions is maintained by ionic pumps which use ATP hydrolysis to obtain energy for their action. Table 6-4 shows the resting state of the cell. The nonequilibrium state is a source of energy when needed, such as, for instance, in the propagation of a nerve signal. Ion channels open and provide a conductance pathway for specific ions at a very fast rate (<1 ms), creating a potential Ψ of about +50 mV.

On both sides of the membrane, the chemical potentials of any ion are the same, because the concentration difference is offset by a potential:

$$\Delta\mu_{Na^+} = 0 = RT \ln\left(Na_{in}^+/Na_{out}^+\right) + \left(\Psi_{in} - \Psi_{out}\right) \tag{6-16}$$

TABLE 6-4

NONEQUILIBRIUM DISTRIBUTION IN THE CELL		
	Cell Cytoplasm	**Ext. Medium**
Free Na$^+$ [M]	0.010	0.140
K$^+$ [M]	0.140	0.004
Ca^{2+} [M]	<10^{-7}	0.002
Potential [mV]	−80	0

The propagation of this potential change based on Na and K channel regulation and ion pump movements of ions upstream is the universal mechanism of nerve impulse conduction. In addition to the signaling function, cell membranes regulate many processes, such as endocytosis, exocytosis, food uptake, trafficking of synaptic vesicles, and secretion, to name a few.

All these processes, and many others, can be studied in proteoliposomes, i.e., liposomes with membrane-embedded proteins, including ion pumps. Such studies have yielded many important insights into the function of living cells (Barenholz and Lasic, 1996). The subtle distribution of ions across the membrane can be perturbed by cationic lipids which can create transmembrane pores. This is another mechanism of their toxicity.

■ LIPOSOME APPLICATIONS

To conclude this liposome chapter, we shall briefly mention their applications. Among nonmedical applications the best known is in cosmetics, where liposomes can serve as a natural, water-based carrier for hydrophilic and hydrophobic ingredients. As it seems now, special colloidal properties of liposomes may result in some agricultural applications as well as in diagnostics, ecology, the food industry, and bioreclamation. A simple example can show their advantage in a diagnostic test, such as ELISA. Normally, one ligand carries one marker molecule while attached liposomes can contain thousands of molecules and appropriately amplify the signal (Lasic and Barenholz, 1996).

Drug Delivery

Due to their biocompatibility, biodegradability, and low immunogenicity, liposomes are extensively used as drug delivery vehicles. They can dissolve (suspend) drugs with peculiar solubility properties (minoxidil, amphotericin B, cyclosporin, taxol, etc.) and act as a sustained-release system for microencapsulated drug molecules. In systemic applications a liposome-associated drug is less toxic because free drug molecules are not spilled all over in the circulation. Typical examples are reduced cardiotoxicity of liposome-encapsulated doxorubicin and reduced nephrotoxicity of amphotericin B. A liposome formulation containing this antifungal agent has been on the European market since 1990 (AmBisome, Vestar, San Dimas, CA, now NeXstar, Boulder, CO). Upon systemic administration, liposomes are, as all foreign colloidal particles, recognized as "non-self" and rapidly sequestered by the cells of the body's immune system, mostly macrophages in the liver and spleen. This eliminates their most-promising application of site-specific drug delivery but represents an effective vehicle to target these cells. As a result, the therapeutic index of drugs used to treat parasitic infections of the reticuloendothelial system can be substantially increased. The same effect can be used also in vaccination. A hepatitis vaccine has been on the Swiss market since 1994 as well (Swiss Serum Institute, Bern). Additionally, liposomes were shown to enhance intracellular accumulation of encapsulated molecules and can act as a penetration enhancer. Only recently were liposomes, which can evade the rapid uptake by the reticuloendothelial system, prepared. Due to evasion of detection by the immune system, they are often referred to as stealth liposomes. This effect is due to steric stabilization by surface-conjugated polymer. Sterically stabilized liposomes, as they are normally called, were shown to circulate in patients for up to a week, and enhanced accumulation in several tumor models was found (Lasic, 1996). This resulted in the first FDA-approved liposomal formulation {Doxil™, anti-cancer agent doxorubicin encapsulated in sterically stabilized liposomes by Sequus Pharmaceuticals (formerly Liposome Technology, Inc., Menlo Park, CA). These liposomes with attached targeting ligands (antibodies or lectins) can have some site specificity, mostly depending on the accessibility of target cells. The immunogenicity of such systems, however, has not been properly addressed yet. It is very likely that they are rapidly cleared after the second administration.

Cationic liposomes have been tried mostly for topical applications in the hope that their charge will increase the adhesion and persistence at the site (Guo et al., 1996). Although the controlled-release systems worked quite well, irritability of skin or eye prevented larger expansion in this area.

Table 6-5 shows some of the medical applications of liposomes.

Because of their ability to improve delivery of the encapsulated substances into the cells, liposomes were tried for delivery of DNA and RNA in the late 1970s. However, the procedures were cumbersome, encapsulation efficiencies very low, and interest relatively rapidly faded away. pH-sensitive liposomes and virosomes have been also tried. The idea is to reduce DNA degradation in endosomes by bypassing lysozomal degradation. pH-sensitive liposomes change their phase upon lowering of pH, which induces fusion with the endosomal membrane, and DNA can be released into the cytoplasm. Virosomes contain viral fusion proteins which become activated in the low-pH environment of the endosome and enter cells upon fusion with endosome membranes. Both systems still have problems with efficient DNA encapsulation, and the use of liposomes for DNA delivery was revived when it was discovered that cationic liposomes can qualitatively bind DNA and that these complexes (genosomes) can be very effective gene delivery vehicles.

■ SUMMARY

Liposomes are spherical colloidal particles, composed of self-assembled lipid bilayers, in which one or several membranes encapsulate part of the solvent in which they freely diffuse. Due to their specific topology and colloidal properties, which can be easily controlled by composition, they

TABLE 6-5

MODES OF ACTION OF LIPOSOMES WITH SOME EXAMPLES OF DRUGS AND OF DISEASES TREATED

Liposome Utility	Example	Disease States Treated
Solubilization	Amphotericin B, minoxidil	Fungal infections
Sustained-release	Systematic antineoplastic drugs, hormones, corticosteroids	Cancer, biotherapeutics
Site-avoidance	Amphotericin B (kidneys), doxorubicin (heart)	Fungal infection, cancer
Drug protection	Cytosine arabinoside, interleukins	Cancer, etc.
Passive targeting	Immunomodulators, vaccines, antimalarials, macrophage-located diseases	Cancer, MAI, tropical parasites
Specific targeting	Cells bearing specific antigens	Wide therapeutic applicability
Extravasation	Leaky vasculature of tumors, inflammations, infections	Cancers, infections
Accumulation	Prostaglandins	Cardiovascular diseases
Enhanced penetration	Topical vehicles	Dermatology
Drug depot	Lungs, subcutaneous, intramuscular, ocular	Wide therapeutic applicability
Intracellular delivery	DNA, genes, antisense oligonucleotides	Gene therapy, bioengineering

Adapted from Lasic, D. D. and Needham, D., 1995.

can be useful in various applications. Cationic liposomes have their surface positively charged and interact strongly with anions and polyanions.

◼ ADDITIONAL READING

Bangham, A. D., Ed., *Liposome Letters,* Academic Press, New York, 1993.
Lasic, D. D., *Liposomes: From Physics to Applications,* Elsevier, Amsterdam, 1993.
Lasic, D. D., Liposomes, *Sci. Am. Sci. Med.,* 3, 34–43, 1996.
Lasic, D. D., Barenholz, Y., *Nonmedical Applications of Liposomes,* Vols. 1–4, CRC Press, Boca Raton, FL, 1996.
Lasic, D. D., Martin, F. J., Eds., *Stealth Liposomes,* CRC Press, Boca Raton, FL, 1995.
Many authors in Festschrift for Demitri Papahadjopoulos, *J. Liposome Res.,* 5, 627–932, 1995.
Wilschut, J., Hoekstra, D., Eds., *Membrane Fusion,* Marcel Dekker, New York, 1991.

7 GENOSOMES (DNA–LIPID COMPLEXES)

DNA internalization into cells is greatly improved if it is encapsulated in conventional liposomes or complexed with cationic liposomes. Although in the long-run encapsulation in neutral or anionic liposomes may be the more prospective approach, currently no data on these have been published and we shall mostly discuss the use of cationic liposomes. Conventional and sterically stabilized liposomes as a gene delivery system will be presented therefore in Chapters 11 and 13. In this chapter we shall discuss DNA–liposome and DNA–lipid complexes, from their preparation, characterization, scaleup, and quality control to their safety.

DNA–lipid complex formation is a very complex process which depends on thermodynamic as well as kinetic factors. Thermodynamic parameters, including charge ratios, concentrations, ionic strength, pH, presence of impurities, and, to a lesser extent, temperature, will be discussed below, after we describe typical methods of genosome preparation.

At lower lipid concentrations complexes are often made by pouring lipid and DNA solutions together and incubating for 5 to 15 min. Some papers report separate addition of plasmids and liposomes to the cell culture. For *in vivo* applications, however, larger concentrations of colloidally suspended DNA are preferred and different protocols are used. Complexes are normally prepared by rapidly mixing the two colloidal solutions. Typically, researchers use adjustable pipettes and quickly inject one solution into the other and then follow with a few quick aspiration–ejection cycles. In many cases speed, as well as the sequence of mixing (DNA into liposomes or vice versa), critically influences the characteristics of the DNA–lipid complex (genosome) formed. Normally, 50 to 200 μL of each reactant is used. Surprisingly, scaling up to milliliter quantities often results in precipitation. Large differences between various operators are typical. In some cases very slow addition of one concentrated solution into the other also results in small complexes. Hydration of dry lipid with a DNA solution yields in general a very heterogeneous population of mostly large genosomes, possibly with a precipitate or flocculae present, which are not advisable for systemic administration.

All these observations indicate that the interaction of DNA with liposomes is clearly also a kinetic phenomenon, and, to reduce operator dependence, automatization is strongly recommended. The easist way is

113

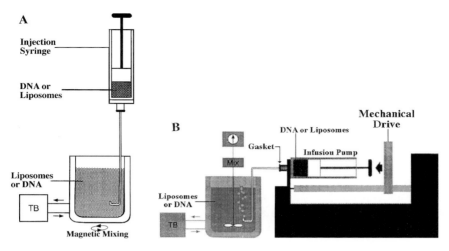

Figure 7-1   Schematic presentation of an apparatus for the intermediate scale complex preparation. (A) hand injection; (B) mechanically driven. Temperature bath is normally not needed. If air in the needle does not separate the two solutions, mixing must be done externally. Such devices can prepare tens of milliliters of complexes. For larger volumes double tangential (or T mixing in the bottom of a mixing vessel) designs can be employed. These may be operated in such a way that the bulk concentration of reactants is constant.

simply to mix one component and quickly inject the other into a stirred solution without dipping the needle into the stirred solution (typically at ½ to ¾ of maximal stirring speed) to prevent slow interaction before injection. A thin needle (gauge 27, for instance) with a cut end (to prevent splashing) is preferred, and in scales from 1 to 20 mL an injection rate of approximately 2 mL/s is recommended (Figure 7-1).

Quick hand injection is practically as good as any commonly used mechanical device. The important difference of pipette mixing is better mixing, especially because a pipette does not suck up all the sample and the concentrations in the pipette tip are typically not characteristic of the bulk. Too vigorous stirring of the recipient solution, on the other hand, also results in precipitation. The precipitate, however, looks more compact as compared with typical slow setting and growing flocculae of normal precipitation and normally cannot be redispersed by vortexing. This probably indicates different interactions or the primary minimum in the DLVO potential. The explanation may involve surface properties of the colloidal solution. Vortexing of liposome solution greatly increases its surface area and surface effects become important. Surface monolayers catalyze fusion and so does the presence of bubbles, foam, and splashing. Large volumes of complexes (10 to 20 mL) can be prepared by injecting one solution into the other, which is magnetically stirred in a beaker/vial. Improvements would make use of a multiple-needle injection head and/or simultaneous mixing of the two reactants in a T mixer or double tangential injector with a head-on beam collision. Optimal mixing and best dispersal are achieved if solutions are mixed equivolumetrically, concentrations permitting.

Slow mixing, with the exception of that at lower concentrations, typically results in precipitation. This can be understood by assuming that local concentrations are different from the bulk and, as we shall see below, can go through the charge neutrality region, where the complexes are the most unstable, slowly and in a relatively rather large volume. Quick mixing, on the other hand, evenly distributes the reactants, and when the reaction is over, all the injected material dissipates in small local volumes and not in a few large ones where large aggregates, which catalyze precipitation, can be formed. An analogy from crystallography would be crystal growth. Close to the thermodynamic equilibrium only a few large crystals grow, while in far from equilibrium conditions numerous crystallization nuclei are formed resulting in numerous small crystallites. In a similar way homogeneous inorganic colloidal particles are formed after a burst of nucleation embryos is created (Lasic, 1993b).

Obviously, thermodynamic factors influence complex properties as well. Typically, scientists create a precipitation curve (as shown in Figure 7-2) to study the complex and select optimal genosomes for transfection. In such a study one chooses a fixed DNA concentration, normally between 5 and 100 μg/mL, and mixes it with lipid at charge ratios in the range from about 3 to 0.25. With the exception of very low concentrations, around charge neutralization ($\rho = 1$) precipitation occurs. The presence of electrolytes drastically increases precipitation and therefore liposomes and DNA are normally suspended in a nonelectrolyte solution (5% dextrose or 10% sucrose). Very low concentrations of salt (<0.03%, introduced normally from diluted DNA solution which is typically 10 mM TRIS, 1 mM EDTA, pH = 8) can be tolerated.

Better characterization of genosomes is obtained by the phase diagram study. In the phase space of lipid and DNA concentration a property, such as precipitation (solubility gap), turbidity, size, ζ potential, as well as transfection activity and gene expression *in vivo/in vitro,* and similar properties, is measured. Figure 7-3 shows a phase diagram of a typical system. Around charge neutralization ($\rho = 1$) the system precipitates. Also, at higher lipid and DNA concentrations there is obviously phase separation or formation of a viscous phase, which is a well-known effect observed by pure lipid and pure DNA which form a liquid crystalline phase at higher concentrations (lipids typically above 30 wt% and DNA, in the 3 to 10 kb size range, above 15 mg/mL). The solubility gap, as well as characteristics of soluble complexes, depends on the nature of cationic and neutral lipids and the size of the liposomes. Preliminary data indicate that complexes are smaller and less turbid at higher temperatures, which may indicate nonelectrostatic contributions.

A phase diagram can also explain the importance of mixing order. Anionic complexes (on the left of the precipitation diagonal) should be prepared by injecting liposomes into DNA, and cationic liposomes by injecting DNA into liposomes. In this way the system does not cross the

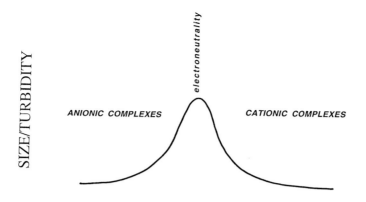

Figure 7-2   A typical precipitation curve of titrating fixed concentration of DNA with liposomes. Researchers study normally anionic or cationic complexes and measure size, turbidity, ζ potential, transfection activity, toxicity, and similar parameters.

precipitation area, at least not in the bulk, during which it can be destabilized. Various cationic lipids and neutral lipids exhibit different phase diagrams. While turbidity values may be similar, the width of the precipitation gap can vary substantially. Normally, larger liposomes and longer DNA plasmids also increase the precipitation gap. Somehow, surprisingly, so do the micelles.

The precipitation behavior for a particular cationic lipid scales with its charge and is neutral rather than independent (i.e., DOTAP, DOTAP:Chol, DOTAP:DOPE yield similar phase behavior if liposomes of similar size are used when plotted in the diagram with positive and negative charge axes). The solubility among different cationic lipids shows different behavior, as can be seen in DODAB:Chol and DODAB:DOPE systems as opposed to X:Chol and X:DOPE systems where X = DOTAP, DMEPC, or DOIC. Solubility gap increases also with increasing ionic strength, larger liposomes, and contamination of DNA with chromosomal segments.

The stability of the complexes depends on the lipid composition, ionic strength, pH, absolute concentration, and charge ratio. In our hands, an empiric observation was that complexes which at cationic lipid concentration of 0.1 mM had adsorbance at 400 nm (i.e., turbidity) >0.35 to 0.4 tended to precipitate within hours. In general, the complexes with τ <0.3 are stable up to several months when stored at 4°C. In general, extruded liposomes of similar size range have a smaller precipitation gap and can therefore form complexes with higher concentration of colloidally suspended DNA. If a subtle precipitate was observed in stored cationic

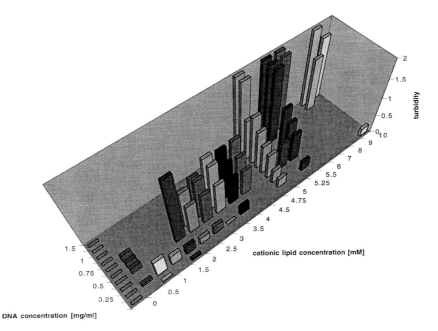

Figure 7-3 Characteristic phase diagram of DOTAP/Chol system condensed with 4.7 kb DNA. Turbidities are measured, and for precipitated complexes a value of 2 is assumed. Different lipids can colloidally suspend DNA to different concentrations. This system can typically dissolve up to 1 mg DNA/mL. Higher values (up to 5 mg/mL) are, however, because of large lipid concentrations toxic (see also Figure 9-3).

complexes ($\rho = 0.5$), it could be normally redispersed by vortexing. This indicates that genosomes aggregated probably in the secondary minimum in the DLVO potential-distance profile (Templeton et al., 1996).

Stability of colloidal systems can be explained by the DLVO theory which states that the balance between ubiquitous van der Waals attraction and electrostatic repulsion determines the stability of the system. Quantitative agreement with the model was observed although preliminary ζ potential measurements at these high surface charges did not obey the Poisson–Boltzmann equation (Lasic, unpublished). Lower than expected surface charges may be due to counterion association (Israelachvili, private communication). It is well known that degree of ionization α can be close to 1 for monomeric surfactants while upon micellization it can drop below $\alpha < 0.3$.

Qualitatively, genosomes follow the DLVO stability predictions; i.e., by increasing electrolyte concentration they precipitate. One must, however, distinguish between electrostatic interaction during genosome formation and stability of preformed genosomes. The complexation itself is an electrostatic phenomenon where electrostatic forces are attractive, while after genosome formation they are repulsive. If genosomes are

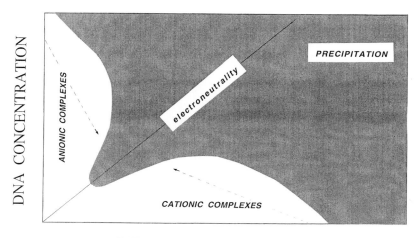

LIPOSOME CONCENTRATION

Figure 7-4   Top view of a typical phase diagram. Solubility gap is hatched and arrows indicate the preferential addition of reactants to prepare cationic and anionic complexes. Dashed lines show the bulk concentration change in the case of equivolumetric addition. More concentrated solutions approach final point (C_{lip}, C_{DNA}) more directly. The addition sequence is important. In general, one doesn't want to cross the solubility gap, as happens, for instance, if one adds liposomes into DNA to prepare cationic genosome.

prepared in 5% glucose they can be stable against freeze-thawing, while for preparations formulated in 10% sucrose lyophilization is possible. Reconstituted genosomes are typically within 20% of the measured size and turbidity. This is not surprising; these are kinetically trapped systems and after formation they can be rather stable. Also, the interaction between lipids and DNA is strong enough that the free energy minimum of the genosome is sufficiently deep. If upon reconstitution the complex ends up in a different free energy minimum, the sample heterogeneity is broad enough that these differences cancel out. Sometimes even smaller or less turbid reconstituted solutions were prepared.

In general, genosomes are rather heterogeneous with respect to size distribution, shape, and density. This is a consequence of the kinetic nature of their formation. Efforts to prepare more homogeneous preparations are based on the optimization of reaction, separation of various fractions (mostly by density centrifugation), and special treatments of genosomes. These include extrusion, sonication, or preparation by detergent depletion. We must be aware, however, of the sensitivity of DNA to mechanical treatments and the inherent irreproducibility of colloidal systems.

Along these lines, a hydrophobic complex, as an intermediary structure for the preparation of homogeneous genosomes, was developed. A hydrophobic complex is formed in an organic phase and the DNA is not condensed, and it is therefore hoped that such intermediates are well suited for the preparation of homogeneous genosomes (Reimer et al., 1995).

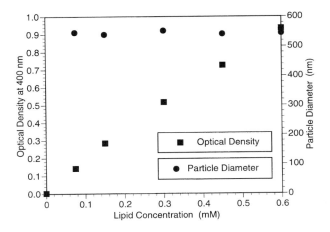

Figure 7-5   Concentration dependence (total lipid) of genosome turbidity of DOTAP:Chol–DNA system at +/– ratio 0.5. On the right side, sizes, as determined by dynamic light scattering are shown. Linearity of turbidity (concentration) function as well as constancy of their size demonstrates that they are colloidally (size and shape) a stable system.

■ REACTIVITY AND STABILITY

Genosomes are stable upon dilution with nonelectrolytes as can be concluded from the linearity of the Lambert–Beer law (Figure 7-5). In the presence of electrolytes, however, they can aggregate and precipitate. However, their stability against aggregation is much higher after they are formed in a low-ionic-strength milieu. Indeed, DOIC-Chol and DMEPC-Chol genosomes at $\rho = 0.5$, for instance, can be diluted to 0.2 mM with physiological saline without aggregation. This indicates a subtle balance between attractive and repulsive forces during interaction. In the case of higher ionic strength during complex formation, therefore, the precipitation is much more pronounced than in the case of the preformed genosomes placed in the same solution. After formation DLVO is qualitatively obeyed, while during complex formation electrostatic forces are attractive and it seems that faster reaction and more intense interaction at low ionic strength prevents large-scale aggregation; i.e., the lifetime of electrically neutral complexes is shorter. Quantitative agreement, however, is much more difficult because of the validity limits of the Poisson–Boltzmann equation at these high surface charges. It is also possible that attractive ion–ion correlation forces play a role and that at higher surface charges counterions are bound closer to the surface.

DC-Chol:DOPE–based genosomes are known to aggregate within dozens of minutes. This can be explained by the fibrillar structures which were observed in these samples (Sternberg et al., 1994) as well as in DOTAP–DNA systems by electron microscopy (EM) (Gustafsson et al., 1993; 1995). Probably the aggregation of the particles occurs via the so-called bridging attraction where one polymer interacts with two liposomes and aggregates them.

Electrostatics of DNA-Liposome Interactions

In previous chapters we have discussed electrostatics of DNA and liposomes. Here we shall briefly review the theoretical aspects of this interaction. While this is an extremely complicated interaction we shall discuss few particular cases. Despite some scepticism with respect to the adequacy of the Poisson Boltzmann equation for these complex cases we believe that it can still yield meaningful results and can avoid the use of various statistical lattice models. One of the reasons is also that electrostatic interactions seem to be the dominant forces in genosome formation.

The very simplest approach would be to use Coulomb Law which states that force between two charges is proportional to the charges and inversely proportional to the separation squared ($F \propto q_1 q_2/r^2$). This expression is equivalent to the interaction of a charge with electric field of another charge. Electric field is therefore force over charge (F/q) and electric potential (V) is defined as scalar product between electric field (E) around point charge times integral over distance, or $dV = E \int dr$. Therefore potential around point charge is proportional to its charge and inversely proportional to the distance from the charge. Proportionality constant includes permittivity constant ε_o

$$V = (1/4 \pi \varepsilon_o) q/r \qquad (7\text{-}1)$$

In contrast to the potential of a point charge in vacuum, potentials around rod-like molecules similar to DNA and spherical particles like liposomes in a solution with dielectric constant ε are described by more complex equations, as shown in Chapters 3 and 6. Interaction potential is therefore a product of two charges times geometrical factors as well as the influence of the solvent and solutes, which are defined by dielectric constant of the medium and Debye length, λ_D, with $\kappa = \lambda_D^{-1}$.

Here we shall discuss four different cases: interaction between DNA and liposomes close together and far apart as well as interaction between DNA helices at different angles. These four examples (R. Podgornik, personal communication) can serve as the basis of a simple theoretical model for modeling DNA-lipid complexes. Additionally, the first three cases we shall describe are in the limit of low and high ionic strength.

A.   Interaction potential between linear DNA with linear charge density u (e_{total}/length) and liposome with charge e at a distance h (far away) can be written as

$$V(h) = (eu/2\ \pi\ \varepsilon\ \varepsilon_o)\ K_o\ (\kappa\ h) \qquad (7\text{-}2)$$

where $K_o(x)$ is Bessel function of zero order. Two limiting cases can be approximated:

- large λ_D and $h/\lambda_D \ll 1$: $V(h) \approx (eu/2\ \pi\ \varepsilon\ \varepsilon_o)\ \ln\ (\kappa\ h/2)$ \qquad (7-3)

- small λ_D and $h/\lambda_D \gg 1$: $V(h) \approx (eu/2\ \pi\ \varepsilon\ \varepsilon_o)\ e^{-\kappa h}$ \qquad (7-4)

B. DNA (with length L) very close to a liposome surface with surface charge density σ

$$V(h)/L = -(u\ \sigma/4\ \pi\ \varepsilon\ \varepsilon_o)\ E_i(x)\ (-\kappa\ h) \qquad (7\text{-}5)$$

where $E_i(x)$ is an exponential integral function. Again, two limiting cases can be defined:

- large λ_D and $h/\lambda_D \ll 1$: $V(h)/L \approx (u\ \sigma/4\ \pi\ \varepsilon\ \varepsilon_o)\ \ln\ (\kappa\ h/2)$ \qquad (7-6)

- small λ_D and $h/\lambda_D \gg 1$: $V(h)/L \approx (u\ \sigma/4\ \pi\ \varepsilon\ \varepsilon_o)\ e^{-\kappa h}/(\kappa\ h)$ \qquad (7-7)

C. Now we shall also define the potential between 2 parallel DNA molecules with linear charge density $u = e_{total}/L$ and separated by h:

$$V(h)/L = -(u^2/2\ \pi\ \varepsilon\ \varepsilon_o)\ K_o\ (\kappa\ h) \qquad (7\text{-}8)$$

For the two limiting cases we can write approximate solutions

- large λ_D and $h/\lambda_D \ll 1$: $V(h)/L \approx -(u^2/2\ \pi\ \varepsilon\ \varepsilon_o)\ \ln\ (\kappa\ h/2)$ \qquad (7-9)

- small λ_D and $h/\lambda_D \gg 1$: $V(h)/L \approx -(u^2/2\ \pi\ \varepsilon\ \varepsilon_o)\ e^{-\kappa h}\ \sqrt{1/(2\kappa\ h)}$ \qquad (7-10)

D. If these molecules are parallel only in one plane and inclined by angle φ in the other, the exact solution was derived (Brenner and Parsegian, 1974)

$$V(h) = (u^2/4\ \varepsilon\ \varepsilon_o \kappa\ \sin\varphi)\ e^{-\kappa h}$$

These equations, along with elementary papers on Poisson Boltzmann equation (Verwey and Overbeek, 1946; Schmitz, 1993; Podgornik et al., 1994) may be a starting point for various calculations of interactions of DNA with liposomes (R. Podgornik, personal communication). In contrast to such mean-field models, quantum chemistry and molecular dynamics allows calculation of electrostatic interactions which depend on the molecular structure for sufficiently small numbers of interacting atoms. Such calculations may be used to evaluate different interactions of various cationic lipids with DNA and shed more light on the obscure structure-activity relationships.

In genosome preparation the majority of workers mixes DNA and liposomes at very low ionic strengths and therefore Debye length may be between 50 and 100 nm. In the case of physiological ionic strength, however, Debye length is around 1 nm. These parameters, however, do not determine only interactions between liposomes and DNA, liposomes and liposomes, and DNA and DNA, but also between all the intermediate structures during genosome formation which includes DNA and liposome structural changes. Obviously many other forces are involved, from many attractive forces, such as van der Waals, which may become important when the above-described electrostatic (and possibly hydrophobic and ion-ion correlation) forces bring particles sufficiently close, to a range of repulsive forces. While on one side the approach described above is far from being a complete description of the system, on the other side, it definitively represents the framework where one has to start in order to get theoretical insight in the genosome formation and structure.

■ STRUCTURE OF CATIONIC LIPID-DNA COMPLEXES

The majority of researchers have been interested in gene expression and not in the structure and characteristics of genosomes. Practically all the papers only compare different lipids at different ratios and the effect on activity. This, coupled with the complexity of genosome structure and properties resulted in the fact that not much is known about genosome structure and physicochemical properties. In addition, practically nothing is understood about genosome structure–activity relationships nor about their stability and fate upon application.

From the few studies published in the literature we can comment on three different models described. The original model by Felgner et al. (1987) assumed that DNA and cationic liposomes simply aggregate because of electrostatic attractive forces and form small stoichiometric complexes. Small liposomes have around 500 to 1000 positive charges on the outer surface and four to five liposomes were thought to surround DNA containing a few thousand negative charges (Smith et al., 1993). The outside of such a complex is positively charged as a result of charges which were not neutralized. However, detailed studies using a variety of techniques have shown a different picture. Minsky and co-workers (Gershon et al., 1993) have shown that cationic lipid induces DNA condensation and DNA induces liposome restructuration and that at a critical ratio DNA becomes encapsulated into an elongated bilayered liposome. EM and the inability of DNA to interact with intercalating agents and digestive enzymes supported their claims. Similar claims of DNA condensation were described previously by Behr (1993). Freeze-fracture EM was used, and partially fused spherical aggregates with a halo of fibers were observed by Sternberg et al. (1994). This gave rise to the so-called

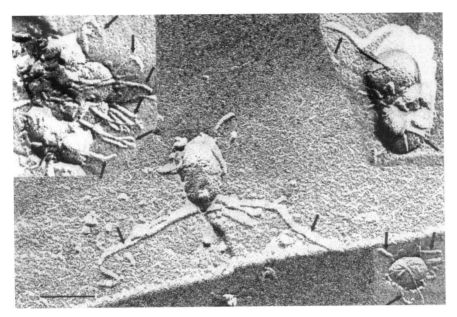

Figure 7-6 Freeze-fracture EM of complexes formed during interaction of plasmid DNA with cationic liposomes made from DC-Chol:DOPE (3:2 molar ratio). The bar represents 100 nm and the shadow runs from bottom to top. Some of the bilayer-covered DNA (spaghetti-like structures) is marked by arrow. (Courtesy of B. Sternberg.)

"meatballs with spaghetti" model, as shown in Figure 7-6, and similar pictures were obtained in other systems by other laboratories as well. Fibers were shown to be strands of DNA surrounded by a lipid bilayer. Fibers were present only in the case of DOPE as a neutral lipid (Xu et al., 1995). Equilibrium centrifugation analyses established that the density of anionic complexes is around 1.05 to 1.08, while the density of cationic genosomes is around 1.02 to 1.05. Recently, Felgner et al. (1996) proposed a model of hexagonally packed DNA in the complex. All these models are schematically shown in Figure 7-7.

It is possible that none or all of the above models are correct. Recent electron microscopic observations (Sternberg et al., 1994; Gustafsson et al., 1993; 1995; Xu et al., 1995; Lasic et al., 1996; Templeton et al., 1996), however, show different images. It is likely that different methods visualized different subpopulations of complexes in a particular sample. Understanding general liposome properties as well as DNA and polyelectrolyte behavior, one would predict that DNA induces aggregation of liposomes which consequently fuse, and in the process, DNA becomes trapped into the aggregate. Some models involve random structures of DNA being sandwiched between concentric lamellae in the multilayered lipid particle. If the charge is sufficiently neutralized (>90%, Equation 3-2), DNA collapses in the process, and one can think of several possible structures. Some of the DNA may not become entrapped into the lipid

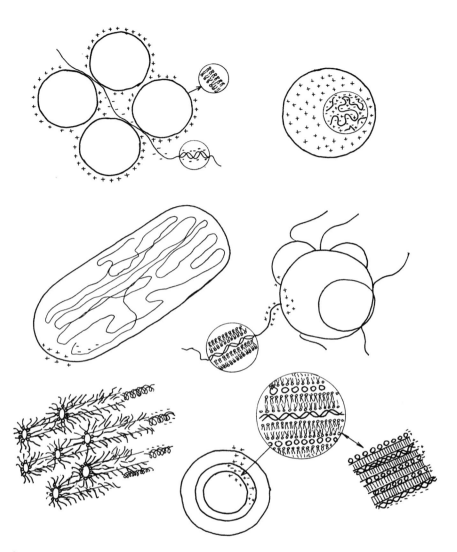

Figure 7-7   Schematic presentation of various models of genosomes proposed in the literature. Some of them will be described in detail on the next few pages. Adapted from the models presented by Felgner, Behr, Minsky, Sternberg, Lasic et al. Top left: Stoichiometric complex of electrostatic aggregates (Felgner et al., 1987). Top right: Cationic lipid condensed DNA coated by a cationic bilayer (Behr, 1993). Middle left: Fused bilayer encapsulates condensed DNA (Minsky, et al. 1996). Middle right: Fused and aggregated liposomes with detached fibers — DNA coated by a single bilayer — model by Sternberg. Bottom left: Inverted hexagonal phase in which water rods are actually a DNA helices model, presented by Felgner et al. (1996); short-range lamellar order model in which two-dimensional bilayers alternate with 2d nematic DNA (see EM and AFM pictures and SAXS reflectogram below) by Lasic et al. (1996). Topology of the structures generated depends on size of the liposome and the stretching elasticity of the bilayers. If liposomes with excess surface area are used, complete encapsulation of DNA can occur (see Figures 7-12 and 7-13) (Templeton et al., 1996).

aggregate and some loops or chains may protrude. Especially at lower lipid concentrations one would expect smaller lipid–DNA clusters bridged by DNA. Similar structures have been observed and theoretically predicted in the studies of polymers and micelles/colloidal particles (Cabane and Dupplesix, 1987). Some EM also show heterogeneous aggregates of fibrillar clusters (Zabner et al., 1995). Another possibility would be hexagonally packed DNA coated with lipid bilayer or two nested hexagonal phases — one lipid and one DNA as was observed in the case of cationic detergents (Ghirlando, 1991). Alternatively, an inverse structure in which water channels contain DNA rods was also proposed (Felgner et al., 1996).

It seems that EM data support some of the predictions. Initial studies were performed using cryoelectron microscopy (cryo-EM) and they revealed aggregates surrounded by a halo of fibers. This picture was confirmed by freeze-fracture microscopy which showed similar aggregates and shorter and stiffer fibers of approximately 6.5 nm diameter, which matches the diameter of DNA and a bilayer (Sternberg et al., 1994). Similarly, recent cryo-EM also showed some aggregates with detached DNA (Gustaffson et al., 1995). These structures, which were shown by using several different cationic lipids and DNA of various lengths, were given various names, due to their appearance. Such names included meatballs with spaghetti, medusas, and sea urchins. Negative stain and metal-shadowing EM (Gershon et al., 1993), however, showed more anisotropic, elongated structures in which condensed DNA is coated by lipid. At present, it is not known if the difference is due to the EM sample preparation or the fact that the first two methods were performed with circular supercoiled plasmids and the latter with linear DNA. In many cases such structures are not very stable. They start as smaller aggregates and grow to larger ones with less "free DNA" on the surface, a behavior sometimes referred to as bridging flocculation. While liposomes themselves already represent thermodynamically difficult-to-understand systems (Lasic, 1993a), the thermodynamics and kinetics of the genosomes and their colloidal stability have yet to be established.

A major question is which structure, a small "sea urchin" or a large aggregate with "less hair," is more effective in transfection. While the answer is still unknown, Bangham (personal communication) pointed out the resemblance between viral spikes and pointed DNA fibers as observed by freeze-fracture and cryo-EM. Both spikes, protein ones from viruses and lipid ones, may contain highly charged and anisotropic regions with high binding ability. Recently, structures with high radii of curvature were also associated with increased transfection efficacy *in vitro* (Xu et al., 1995). *In vitro* data, however, show better transfection at larger genosome sizes, and this may be due to a higher degree of phagocytic action seen by cells in culture (Felgner et al., 1994). Because it is not likely that such a structure is preserved upon systemic administration, we do not believe that these are relevant for *in vivo* transfection.

Certainly, genosome formation is a thermodynamic as well as a kinetic phenomenon that results in a broad distribution of sizes and shapes of particles formed. Each picture and each study may emphasize only a particular structure and ignore many others. Here, we shall describe anionic and cationic genosomes which we studied by microscopies, small-angle X-ray scattering (SAXS), analytical ultracentrifugation, size and ζ-potential analysis, size exclusion chromatography, and agarose gels. Similar results were observed in six different liposome systems. Optical microscopy observation reveals that a (small) fraction of the sample is always visible indicating that some particles are larger than 400 nm. The fraction of these particles is rather small, however. A similar broad size distribution was observed by EM as well. Typically, particles which are 200 and 300 nm in diameter as measured by dynamic light scattering (DLS) show a heterogeneous population in the range from 100 to 500 nm.

Velocity ultracentrifugation revealed a broad distribution of geno-somes with respect to the sedimentation coefficient, indicating large differences between particles in molecular weight, density, and shape (friction coefficient). Typically, cationic genosomes travel down the centrifuge cell in a broad boundary without any clear boundary between very heavy particles and unreacted liposomes which are spun down with a boundary characteristic for free liposomes (Figure 7-8). These particles have sedimentation coefficients in a continuous range from S > 1000 to 5 Svedbergs (Sv). High values of S indicate very tight packing. For instance, DNA in chromosomes has S around 1000 and DNA packed in viral heads has S normally around 800 S^{-1}. Sedimentation coefficient values of empty liposomes depend on the lipid structure and composition and can vary between 50 Sv to negative values for liposomes which are less dense than water and float. Naked DNA has apparent values of S around 5 Sv and this band trails anionic complexes. Exactly the same distribution of S was observed by simple pelleting of genosomes on a tabletop centrifuge. These values can be estimated from the equation

$$S = v / 4\pi^2 (vps)^2 \qquad (7\text{-}12)$$

where rpsare rotations per second (rpm/60), r radius, and v is measured velocity in meters per second.

EM supported the broad size and shape distribution as observed by centrifugation. High-resolution cryo-EM revealed several different particle shapes. In the case of DOTAP and DOTAP/Chol liposomes spherical genosomes with encapsulated DNA were observed (see below), while in the case of DODAB/Chol, DODAB/DOPE, DOIC/Chol, DMEPC/Chol, and DMEPC/DOPE, DOTMA/DOPE, and DOTMA/Chol liposomes particles with periodic structure were observed. Despite marked differences in the appearance we still believe that the major difference is in colloidal preparation and not in the nature of cationic lipid. DOTAP liposomes were very dilute and complexation was done at physiological ionic strength. On the other hand, DOTAP:Chol liposomes were extruded and contained a large excess surface area (see Figure 7-13). Figure 7-9 shows

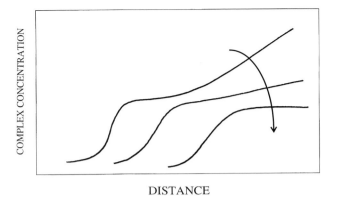

Figure 7-8 Qualitative presentation of analytical ultracentrifuge profiles of a typical genosome sample. Genosome samples do not show any distinguishable component. Basically, everything is spinning down, in a continuous pattern, from the very densest and heaviest, most compact complexes (S > 1000 Sv) to the trailing band of reactant in excess. Typically, one spins at 5 to 10 k rpm (distance from 6 to 7 cm), then cranks up to 15 to 20 k rpm for 1 h, and then analyzes the remaining fractions and trailing band at 40 or 50,000 rpm. Measuring either interference or adsorption mode yields identical results. (From McRorie, D., and Lasic, D. D., unpublished.)

various complexes prepared from small liposomes. Identical pictures were shown in the DODAB:Chol–DNA system (Lasic et al., 1996). They do not have excess surface area and upon interactions break and restructure.

When minimal-size liposomes are used, stacks of lamellae are typically observed. The periodicity between lamellae which are flat, open and stacked in columns (Figure 7-9a), open, and bent into horseshoelike structures (Figure 7-9b) or self-closed into concentric spheres is 6.5 nm (Figure 7-9c). No free fibers were observed. Superposed onto the lamellae a second periodicity with a period between 3 and 4 nm could be observed.

SAXS measurements revealed exactly the same periodicity of 6.5 nm with higher-order reflections at d/n (d = periodicity, n = order of reflection) positions, which are characteristic for lamellar symmetry. From the line width of X-ray reflections, the size of the scattering domain can be estimated to be around 300 nm, in agreement with cryo-EM (Lasic et al., 1996). A weak periodicity with a period of 3.6 nm, in agreement with cryo-EM data, could be observed.

As a control, unreacted liposomes (including the unsized LMV) and DNA solution did not show any reflections. DNA condensed by PEG and high salt, however, showed a hexagonal array with interaxial periodicity of 2.5 nm. No reflections were observed in precipitated complexes of cationic liposomes and polyglutamic acid. If one assumes strong binding of DNA on the bilayer surface, the observed periodicity matches a

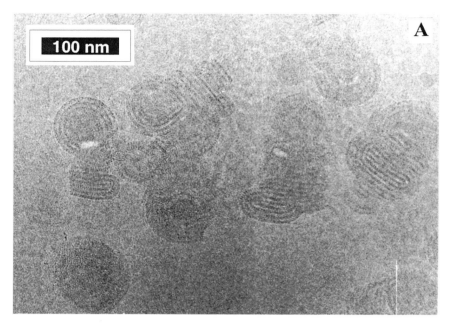

Figure 7-9   Cryo-EM of various liposomes and genosomes, all at ρ = 0.5 and for 4.7 kb DNA. (Courtesy of P. Frederik.) (A) and (B) DOIC:Chol–DNA and (C), DME-PC:Chol–DNA systems. This is a collage to show different shape distributions. Typically these particles are between 200 and 500 nm in diameter. In the DOIC system a long and short periodicity can be clearly observed (arrows).

thickness of a bilayer (4 nm) with adsorbed DNA (2.5 nm). Indeed, atomic force microscopy observations of DNA plasmids adsorbed on supported cationic bilayers showed aligned and parallel fibers without any knots and crossings, indicating strong electrostatic interaction, as shown in Figure 7-11. The lateral periodic spacing between aligned DNA helices was around 4 nm.

We have observed this pattern in many different genosome systems, rather independently of neutral and cationic lipid. The main difference seems to be in the absolute concentrations of reactants. At low concentrations the structures formed may be less dense and more diffuse. Occasionally, an unreacted liposome is bound in the structure, and in cationic samples (ρ = 0.5) many unreacted liposomes may be observed. Analogously, anionic complexes (ρ = 2) show that approximately one third of the DNA travels with a boundary which has S = 5 Sv, which is characteristic for naked DNA.

The periodicity of around 6.5 nm indirectly tells us that charges are not dehydrated. If this happened, DNA would contribute around 2 nm, lipid bilayers would tilt, and overall periodicity of ~4.7 to 5 nm would be observed. This observation may indicate that fluid lipid bilayers are important for transfection. Recent data obtained by the Barenholz group

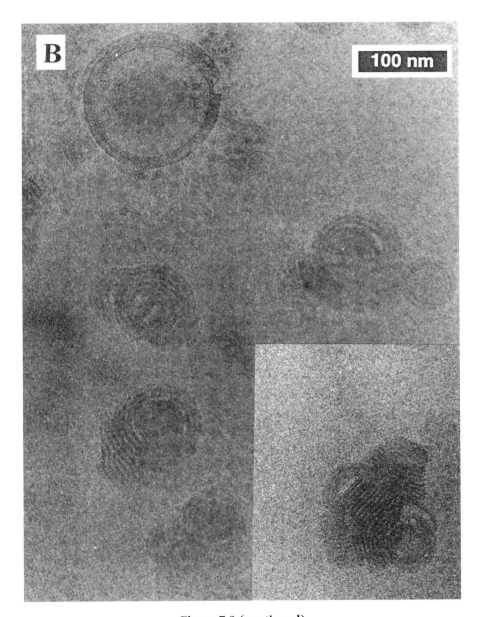

Figure 7-9 (continued)

are in agreement with this conclusion (Zuidam et al., 1997). They have used fluorescent probes to monitor changes on the lipid surface and in the hydrocarbon chain region of the bilayer during DNA-lipid interaction. Although the ordering of chains in DOTAP and DOTAP:DOPE bilayers increases upon DNA adsorption chains remain fluid. Order parameter of

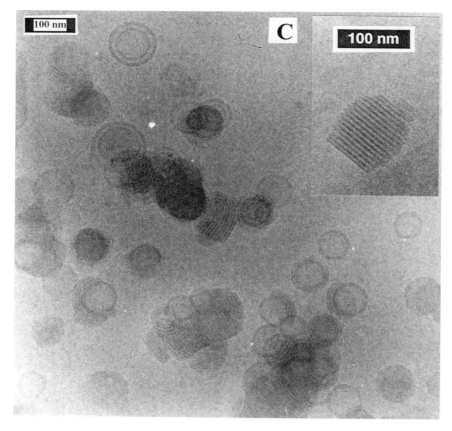

Figure 7-9 (continued)

DOTAP liposomes S_{33} = 0.206 increased to 0.245 in anionic complex (ρ = 1.4) and to 0.345 in cationic complex (ρ = 0.44). By using the surface attached probe they could monitor surface pH and potential. 3 to 4 units higher surface pH was measured and theoretical calculations have shown nice agreement with the Gouy-Chapman model. This is somehow surprising because measured and calculated surface potentials were around 200 mV where the validity of this formalism has not been established. Indirectly they could monitor pK of lipids and they found that DC-Chol has pK between 7 and 8. Circular dichroism measurements have shown that DNA conformation changed upon interaction, leading to condensed ψ-DNA. They have measured also phase transition temperatures of DOTAP (T_c = –12°C, and –15°C for DOPC and –21°C for DOPE) and estimated that these lipids have 8.7, 11 and 3 bound water molecules in excess water, respectively. An important measurement is also critical micelle concentration of DOTAP for which measurements of surface tension has shown cmc = 7 10^{-5} (Zuidam et al., 1997). This confirms the fact that diacylcationic surfactants have higher aqueous solubility than anionic

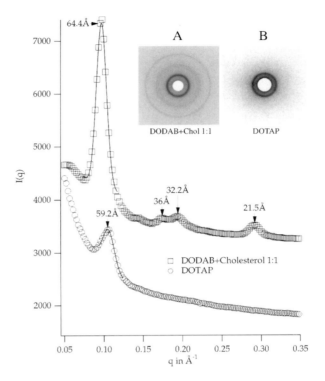

Figure 7-10 SAXS refractograms of DODAB/Chol liposomes complexed with DNA at ρ = 0.5. Many different complexes yielded similar reflections. DOIC:Chol–DNA genosomes gave similar periodicities (6.5 and 3.7 nm), while the DOTAP system gave shorter periodicity. Some genosomes, such as commercially prepared DOTAP complexes, did not yield any reflections. (Courtesy of H. Strey.)

lipids. This brings important question of size growth of such particles due to Ostwald ripening (Lasic, 1993). In Lifshitz-Slezov-Wagner approximation the cube of the mean number droplet radius increases linearly with time and proportional constants include interfacial tension at amphiphile-water interface, solubility of the dispersed phase and its diffusivity in the continuous phase (Weers and Arlauskas, 1995). At these high cmc values the growth may be in the order of 20–50% of the radius per month at room temperature. Such size growth may therefore be expected by some cationic liposomes as well as genosomes. This is in contrast to phospholipid liposomes for which we know, that this mechanism of growth in is not important (Lasic, 1993). Furthermore, in my opinion, at these very low solubilities (<10^{-8} M) the term cmc, or critical bilayer concentration, as referred to by some, really does not have any physical meaning. It does not describe a dynamic micellar process but simply reflects solubility of the compound.

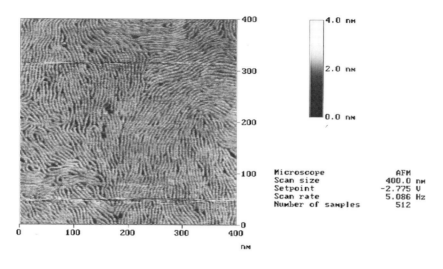

dsdna1.09

Figure 7-11   Atomic force micrograph of DNA adsorbed on a solid cationic bilayer, deposited on mica (incubation at 45°C for 30 min in 20 mM NaCl). The images were obtained with a Nanoscope E AFM from the Digital Instruments (Santa Barbara, CA) using a homemade fluid cell and Si_3N_4 tips with k = 0.06N/m. (Courtesy of J. Yin.)

Cryo-EM, SAXS, and analytical ultracentrifugation have shown that genosomes are rather heterogeneous with respect to size, shape, and density. Cationic complexes ($\rho = 0.5$) contain unreacted liposomes, while anionic complexes ($\rho > 2$ to 3) contain naked DNA. The system is stable as a heterogeneous coexisting state. Our limited efforts to separate particular structural populations or prepare samples without the excess of empty liposomes, for instance, were not successful. This may be due to dynamic changes during filtering and increased local concentration and osmotic effects during sucrose gradient centrifugation.

Using the data presented above, we can propose a model of these genosomes. They contain alternate stacks of lipid bilayer with adsorbed DNA which forms a two-dimensional ordered array on the surface between two lipid bilayers. At the edges the structure may be less well defined because topologically DNA must form a continuous spool. Complexes prepared from small cationic liposomes in low-ionic-strength solutions are normally very dense, small (200 to 400 nm) complexes which contain 5 to 15 condensed DNA molecules. They are characterized by a short-range lamellar order. The long periodicity reflects the stacks of bilayer–DNA sandwiches while the short one shows in plane organization of DNA helices. Charges are not dehydrated and lipid bilayers are in a fluid state.

Genosomes prepared from large DOTAP and DOTAP:Chol and DOTAP:DOPE vesicles (diameter 250 nm) are somehow different. They

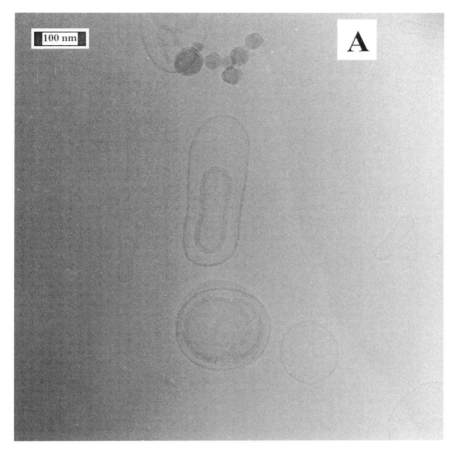

Figure 7-12   Cryo-EM of DOTAP:DOPE (0.75 mg/mL DNA at ρ = 0.5) and DOT-AP:Chol (0.5 mg/mL at ρ = 0.5) genosomes (A and B, respectively). DLS gave the following sizes: DD liposomes, 240 nm; DC liposomes, 215 nm; sample (A) 450 nm; (B) 420 nm. (Courtesy of P. Frederik.)

look like vesicles that have entrapped dense material of tightly wound DNA. It seems that in the case of cholesterol being a neutral lipid that these particles protect DNA better than in the case of DOPE. Figure 7-12 shows cryo-EM of these liposomes and genosomes.

I believe that the major difference between the encapsulated DNA and stacks of lipid–DNA lamellae (see Figure 7-9) is in the size and preparation method of vesicles. On some previous slides we have seen that some large spherical liposomes may be trapped in the structures. If liposomes are small, strong interactions with DNA lead to their disintegration. However, if they are larger and nonspherical (as seen in Figure 6-9B) and, which is often characteristic for the extruded liposomes, if they possess an excess of free surface area, they can restructure without disintegration. As can be seen from the micrograph, the majority of

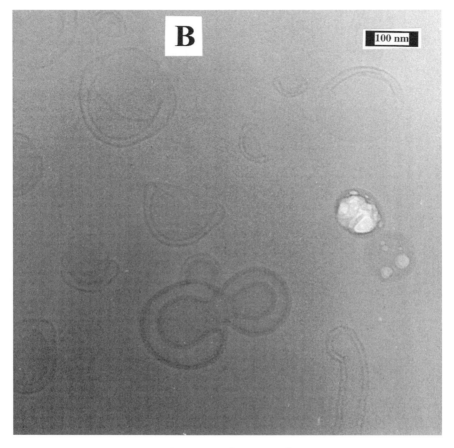

Figure 7-12 (continued)

liposomes are completely invaginated liposomes with a small orifice. When DNA is added it starts to spool around the outer monolayer. Due to the charge neutralization and lipid ordering the outer monolayer surface area is reduced, and this mismatch with the inner monolayer causes negative curvature. Because the liposome has a large excess of free membrane it relaxes the stress by inversion, and in the process DNA becomes encapsulated in the interior. The difference between the dioleoyl (DO, as in DOTAP/DOPE bilayers) and DO/Chol bilayers is in the mechanical strength of the bilayer. Cholesterol increases mechanical cohesivity for an order of magnitude (Lasic and Needham, 1995) and such a strong bilayer can undergo the inversion process while soft dioleoyl bilayers break. This indicates that mechanically cohesive liposomes with excess surface area are able to encapsulate DNA effectively. The driving force is the mismatch of the two surface areas on the opposed leaflet of the bilayer. Similarly, DNA is frustrated because only one side of the charges is neutralized, and therefore in the process of encapsulation it normally obtains another lipid coating resulting in concentric lamellar structures. The process of inversion of liposomes with excess of surface area (i.e., the encapsulated volume is well below the maximal volume the same number of lipid molecules in a bilayer can enclose if forming a sphere) is schematically shown in Figure 7-13A. Size analysis of complexes shows that they contain approximately 5 to 15 plasmids (~5 kb). All these indicate that several liposomes have to fuse to produce the complex (a typical invaginated 100-nm liposome contains ~120,000 molecules and a complex around 750,000). The schematic presentation of adsorption, induction of negative curvature, fusion, inversion, and self-encapsulation is shown in Figure 7-13B.

The ability of DNA to disintegrate bilayers can be proved by another example: a turbid solution of LMV becomes clear immediately upon addition of excess DNA ($\rho > 3$-5).

Following the above analysis we can describe complex formation as a sequence of several steps:

DNA adsorption

Lipid frustration $\rightarrow$ curvature change, breakage/restructuring/adhesion/fusion/inversion

DNA frustration $\rightarrow$ seeking of another coating — sandwich formation

Relaxation $\rightarrow$ restructuring and genosome formation

This process is governed by electrostatic, van der Waals (possibly ion correlation) attraction, intercalation, hydrophobic interaction as energy-minimizing interactions, and steric, hydration, electrostatic, and, possibly, undulation repulsive forces which interact with the bilayer via its bending and stretching elasticity as well as energy to create pores and break bilayer (critical tensile strength). Because of the size mismatch between liposomes in DNA, it is more likely that DNA starts to spool around liposomes than the formation of necklace structure observed in micelle–polymer systems. As discussed above, liposome size as well as the possibility of liposomes having excess surface area and flexibility and the mechanical strength of bilayers play also a major role in this process.

■ CHARACTERIZATION

Genosomes can be characterized by the same methods as are used for liposomes. The most frequently measured parameters and their typical values are shown in Table 7-1.

Despite numerous new techniques and because of the large heterogeneity of these samples, careful naked-eye observation (possibly aided

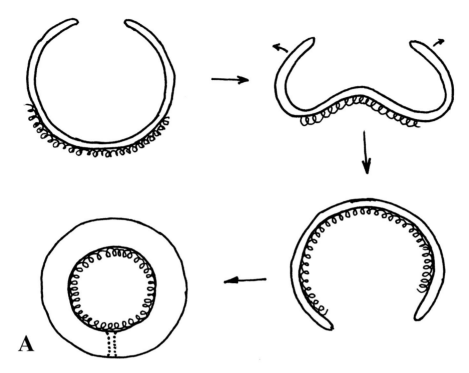

Figure 7-13   Schematic representation of DNA encapsulation by liposomes with excess surface area in the condition of mechanically strong bilayers. (A) Upon DNA adsorption both reactants are frustrated: bilayers because the outer surface area mismatches the inner one and DNA because only one side has its charge neutralized. Lipid relaxes the stress by changing the (sign of) curvature while DNA, in addition to spreading to a maximal surface, tries to obtain another coating with the opposite charge. During this process liposome with excess surface area undergoes inversion and DNA binds more bilayers which can result in physical disconnection of the inner (previously outer) part of the invaginated liposome. When the geometries are not matched, random disintegration and reaggregation occur. While lipid can relax its frustration by bending (negative curvature), DNA adsorbed on the invaginating liposome can relax its stress if another, smaller liposomes adsorbs (B). In this process the primary vesicle with excess surface area undergoes inversion and in the process DNA sandwiched between two bilayers becomes encapsulated (thickness of the inner circle of 10 nm may indicate 2 bilayers and one layer of DNA). Indeed, the thicker internal circle seems to be composed of DNA trapped between concentric bilayers which are, due to the positive surface charge, centered in the middle of the particle. Excess area of the primary vesicle forms attached tubular structures.

by a magnifying lens or optical microscope) can still be the most crucial observation. For *in vivo* applications no flocculation or precipitation should be observed. In the optical microscope some large particles (up to 10 μm, in more turbid samples up to 20 to 50 μm, depending on the concentrations) can practically always be observed (Figure 7-14). However, this is normal with colloidal suspensions and does not seem to

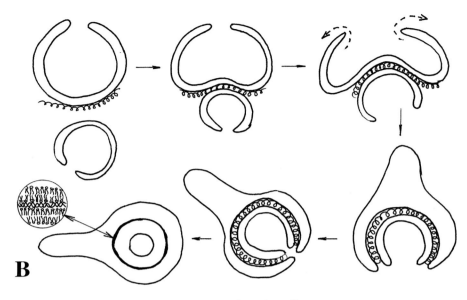

B

Figure 7-13 (continued)

TABLE 7-1

MOST IMPORTANT PARAMETERS FOR QUALITY CONTROL OF GENOSOMES

Turbidity
Size
Shape
Lipid and DNA concentration
pH
Surface charge (ζ potential, i.e., electrophoretic mobility)
Conductance
Density profile
Stability upon dilution (water, nonelectrolyte, saline, plasma)
Phase diagram
Endotoxin contamination
Transfection *in vitro, in vivo*

interfere with sample performance. Another simple and useful check is sample turbidity. Normally, it is measured at 400 nm at lipid concentration between 0.1 and 0.3 mM. This value must follow the Lambert–Beer law; i.e., turbidity must be linear with respect to concentration and intersecting ordinate at 0. If this is not the case the genosomes are unstable and not useful for applications. In some cases turbidity decreases with time, and

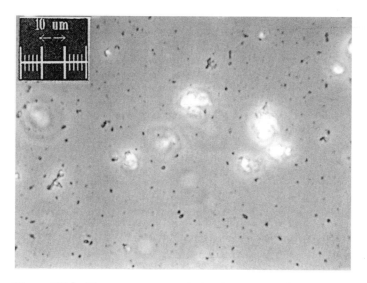

Figure 7-14 Phase contrast optical microscopy of genosomes (same sample as shown in Figure 7-12A). A few larger aggregates can be observed. The majority of the sample is below the resolution limit. Bar represents 10 μm.

these samples must be carefully inspected to see if this is not due to particle precipitation. Other measurements employ more-sophisticated experimental techniques.

Briefly, size can be measured by DLS. One has to be aware, however, that the method may not be too reliable for heterogeneous samples and nonspherical particles larger than 0.5 to 1 μm. If Gaussian analysis and bimodal distribution analysis yield similar size distributions, one can reduce the doubt of an artifact. Size should not depend on the genosome concentration in the working concentration range.

A simple test for aggregation (which is normally followed by precipitation) is phase contrast optical microscopy. Two stages of aggregates are shown in Figure 7-15 where (self) similar morphology can be observed also at higher magnifications. A thorough hydrodynamic analysis of such systems is extremely complex and few solutions for various shapes are given by Harding (1995).

Another method for size characterization is gel chromatography. However, in positively charged systems it is normally very difficult to elute particles. When one wants to suppress electrostatic attraction with high salt, the complex often precipitates and clogs the column. Heterogeneous samples also reduce the applicability of analytical ultracentrifugation. This method, however, can yield useful data on the distribution of the complexes with respect to their density, size and shape (friction coefficient), and molecular weight. Size and shape of the particles can be determined by EM. Cryo-EM is undoubtedly the least prone to artifacts.

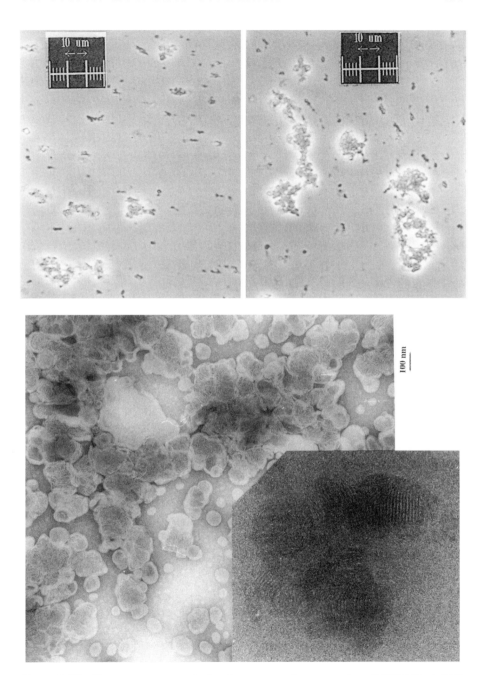

Figure 7-15 Phase contrast optical microscopy of aggregating DOTAP:Chol–DNA (0.75 mg DNA/mL, ρ = 0.5) genosomes during drying. For comparison, negative stain and cryo-EM are shown as well. The structure of aggregates in the optical micrograph can be deduced with the help of EM. (Courtesy of P. Freden'k)

The surface charge of colloidal particles can be measured by ζ potential. Quantitative predictions, however, are at present still nonexistent because of the inapplicability of the Poisson–Boltzmann equation to these highly charged systems and because of surface charge–dependent counterion association with the bilayer.

Lipid and DNA concentration can be measured similarly to the procedures discussed in liposomes and DNA (adsorbance at 260/280 nm). In the complexes, however, lipid and DNA must be separated, which is most easily done by Blight–Dyer extraction. TLC may separate lipid from DNA, especially if the complex is bathed at very high NaCl concentration (>1.4 M). TLC and especially HPLC can show degradation products. The DNA degradation can be followed by agarose gel electrophoresis. pH, conductance, and tonicity can be measured by standard laboratory techniques.

Various lipids and liposomes can be characterized by precipitation curves or phase diagrams. On such templates transfection activity can also be plotted. For applications, stability in distilled water, saline, CaCl$_2$ solution, serum, plasma, and whole blood may be important. Additionally, one expects more physicochemical studies of these complexes and interactions to appear, from NMR and EPR studies of lipid order, surface force apparatus measurements (Campbell, Kuhl, Lasic, Wong, Israelachvili, unpublished), surface reflectivity (Cevc, unpublished), monolayer studies, and others. Interaction between the charges can be also followed by IR and R spectroscopy, especially if the charges are on nitrogen and phosphorus atoms.

For *in vivo* applications pharmacokinetics and biodistribution are very important parameters which are too often completely neglected.

■ PHARMACOKINETICS AND BIODISTRIBUTION

Despite the fact that many *in vivo* studies have been performed, not a single thorough biodistribution study has been published although this is, in the liposome field, a very routine experiment. Complexes can be labeled with fluorescent probes which can interact with DNA, lipid bilayers, or both, radioactive lipids or DNA, as well as with paramagnetic ions for NMR imaging. In such cases lipid chelators are normally mixed in liposome bilayers. Especially with markers which intercalate in the lipid bilayer or in DNA a caution must be taken not to measure the biodistribution of the label itself. Some of them are known to quickly dissociate from liposomes and experimental artifacts can be observed. In the case of fluorescent probes and confocal optical microscopy, care should be also taken to take into account quenching effects for quantitative analysis.

Early biodistribution studies used the polymerase chain reaction (PCR) technique to follow mRNA expression in many tissues (Nabel et al., 1992). This method lacks quantitation and classical methods are recommended. A thorough study of biodistribution and pharmacokinetics of DC-Chol genosomes *in vivo* and toxicity *in vitro* was presented by Gabizon and collaborators (Rosengarten et al., 1994). DC-Chol:DOPE (1:1) liposomes (150 to 200 nm) were prepared in dextrose (4.3%)–NaCl (0.18%)–HEPES (15 mM, pH = 7.4) buffer. In the *in vivo* studies pharmacokinetics and biodistribution were followed via radioactively labeled tracer ([³H]choles-teryl-hexadecyl ether). After intravenous administration cationic liposomes were cleared from the circulation within minutes. The majority of radio-activity accumulated in the lung, from which it was quickly cleared. After 15 min 18% of the injected dose was in the lung, 5% in the heart, 27% in the spleen, and 1% in the liver. The fraction in the lung decreased to 4% after 1 h and to 2.5% after 1 day. The fraction in the heart did not change appreciably while that in the spleen increased (14% after 1 h, 20% after 4 h, and 18% after 1 day). The fraction in the liver remained steady from 15 min to 1 h (27%) and started to decrease (25% at 4 h and 22% at 1 day). After intravenous administration of the DNA–liposome complex the results were similar. Lungs had the highest uptake after 15 min (27% of the dose). This decreased to 6% at 1 h and 2% after 1 day. Liver increased from 18% at 15 min to 23% after 1 h and this amount gradually decreased to 17% after 1 day. Accumulation in the spleen grew from 14% (15 min) to 21% at 4 h and 19% after 1 day, while accumulation in the heart was steady at all time points around 3 to 4%. After intraperitoneal administration the majority of labeled liposome and genosome label ended up in ascitic cells (around 50% at 1 to 24 h) for liposomes and 60 to 70% in the same time interval for genosomes, while ascitic fluid contained around 1% of the label, liver about 2%, and spleen about 2.5% for both samples at 1, 4, and 24 h time points. This label is considered in the liposome field to be a reliable indicator of liposomes in the time frame of hours. In this case, however, its biological fate is not yet known. We do not know what happens to the complex after adsorption and if later points show only the biological fate of the label. In any case, the fact that everything happens in the first minutes, and that at that point lungs are the primary site of accumulation, is not surprising. After tail vein (i.v.) administration, the lungs are the first capillary bed encountered and have large surface area. It is likely that the complex adsorbs on the lung endothelia even if we can discount complex aggregation and physical trapping in the thin capillaries (diam-eter 7 to 10 μm). This study concludes that enhanced cytotoxicity of cationic lipids complexed with DNA is perhaps due to the larger liposome aggregates that interact with cells causing greater focal damage. Systemic uptake by liver and spleen, and short residence times in the lung probably do not allow effective systemic delivery of this formulation while accu-mulation in the ascitic cells after intraperitoneal administration points to the possibility of effective DNA targeting to intracavitary tumor cells.

Using different labels, Litzinger et al. (1996) obtained similar results. DC-Chol:DOPE cationic liposomes followed typical biodistribution as observed by anionic liposomes. Practically independently of charge ratio from 4:1 to 1:4, the majority of liposomes (75 to 80%) accumulated in the liver within minutes. Spleen accumulated 4 to 8% and skin about 3%.

With the exception of the intestine, all other organs accumulated less than 1% of the ^{111}In label. In contrast, when these liposomes were complexed to oligonucleotide (+/− ratio 4:1), liver accumulation increased slowly from 10 to 50% in 3 h while in the same time lung accumulation decreased from 80 to 50%. Immunohistochemical studies revealed large aggregates within pulmonary capillaries at 15 min postinjection suggesting that the early accumulation was due to embolism. Immune EM revealed that at 15 min oligonucleotides were localized mostly in the lumen of pulmonary capillaries and at 24 h in the phagocytic vacuoles in the Kupffer cells in the liver.

■ TOXICITY

Cytotoxicity of DOTMA:DOPE and DC-Chol:DOPE liposomes complexed to DNA was tested in the A431 cells. IC_{50} values of Lipofectin/DNA complex were around 6 µg/mL while complex containing DC-Chol liposomes exhibited IC_{50} of 25 µg/mL. Presence of DNA was shown to reduce toxicity (Gao and Huang, 1991). IC_{50} values of around 15 µg/mL for a series of imidazol cationic lipids were observed in CV1-P cells (Solodin et al., 1995).

Toxicity was examined also in three human tumor cell lines (Rosenberg et al., 1994). Rapid binding to all tumor cell lines was observed. Morphologically, severe cell damage and necrosis as well as liposome aggregates on the cell surfaces were noticed. IC_{50} of 5 to 20 mg lipid/mL were obtained, depending on the cell line. Surprisingly, cytotoxicity increased when DNA was complexed with liposomes. The growth rate of the cells decreased approximately from 3%/mg lipid in N87 cells (1.5%/mg in SaSO2 cells) to 9%/mg at DNA/lipid = 0.1 (w/w) in N87 cell line and SaSO2 cells. With a higher ratio of DNA to lipid (0.5), cytotoxicity decreased.

The cytotoxicity of Genzyme lipids was measured by a cell proliferation assay. The 50% death of cells was compared to DMRIE:DOPE liposomes, and relative cytotoxicity varied from 3 to 0.5. DC-Chol:DOPE liposomes were found to be far less cytotoxic (<0.05) (Lee et al., 1995). When the cytotoxicity of identical and similar lipids were compared to DOTMA, lower cytotoxicity was found (Guy-Chaffey et al., 1995).

The first studies of DNA complexes *in vivo* normally concluded that preparations were safe because no adverse effects in animals were observed and that animals tolerated treatment well.

The safety of DOTMA/DOPE–DNA complexes was studied in rabbits. Animals received four weekly injections or inhalations (pediatric face mask) of 500 µg plasmid complexed with 2.5 mg of cationic lipids. No adverse effects on pulmonary histology, lung compliance, lung resistance, and alveolar–arterial oxygen gradient were observed. The authors concluded that the system is safe (Canonico et al., 1994).

Toxicity in mice was studied by Stewart et al. (1992). DC-Chol:DOPE complexes were administered intravenously and in the tumors. No inflammation, no major abnormalities, no liver malfunction as measured by blood chemistry of various enzymes and no changes in electrocardiogram were observed. This study supported application of these complexes in human studies. Similar is the situation for inhalation of aerosols. While reversible inflammation was recently reported (Chen, 1995), exogeneous lipid pneumonia is another problem with lipid administration via airways (Malone, personal communication) which has not been addressed yet.

In general, however, a systematic, dose escalation study is still missing. Current studies have mostly shown that a particular application, at low concentrations, was safe. Longer studies at higher doses with follow-up of blood chemistry, spleen, lung, liver, and other organ necroscopy should be performed as well. Upon measuring CAT expression in the lung, some researchers mention that they detect CAT enzyme in blood which may indicate death of lung cells because this is an intracellular protein. A 1-day study may therefore be too short to see all the consequences. Therefore, the safety of cationic liposomes and complexes still remains to be adequately addressed. Short-term toxicity may be masked by quick colloidal neutralization of positively charged genosomes, and only biodegradable cationic lipids can reduce the molecular toxicity of positively charged lipids.

We must also be aware that large doses and volumes (in mice up to 0.2 mL i.v., 0.5 mL i.p., and 0.1 mL i.t. and in rats from 3 to 10 times more) cannot be scaled to larger animals, especially not to humans.

◼ SUMMARY

DNA–lipid complex formation depends on thermodynamic and kinetic factors. Structurally these complexes range from large, amorphous, and loose aggregates to smaller and denser structures containing around 5 to 15 condensed plasmids which are characterized by a short-range lamellar order. In none of the complexes investigated was a hexagonal symmetry observed. Lipid and DNA charges are not dehydrated.

◼ ADDITIONAL READING

Lasic, D. D., Barenholz, Y., Eds., *Liposomes: From Gene Delivery and Ecology to Diagnostics,* CRC Press, Boca Raton, FL, 1996.

Felgner, P. L., Ed., Issue on cationic lipids, *J. Liposome Res.,* 3, 3–106, 1993.

Schreier, H., Sawyer, S. M., Liposomal DNA vectors for cystic fibrosis gene therapy. Current applications, limitations, and future directions, *Adv. Drug Del. Rev.,* 19, 73–87, 1996.

Weers, J. G., Arlauskas, R. A., Sedimentation field-flow fractionation studies of Ostwald ripening in fluorocarbon emulsions containing two disperse phase components, *Langmuir,* 11, 474–477, 1995.

Zuidam, J. K., Hirsh-Lerner, D., Barenholz, Y., New insights into DNA interaction with cationic liposomes, in preparation.

8 GENOSOMES FOR GENE DELIVERY AND TRANSFECTION

Gene transfection can have several applications. In addition to genetic engineering and gene therapy, a major interest in modern biology is to understand the function of various genes. Therefore, gene expression or its blockage can yield important data on gene and protein functionality. Answers can be sought in two different approaches: the gene function can be "knocked out" from the cell or the gene can be introduced into the cell.

After we briefly mention first attempts to transfect bacterial, animal, and plant cells with DNA encapsulated in conventional liposomes, we shall concentrate on the use of cationic genosomes for *in vitro* and *in vivo* transfection. In this chapter we shall mostly describe the results and in subsequent chapters I shall try to explain the mechanism of transfection and draw some conclusions on the structure–activity relationships and correlations between *in vitro* and *in vivo* experiments which are difficult to see and prompt most of the researchers in the field to state that there is none, or, at best, an inverse one.

EXPRESSION *IN VITRO*

In vitro transfection is a procedure in which a cell culture is incubated with a plasmid and after a certain time the expression of the encoded gene is measured via the activity or concentration of the synthesized protein. A typical experiment consists of selecting cells of appropriate confluence (normally one half million to one million cells are plated in a 60-mm dish and grown in special medium with heat-deactivated fetal calf serum) and adding plasmids (1 to 10 µg DNA normally complexed to selected transfection agents) for 1 to 5 h incubation. After that a growth medium is added which is after 12 to 24 h replaced with a fresh one. Gene expression can be measured as a function of time and has to be normalized to the total protein concentration which indicates the amount of the cells. DNA plasmids can be added in various forms. Most frequently, precipitates with calcium or complexes with polymers and liposomes are applied. Naked DNA cannot be inserted into cells spontaneously and physical means have to be employed. Factors, like the presence of plasma in the growth medium, liposome incubation with the medium prior to application, and many others, were found to have significant influence on the expression levels. Different liposomal formulations, including cationic and neutral lipids, are known to behave very differently in different conditions. Parameters such as DNA and liposome concentration, liposome composition, charge ratio, confluence, age and type of cells, incubation and growth times, and presence of particular agents are studied to optimize a particular system. A wide variety of cell lines can be used. Typical cell lines are L cells (mouse connective tissue), CHO-K1 (hamster fibroblasts), BHK-21 (hamster kidneys), HeLa (human cancer epithelial cells), NIH 3T3 (mouse embryo fibroblasts), PC 12, Jurkat (human lymphoma), many fibroblasts with various genes, CV-1 (simian kidney cell line), COS-7 (fibroblast derivative of CV-1), psi-2 (murine fibroblast line), MSC.1 (rat hepatoma line), JZ.1 (rat hepatoma line with one integrated copy of mouse mammary tumor virus), TA1 (derived from murine fibroblast line), L-M(TK⁻) cells which are derived from murine L cells and are thymidine kinase deficient, NCI-H146 (human small cell lung cancer), many epithelial and endothelial cell lines, and many others.

With HeLa we can also mention cell immortality and molecular origin of cancer and aging. These cells are named for the donor, Henrietta Lacks, who donated her cells a few months before her death in 1951. These are the first human cells to successfully grow in culture and are immortal because they divide well beyond the 50 or so times characteristic for normal cells. This property of cancer cells also offers a possibility to study the molecular origin of uncontrolled cell division. Chromosome tips, or telomers, which are a six-building block sequence repeated many times, shrink with each cell division until they reach a certain point and cells are signaled to stop dividing. In cancer cells, however, the telomers do not get shorter and shorter and the cells never stop dividing. Telomerase, an enzyme, constantly attaches new telomere sequences. On the other side, aging may be related to a too quick loss of telomers and a slowdown in cell division. It is therefore obvious that the molecular biology of telomers may add important breakthroughs in our understanding of life and death.

Due to their ability to protect encapsulated DNA molecules against nucleases and to deliver the encapsulated material across cell membranes, conventional liposomes were tried as delivery vehicles for DNA and RNA. The best results were obtained with phosphatydylserine-cholesterol liposomes with a highly negatively charged surface. Although approximately 100-fold improvement in gene delivery over naked DNA was observed, the transfection yields were still orders of magnitude smaller than that by calcium or polycation precipitation and the interest in liposome-encapsulated nucleic acids quickly dissipated, especially because the preparation procedures were rather cumbersome. Improvements thought to enhance cytoplasmic delivery, either via the endocytotic pathway by using pH-sensitive liposomes or via direct entry into the cells by fusion of fusogenic liposomes, did not bring satisfactory results that would change the trend at the time. This work, however, established that bacterial, yeast, and mammalian cells as well as plant protoplasts (cells stripped of cellulosic wall) can be transfected by DNA encapsulated into the aqueous cavity of liposomes. Cationic liposomes tried at that time were toxic, because stearylamine was used to induce the charge. Also, due to low surface charges DNA was probably not sufficiently complexed and condensed. For instance, a typical liposome (single charged lipid, 1:1 w/w with DOPE*) has a surface charge density of approximately 0.2 Cb/m² (LipofectAMINE has 12 times higher) which is 2 to 3 times more than the stearylamine-doped neutral liposomes had, even if none of the cationic detergent had dissociated from the bilayer.

Following DNA transfection by using cationic polymers and DNA condensation by cationic micelles and liposomes, as well as several unsuccessful tries to use cationic liposomes for effective transfection in the early 1980s, positively charged liposomes were shown to transfect cells with complexed DNA *in vitro* (Felgner et al., 1987). DOTMA:DOPE (1:1, w/w) SUV complexed with the CAT plasmid were shown to transfect just-confluent cells. Around 100-fold improvement as compared with DEAE-dextran was observed in the JZ-1 cell line and around tenfold improvements in COS-7 and CV-1 cells were reported. No dose response was observed, but it was noted that liposomes were cytotoxic. Almost simultaneously, plant protoplasts were transfected by tobacco mosaic RNA upon complexation with lecithin–cholesterol liposomes containing cationic quaternary ammonium detergent. Up to 30% of cells were transfected while neutral liposomes were not efficient (Ballas et al., 1988).

To reduce cytotoxicity many novel cationic lipids were synthesized. An investigation of a series of molecules having different positive charges attached to the cholesterol anchor showed that tertiary amino groups were 4- to 20-fold less inhibitory to protein kinase C activity than quarternary amine derivatives of cholesterol and less cytotoxic than DOTMA (Gao and Huang, 1991). Since then, numerous novel lipids have been synthesized and tried for their transfection activity and cytotoxicity, as reviewed by Lasic and Templeton (1996).

Following the satisfactory transfection efficiency and relative ease of experimentation, the DOTMA:DOPE formulation became commercially available as a transfection kit with the name Lipofectin®. The prospectus claims that it is efficient in transfection of various human, monkey, murine, cow, bird, insect, and plant cells. One milliliter is sufficient for approximately 50 to 200 transfections in 35-mm tissue culture dishes or a third of that number in 60-mm dishes. This kit was soon followed by DOTAP, LipofectAMINE™, LipofectACE™, Transfectam™, CellFectin™, TFX-50, DOSPER, and some others. Table 6-1 shows the composition, manufacturer, some physicochemical characteristics, and price as of the end of 1995. LipofectAMINE is a highly active reagent (3/1 w/w ratio of DOSPA which has four positive charges at physiological pH with DOPE) and was shown to be from 2- to 100-fold more efficient in HeLa, BHK-21, CHO-K1,

---

* Abbreviations and chemical structures are shown in Figure 6-8 as well as in Appendix E.

PC 12, NIH3T3, and COS-7 cell lines. LipofectACE, which is a mixture of DODAB and DOPE (1/2.5), was a few times less effective than Lipofectin in these cell lines. The mechanism of action of all these systems is believed to be, in addition to quantitative DNA encapsulation, also in the ability of DOPE to induce lamellar–hexagonal phase transition and allow DNA to escape the endosome before lysozomal degradation (Farhood and Huang, 1996; Felgner et al., 1996; Friend et al., 1996). The fact that there are many mechanisms at work exemplifies DOTAP, which is a formulation of pure cationic lipid and works better with some cell lines than DOPE-containing complexes. Transfectam can give rise to transient expression in many cell lines, from human HeLa epithelial cells, hepatocytes (Hep G2, HC 11), lymphoblasts (IM9), and fibroblasts, as well as stable transfection in mouse (NIH3T3) and hamster (CHO) fibroblasts. Most of these kits are ineffective in the presence of plasma. This may be due to plasma-induced aggregation and precipitaton into large particles which are too large to enter into cells. In preliminary studies large differences between different cationic liposomes and genosomes were observed. Some liposome systems, such as DOIC/Chol liposomes showed immediate flocculation and precipitation within minutes (in 50% bovine plasma at 0.3 mM) while others were more stable (DMEPC:Chol 1/1). No flocculation was observed but some precipitate was formed at 24 h. Cationic genosomes prepared from the two liposomes have shown similar stability. Due to lower charge they were more stable, but flocculation followed by precipitation within minutes and hours, respectively, was observed.

According to producer's manuals, some of the kits can also be active in the presence of serum, including the TFX-50 kit, which comes as a dry lipid film and is hydrated to form larger vesicles before use. It is active in human hepatocyte and monkey fibroblast lines also in the presence of serum. This lipid has two positive charges which may provide better electrostatic stabilization than univalent cationic lipids. Similarly, a new double-charged lipid was introduced recently which was shown to be able to deliver antisense oligonucleotides and plasmid DNA into cells in the presence of plasma (Lewis et al., 1996).

Hundreds of articles describing transfection of various cells with various liposome preparations at various charge ratios have been published. To my knowledge, however, no comprehensive review exists and the interested reader is directed to data search. One has to be aware, of course, that it is very difficult to compare even parallel, not to mention different, experiments because of inherent and practically unavoidable biological and colloidal irreproducibility of experimental parameters.

Recently, structure–activity variations on DOTMA and neutral lipid were performed. *In vitro* work did not find a more effective neutral lipid than DOPE (Litzinger and Huang, 1992; Felgner et al., 1994), but exchange of the methyl group on the polar head with a hydroxyethyl group resulted in a very efficient lipid, DMRIE or DORIE, depending on the attached dioleoyl or dimyristoyl chains. In a typical *in vitro* assay (COS-7 cells,

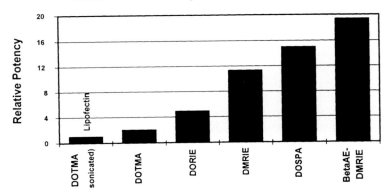

Figure 8-1 Relative potency of various liposome formulations in COS-7 cells. (From Felgner, P. L. et al., in *Liposomes: From Gene Therapy to Diagnostics and Ecology*, Lasic, D. D. and Barenholz, Y., Eds., CRC Press, Boca Raton, FL, 1996. With permission.)

pRSVlacZ plasmid DNA) DMRIE, for instance, shows more than double the activity of DORIE, which is in turn twofold more potent than DOTMA (Felgner et al., 1994). By converting the alcohol to the amine, even more effective lipid–β aminoethyl DMRIE was synthesized. This lipid was found to be more effective without neutral lipid (Wheeler et al., 1996).

A typical study is shown in Figure 8-1 where the transfection activity of several different liposome–DNA complexes is compared in COS-7 cells.

A bottom-line conclusion is that conditions for effective transfection can be optimized and that practically any cell type can be transfected. Optimal lipid compositions, liposomes, and charge ratios of genosomes as well as concentrations have to be determined for each particular cell line. It is very likely that at present no general rule can be applied as a result of differences in phagocytic activity, resistance to toxic lipids, and membrane composition of different cell lines.

While the exact mechanism of transfection is not known, *in vitro* expression is not affected by turbidity increase or slight precipitation in the DNA–lipid complex colloidal solution. It seems that transfection efficiency increases with increasing lipid concentration. Obviously, this increases cytotoxicity and optimal expression has to be determined for each cell type. It seems that the balance between cytotoxicity and transfection activity determines the optimal ratio. Even this may vary with the age and confluence of the cells. At present, therefore, it seems that an effective transfection procedure is still both a science and an art.

Not many mechanistic studies were performed. In the beginning it was thought that the ability of lipid to induce fusion with the cell membrane was responsible for transfection. Subsequent studies using endosome-disrupting agents such as chloroquine showed that transfection can be enhanced pointing to an endocytotic pathway. So did the observations of fluorescently labeled genosomes and EM observations. From the toxicity/activity balance, however, and knowing that large aggregates do not seem to interfere with transfection, as well as the fact that single chain cationic surfactants are known to induce holes in the bilayer (they were used as pesticides in the 1960s, Jungerman, 1970), we can speculate that DNA entry into cells may be also a consequence of lipid-mediated poration of the cell membrane. If the pore is transient, the hole can be resealed from the remaining pool of cell membrane lipids and the transfection is efficient. When the cell cannot repair the damage, the cytotoxicity reduces the transfection activity. Such a mechanism should depend on the confluence of the cells, which is indeed experimentally observed.

In parallel to these studies using cationic liposomes, several groups also investigated conventional liposomes or their variations. Legendre and Szoka (1992) used pH-sensitive liposomes, but higher transfection activity was observed when a cationic system was used. In contrast, *in vitro* transfection of vascular smooth muscle cells was only effective in the case of conventional liposomes containing hemagglutinin from Sendai virus (Morishita et al., 1993). Genes for the renin angiotensin system were used because of the important implications these proteins have in the growth of vascular smooth muscle cells and in hypertension, atherosclerosis, restenosis, and congestive heart failure.

Besides standard calcium phosphate transfection, it seems that among many systems cationic liposomes, either prepared in the laboratory or bought as a kit, are currently the most popular transfection system.

■ GENE TRANSFECTION AND EXPRESSION *IN VIVO*

Soon after successful *in vitro* gene expression, attempts were made to achieve transfection *in vivo*. This proved to be a much more difficult task. At present, there is still apparently no correlation between *in vitro* and *in vivo* expression. After reviewing the data, however, we shall propose a model of transfection and try to correlate these data.

While *in vitro* transfection is a powerful tool in genetic engineering to produce large quantities of proteins and in molecular biology to study the function of genes, *in vivo* work may have significant benefits in gene therapy. In principle, human diseases can be eliminated as well as human traits altered. Obviously, numerous scientific as well as many ethical and social problems will have to be solved before the color of the eyes and other human traits could be changed at will. What follows, however, is the beginning of this quest.

Genosomes can be administered by the same routes as liposomal formulations. These include systemic, local (intramuscular, intratumor, subcutaneous, intracerebral, intra-articular, etc.), and intraperitoneal injection, as well as topical (skin and inhalation of an aerosol, intratracheal instillation) application. Regular and double-balloon catheters can be used as well for direct delivery to arterial walls. The portal artery can be used for the delivery of complexes to the liver. Currently, studies concentrate on a tail vein injection in mice and rats, intratracheal administration, direct injection into muscle and tumors, as well as inhalation of a genosome aerosol. Especially for aerosol administration and genetic vaccination larger animals were also used, from rabbits, dogs, monkeys, primates, and sheep to cows and horses. When performing such studies, researchers must be aware that not only geometry of the airways but also various cell proportions and their physiology can cause significant changes between species and, for instance, high expression in the sheep lung cannot be generalized to other animal species.

A typical murine experiment consists of genosome administration, gestation period, organ harvesting, and analytical measurements. Normally, 10 to 100 µg DNA with lipid in a charge ratio $-/+$ from 3 to 0.1 (often >1 for aerosolized complexes and <1 for parenteral administration) are applied in 50 to 200 µL/mouse. Animals are left in the cages and food and water are supplied *ad libitum* for a period of 1 to 3 days. Thereafter, they are sacrificed and dissected. Tissues are analyzed either by slicing and immunostaining or for protein concentration and/or activity after tissue homogenization and possible extraction.

As in the cell culture work, the beginning of a liposome-mediated transfection goes back to conventional liposomes. Rat insulin gene injected in egg yolk lecithin:ox brain phosphatidylserine to cholesterol (8:2:10) large liposomes prepared by reverse phase evaporation was expressed and lowered the blood glucose levels. Furthermore, liposomes could be targeted from Kupffer cells to hepatocytes by inclusion of lactosylceramide which is a ligand for hepatocyte asialoglycoprotein receptors (Nicolau and Cudd, 1989). Due to low efficiency and demanding preparation, such experiments were not continued until the field of liposomal gene delivery became revived after the introduction of high-surface-charge cationic liposomes and the mounting safety concerns of viral vectors.

Early work, as will be described in more detail below, showed that CAT and luciferase activity could be recovered from frog embryos following direct injection into neural tissue (Malone, 1989). Expression in mouse lungs after pulmonary application of genosome aerosol and expression in various organs following a tail vein injection in mice were reported (Brigham et al., 1989). Similarly, expression in the mouse brain as well as in mouse lung after tail vein administration and in the arterial walls in the space between the two balloons of a special double catheter were reported in the late 1980s. Currently, many laboratories are trying to repeat some of these measurements and optimize transfection. Novel lipids, liposomes, DNA plasmids, as well as condensing, targeting, endosomicidal, or fusogenic moieties, can be coformulated into genosomes, and this work will be reviewed below.

It is very difficult to extrapolate some conclusions from these early studies. Scientists mostly studied gene expression as a function of the nature of cationic lipid, neutral lipid, and DNA/lipid ratio. Structures, stability, interaction characteristics, and physicochemical properties of the complexes were not determined. Additionally, no stability data in more demanding conditions (incubation in NaCl, $CaCl_2$, serum, plasma, or whole blood) were reported nor were pharmacokinetics and biodistribution of these complexes upon application *in vivo*. Furthermore, authors use very different units when describing DNA and lipid concentrations, ratios, as well as reporting data normally in relative units (see Appendix C), so that different articles are difficult or impossible to compare. Additionally, many of the results reported in the literature are impossible or difficult to reproduce. It is not only a result of the zeal of some scientists to rush with unrepeated and possibly artifactual results to the press, but also a measure of the complexity of the systems. From chemical and colloidal purity of liposomes and DNA, to numerous contaminating factors in animals and analyses, all these make these measurements rather difficult.

We shall review *in vivo* applications of genosomes via parenteral, including systemic and localized delivery, and pulmonary delivery. Other applications, such as topical and oral, will also be mentioned and we shall briefly start with uncomplexed DNA.

In light of extracellular instability as well as low permeability of cell membranes to large and charged molecules, it was surprising when it was shown that naked DNA could elicit some gene expression upon direct injection in some tissues. The best-known example is muscle cells. Intramuscular injections can be used to prime the immune system to recognize and attack the invading pathogens. This offers cheap, safe, and effective vaccines. An example is influenza A vaccine in which a gene for nucleoprotein of the virus, reconstituted into a plasmid, is injected intramuscularly. The expression of the gene was proved via antibodies to the protein and the 90% survival of the animals subjected to a lethal dose of the virus (Wolff et al., 1990).

On the other hand, systemically administered naked DNA is quickly degraded and eliminated by the cells of the reticuloendothelial system (RES). *In vitro* stability tests show a half-life of plasmid DNA in whole blood of 10 min while pharmacokinetic and biodistribution studies of plasmid DNA in mice showed a plasmid half-life of around 10 to 15 s. After initial higher accumulation in the lung at 15 s, liver became the major organ of the uptake of (degraded) DNA radioactivity at 30 s. Some radioactivity was found also in the spleen, kidneys, and lung. Most of the DNA was degraded within ½ to 1 min (Kawabata et al., 1995) Ca-precipitated DNA injected intraperitoneally was shown to express in the liver and spleen while not many reports describe the use of other delivery systems before the advent of cationic liposomes. This indicates a need for DNA delivery vehicles.

■ PARENTERAL APPLICATIONS OF GENOSOMES

Gene delivery by cationic liposomes *in vivo* was first described in 1989 (Brigham et al.) in a mouse model. They used intravenous (i.v.), intratracheal (i.t.), and intraperitoneal (i.p.) administration of genosomes containing a marker gene complexed with commercial cationic preparation Lipofectin at a DNA–lipid ratio of 1:5 (w/w). Gene expression persisted in the lung up to a week upon i.v. and i.t. administration, while expression was not observed in the RES; i.p. treatment did not show any expression; i.t. administration was 50% more efficient than i.v. Similar experiments were also performed in rats (Hazinski et al., 1991). CAT protein, driven by two different promoters (RSV and mouse mammary tumor virus), was expressed in lungs after i.t. instillation. Transfection of mRNA complexed with Lipofectin into *Xenopus* embryos and expression of luciferase was also reported (Malone, 1989).

Transfection can be also probed by infecting organisms. To study the bovine leukemia virus genetic determinants in the induction of leukemia in ruminants, sheep were infected with viral DNA complexed with DOTAP by intradermal injection. This showed that no viruses were needed for the infection. Such experiments can help to understand the function of different viral proteins and in the preparation of vaccines (Willems et al., 1992). Stewart et al. (1992) and Nabel et al. (1992) used DC-Chol:DOPE liposome-based genosomes to determine their toxicity and biodistribution in mice. DNA was detected in the lungs and heart upon systemic application but also in tumors after intratumoral injection. No toxicity of the genosomes was detected after histological examination, biochemical assays, serum enzymes tests, and electrocardiograms of the treated mice. To confirm these findings, safety tests were also performed in pigs and rabbits and no toxicity was observed. Furthermore, no autoimmune damage was observed and no gonadal (testes and ovaries) localization of injected complex was detected by quantitative polymerase chain reaction (PCR) which could detect levels of DNA in lung, kidney, spleen, and liver. These data supported the use of DC-Chol genosomes in a human cancer therapy trial and later in a cystic fibrosis trial.

A series of papers by Debs' group deals with gene expression in various tissues after tail vein injection into mice. The DOTMA:DOPE system was found to be effective in CAT gene expression in the lung, spleen, heart, liver, kidney, and lymph nodes and dose response was found in the lung, heart and liver. Similar expression was found also with DODAB:Chol (Zhu et al., 1993) and DOIC:Chol liposomes (Solodin et al., 1995). Similar levels of expression in all experiments, as can be deduced from the transfection efficacy data, is in disagreement with many current studies which show that cholesterol liposomes are much better for *in vivo* applications. CAT activity was measured 24 h after administration and expression dropped 20- to 150-fold after 3 weeks. Such animals were reinjected and similar expression, as compared with the first one (after 1 day), was observed after the second administration (Liu et al., 1995). Variation of expression as a function of a 375-bp intron sequence (from rat preproinsulin gene) was studied. It was shown that intron 5' to the CAT gene was as much as tenfold more effective than at 3' to the CAT gene while in the absence of intron the expression was between the two. The variation of expression as a function of different viral promoters showed as much as 100-fold variability in the expression: the highest efficiency was observed by using the CMV immediate early promoter, SV40 early promoter, the herpes simplex virus thymidine kinase promoter, and the adenovirus 2 major late promoter fused to the adenovirus tripartite leader. The first two promoters, especially the first one, give in general more than 50-fold higher expression than the last three. The use of 1,3-dialkyl fatty acid derivatives of 2-imidazolinium salts as a novel family of cationic lipids with heterocyclic polar head again shows that, according to many other reports, there is no correlation between *in vitro* and *in vivo* activity (Solodin et al., 1995). All the different liposomal systems, however, show the highest expression in the lung, which is followed by spleen, heart, lymph nodes, liver, and kidney. Lung expression is approximately two to three times the expression in the next highest expression tissue. Dimyristoyl derivative was the most effective *in vitro*, while dioleoyl compound was by far most effective *in vivo*. Cytotoxicity studies show that 50% growth inhibition (GI_{50} in CV1-P cells) occurs between 15 and 20 μM cationic lipids complexed to DNA (ratio ~0.8), rather similar for dioleoyl, dimyristoyl, and dipalmitoyl chains. This number can be compared with DOTMA:DOPE and DC-Chol systems, where GI_{50} of 6 and 25 μM were observed (in A431 cells at <1 and 0.25), respectively (Gao and Huang, 1991).

Long-term expression in lungs, liver, and spleen was observed upon systemic application of dioctadecylamidoglycylspermidine-DOPE liposomes complexed with luciferase gene inserted in a episomally replicative vector (Thierry et al., 1995). Luciferase gene was detected by PCR in liver, lungs, spleen, and heart 3 months after treatment, while expression in brain and ovary lasted 1 month. Expression in the lungs showed an approximately linear dose dependence, while at higher DNA concentrations expression in liver decreased. This study showed that transgene expression depended on the promoter element, formulation, DNA dose, route of administration, and the plasmid construction. Only human papovavirus (BKV)-derived episomal vectors replicated extrachromosomally in lung 2 weeks postinjection. In this study the differences between tissues are smaller than in the studies shown above. Upon intravenous administration the largest expression is in the lung, followed by the spleen and liver, but the differences are within 50%. Upon i.p. administration spleen has four to five times the expression in the other tissue while subcutaneous application yields smaller differences. After administration of 25 μM of DNA (at $\rho = 1/5.6$) about 100 to 200 fg of luciferase/mg of protein was produced while maximal transfection yielded 7.5 pg (lung at 300 μg DNA plasmid), 1 pg (spleen at 100 μg), and 700 fg (liver at 50 μg). We must keep in mind that other reports typically report much higher levels of expressed proteins. Published literature shows a few nanogram (Zhu et al., 1993; Solodin et al., 1995) to 200 ng/mg protein (Templeton et al., 1996). The complexes discussed above, however, were very large (0.2 to 3 μm) and prepared by hydrating dry DOGS:DOPE (1:1 w/w) with DNA solution.

None of the studies reported parallel pharmacokinetic and biodistribution studies, which makes interpretation of the results much more difficult. Also, the toxicity and immunogenicity issues in most of the reports are treated only marginally, if at all.

Stable genosomes which yielded reproducible expression levels were prepared also by the Papahadjopoulos group (Hong et al., 1997). DODAB/Chol and DOTAP/Chol liposomes were stabilized with small amounts of PEG-lipid and/or DNA was precondensed with polyamines prior to the formation of complexes. These formulations were stable for months at 4°C and could also be lyophilized. Nonstabilized formulations lost their transfection activity in 4 days. Up to 2 ng of enzyme luciferase per mg of tissue protein was expressed in the lung upon i.v. administration in mice. Other tissues showed less expression indicating characteristic biodistribution of positively charged genosomes.

Following our studies, which indicated that colloidal properties of the complex seem to be more important than molecular characteristics of cationic lipid (Lasic et al., 1996), we have tried to optimize transfection by using commercially available lipids. Based on colloidal structure–activity relationships we were looking for the highest concentration of colloidally suspended DNA at the lowest cationic lipid content at overall positive charge. We wanted to have small and dense genosomes which would protect DNA. Because these are the highest reported values of gene expression we shall present the data from Templeton et al. (1996) in more detail.

First, we have compared two different cationic and neutral lipids. Figure 8-2A shows that DOTAP is a much more efficient cationic lipid and cholesterol a much more efficient neutral lipid. Transfection of the DOTAP:Chol system shows nice dose dependence, while in DNA concentrations above 0.75 mg DNA/mL (150 μg/mouse) the efficiency is lower probably due to sample aggregation. Moreover, toxic effects are observed at higher concentrations. Panel C and D show charge range optimization for two different concentrations in the lung and heart (Panel F). The expression follows the typical pattern of lung > heart > muscle while the expression in the organs of the RES (liver and spleen) is low, probably due to low efficiency of CAT plasmid in the macrophages of these tissues (Panel E). Panel G shows expression at various concentrations and ratios while the influence of neutral lipid on transfection is shown in panel H. These studies were done with tissues which were not bled. Expression in the blood is negligible, less than 1% of the one observed in the lung. Therefore, exsanguinated lung showed 30% larger expression. This is due to the fact that there was less protein in the analysate.

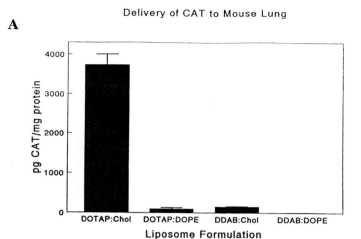

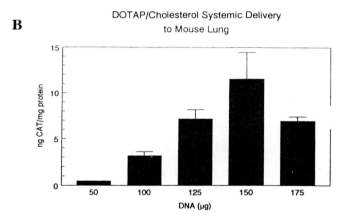

Figure 8-2   CAT protein expression of DOTAP:Chol–DNA system. Most of the samples had positive/negative charge ratio of 2 (ρ = 0.5). Panels: (A) effect of different lipids; (B) dose response of DOTAP:Chol system at ρ = 0.5; (C) effect of charge ratio at 50 µg DNA plasmid/mouse; (D) effect of ρ at 100 µg DNA/mouse; (E) expression of 100 µg DNA/4 mM DOTAP:4 mM Chol sample (= 100 µg plasmid and 0.8 µM each lipid per mouse) in various tissues; (F) slightly different charge ratio is optimal for expression in the heart; (G) gene expression in the phase space of DNA and lipid concentration. Dose dependences can be observed parallel to the axes. Lipid axes show that increasing lipid concentration above some value decreases expression; (H) expression as a function of neutral lipid. (Adapted from Templeton, N. S. et al., 1996 and 1997. With permission.)

As already mentioned, several other studies found high expression in mouse lung after tail vein injection. These data, coupled with pharmacokinetics and biodistribution described above, can give a possible

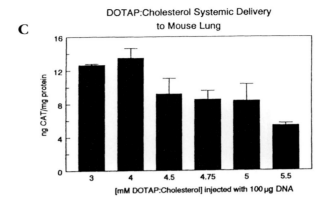

DOTAP:Cholesterol Systemic Delivery to Mouse Lung

C

y-axis: ng CAT/mg protein
x-axis: [mM DOTAP:Cholesterol] injected with 100 µg DNA

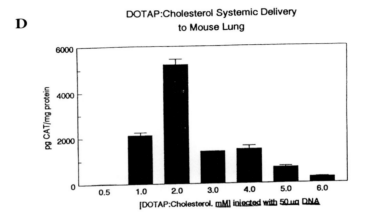

DOTAP:Cholesterol Systemic Delivery to Mouse Lung

D

y-axis: pg CAT/mg protein
x-axis: [DOTAP:Cholesterol. mM] injected with 50 µg DNA

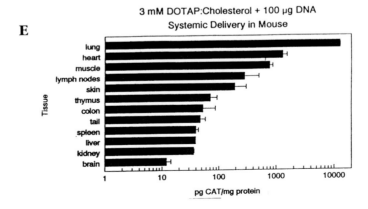

3 mM DOTAP:Cholesterol + 100 µg DNA Systemic Delivery in Mouse

E

y-axis: Tissue
x-axis: pg CAT/mg protein

Figure 8-2 (continued)

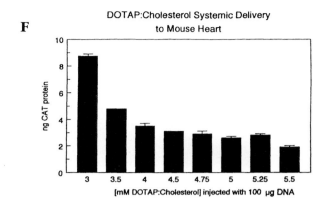

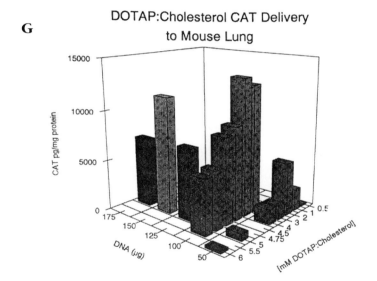

Figure 8-2 (continued)

explanation of the effect. High expression in the lung can be a first-pass phenomenon as a result of the fact that lungs are the first organ genosomes encounter in circulation and that their surface area is so large. Possibly, reversible blockade of some capillaries occurs, in line with above-mentioned pharmacokinetics, which would explain decreased transfection in liver with increasing dose as observed by Thierry et al. (1995). As discussed before, lipid-mediated (transient) poration or the damage to the cell walls during trauma and damage repair can also account for transfection. It is known that the body can reverse/neutralize toxic effects at lower amounts of lipids which can reversibly clog some capillaries and induce transient lipid-mediated poration of cell membranes. Heart is the second organ through which blood flows from tail vein.

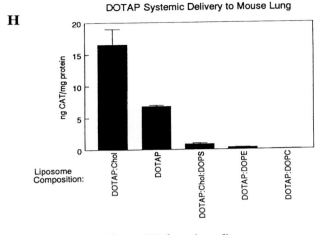

Figure 8-2 (continued)

A very important mechanism for the expression can be also complement activation. Cationic liposomes, genosomes, and especially naked DNA activate complement (Szebeni, Alving and Lasic, unpublished; Planck et al., 1996; Szebeni et al., in preparation; Templeton et al., 1997). Care has to be taken to obtain endotoxin-free DNA which can activate complement several times more than any liposome.

Complement protein consumption indicates that the inflammation which follows results in increased vascular permeability and some of the complexes may enter cells in the area, especially in the lung. Complement activation by cationic DNA complexes was confirmed by hemolytic assay by Planck et al. (1996). However, as this work has shown, the complement activation may not be a limiting factor for gene delivery, because it was found that some complexes coated with PEG could substantially reduce complement activation.

Measurable and lasting gene expression after injection of marker genes complexed with Lipofectin was reported for several other models. Local injection into mouse brain caused local expression lasting for 9 days to 3 weeks (Ono et al., 1990; Roessler et al., 1994). Transfectam (DOGS) was effective in transfection in the brains of newborn mice. After intraastrial injection of 2 µg of plasmid the optimal ratio of 1:1.8 was found. DOPE-containing formulations were fivefold more effective than lipid micelles alone. Dose-dependent expression was observed with an optimum at 1 µg. Higher concentrations resulted in complex aggregation and reduced activity. The superior transfectivity of relatively low charge ratio (five- to eightfold higher luciferase luminosity at 0.6 than at 0.33 and 0.25) was explained by improved diffusivity of the complexes; i.e., at higher charges of the complexes it was speculated that the majority of the complexes adsorbs in the vicinity of the injection site (Schwartz et al., 1995).

In some of the above studies, germ cells were assayed for transfection. No activity was found. Contrary to these results, however, gene transfer into fetuses was observed after a single i.v. injection of plasmid complexed to lipopolyamine into pregnant mice. The transgenes were expressed into fetuses and in the newborn progeny. SV40-CAT plasmid (133 μg) was complexed to 400 nmol DOGS and injected in tail veins of pregnant mice (Tsukamoto et al., 1995). Such experiments open the possibility of the questionable genetic engineering of life forms. In principle, genetic changes can be introduced into sperm cells. One can transfect stem cells in testes which are the source for sperm cells after differentiation. The change in the genes of sperm stem cells therefore alters the genes of an animal's entire lineage. Of course, such manipulation is possible only with sperm cells because there are no stem cells for eggs which are made only during the fetal period.

While studies using marker genes are necessary to optimize systems, the real goal is the expression of functional genes and measurements of biological end points.

In addition to cystic fibrosis, cancer immunotherapy is one of the primary interests of preclinical work. A strategy is that therapeutic DNA, which is normally injected directly into the tumor, encodes the foreign major histocompatibility antigen which, after expression, triggers an autoimmune attack. Results showed hindered tumor growth and complete tumor regression in a few cases (Plautz et al., 1993). In an analogy to the treatment with recombinant proteins, other treatments include gene transfer for cytokine genes, which can help to combat neoplastic tissue growth, and genes for various blood factors and proteins involved in cholesterol removal from the blood circulation in order to prevent arteriosclerosis.

Lung endothelium was targeted by small genosomes (<100 nm) containing the gene for the synthesis of prostaglandins (P G/H Synthase) to treat pulmonary hypertension. Vasodilatory effect was observed in a pig and rabbit model (Tomlinson, 1995). Animals pretreated with such formulations did not show any increase in blood pressure after endotoxin stimulus.

While many laboratories are working with cDNA encoding various cytokines, factors VIII and IX, tumor-suppressor genes, and others, not much information has been published. In order to destroy tumors foreign major histocompatibility complex proteins can serve as potent stimuli to the immune system. Expression of the murine class I *H-2K^s* gene within the CT26 mouse colon tumor (*H-2K^s*) or the MCA 106 fibrosarcoma (*H-2K^b*) induced immune response to the introduced antigen (*H-2K^s*) and also other genes present in unmodified tumor cells. As a result tumor growth was attenuated and in some cases remission was observed. The immunotherapeutic effect due to gene transfer–induced cell-mediated immunity can be therefore applied to the treatment of cancer (Plautz et al., 1993). This, as well as safety, supported the first nonviral gene therapy study in humans as will be shown below.

■ PULMONARY DELIVERY

The transfection values reported in the literature are rather confusing, especially for intravenous or topical delivery to the lung. While researchers, after years of presenting expressions in arbitrary units, relative counts per minute, and similar noncomprehensive ways, are finally starting to report more meaningful numbers — mass of protein expressed. Their normalization still varies substantially, thereby making comparisons between different experiments very difficult. Typically, this number (grams of expressed protein) is reported either per lung, lobe of lung, mass of lung tissue, or milligrams of protein from lung extract. To allow comparisons we shall review these numbers. Typical wet tissue weight of mouse lung is around $0.17 \text{ g} \pm 0.07 \text{ g}$ and it contains on average 11 ± 5 mg of protein (Templeton, personal communication) while the one from rat around 100 mg (Belloni, personal comunication). The proper way to normalize gene expression is therefore in mass of protein produced per milligram of total protein.

After i.t. instillation of $pRSV_2$-CAT complexed to Lipofectin and subsequent expression of the protein in mouse lungs, a similar system was used in nebulization. It was reported that delivery of aerosolized genosomes, pCIS-CAT marker gene and DOTMA/DOPE (1/1 mol/mol, 100 nm) liposomes, to the lung after pulmonary application resulted in expression lasting 3 weeks. Immunostaining for intracellular CAT protein revealed that the majority of airway epithelial and alveolar lining cells are transfected *in vivo* (Stribling et al., 1992). At present, however, the specificity of histochemistry has been severely questioned, and it is not impossible that there is substantial cross-reactivity in histochemical assays, especially in *CFTR* gene experiments between exogenous and endogenous CFTR protein. Aerosolization of Lipofectin-complexed $pCMV_4$-AAT resulted in expression of human α_1-antitrypsin in rabbit lungs for as many as 7 days (Canonico et al., 1994).

Canonico et al. (1994) described i.v. and pulmonary delivery of marker genes complexed to Lipofectin in rabbits. Expression persisted, irrespective of the administration route, for 1 week. Aerosolized delivery led to the expression in alveolar epithelium while the i.v. route caused transfection in pulmonary endothelium, indicating route-specific delivery.

These and several other studies that mainly used marker genes were followed by gene therapy studies in model animals. Hyde et al. (1993) tried to correct the ion transport defect in cystic fibrosis transgenic mice by administering *CFTR* gene to mice. Lipofectin-based genosomes were delivered to airways and deep alveoli via i.t. instillation. The authors concluded that this approach should be efficacious in humans. Another article describes delivery of human *CFTR* gene to mutant mice by nebulization and 50% correction of ion transport in the same mice was reported (Alton et al., 1993). CFTR expression in rats was followed after i.t. instillation. DNA was complexed with various lipids. Using DMRIE:DOPE liposomes, mRNA was detected after 72 h by reverse-transcription PCR (Logan et al., 1995).

In contrast to i.v. delivery, in these studies the overall charge of the complexes varies from study to study. Mostly, anionic complexes are used. Table 8-1 shows various experiments and the ratios used.

Scientists at Genzyme have synthesized more than one hundred different cationic lipids and extensively studied their *in vitro* and *in vivo* behavior (Chen, 1995). Transfection, comparable to adenoviral constructs (Ad-2-CFTR5, 10 to 50 moi) were shown: 400 ng CAT protein/mouse lung 2 days after i.t. instillation, while i.v. delivery was four times less efficient. Expression lasted 3 weeks. An important observation was that transfection efficiency is not correlated to lipid toxicity. Recently it was disclosed that the most effective lipid in their series was cholesterol with attached spermine and spermidine. A recent report shows even higher transfection activity and discloses many details. An optimization of lipid and complexes and molecular structure-transfection activity studies are shown (Lee et al., 1996). The synthesis of many cationic lipids is described and their structure activity relations in *in vitro* and *in vivo* transfection and toxicity studies are presented. The most efficient lipid yielded 1000-fold higher expressions as compared to the naked DNA as well as 100-fold higher as compared to DC-Chol-DOPE based complexes. Transfection level in the mouse lung was comparable to adenovirus vector administration at multiciplicities of infection ranging from 1 to 20. Cationic lipids were mixed with DOPE and optimal ratio had to be determined for each lipid. Typically it was 50 mol%, but it could vary from 66 to 33 mol% of cationic lipid. *In vitro* data did not correlate with *in vivo* results, but high *in vitro* activity was a necessary condition for *in vivo* activity. Cytotoxicity was not related to activity.

Liposomes with diameters between 200 and 400 nm were prepared by vortexing thin lipid films. Complexes were formed upon equivolumetric mixing with appropriate concentration of DNA and incubated for 15 min. *In vivo* activity was measured upon intranasal instillation in mice. The optimal expression yielded (lipid#67:DOPE 1:2, neg./pos. charge ratio 8) approximately 1 µg of CAT protein per 100 mg of lung tissue. Staining the lungs for β-Gal activity indicated that mostly alveolar cells were transfected while very few airway epithelial cells showed positive staining. Highest expression was detected 2 days after administration and declined rapidly to 20% of the highest transfection after a week and to 0.5% after 3 weeks. Repeated administrations yielded similar expression levels as the first administration if performed after a 2-weeks period when inflammation and neutralizing host immune system subsided. Some loss of expression was attributed to the development of the immune response to marker protein while the antibody or cytotoxic T cell-mediated clearance of the epithelial cells probably did not cause the loss of expression. The cause for rapid decline may therefore be in the loss of plasmid, death of transfected cells due to necrosis or apoptosis, or down regulation of the promoter. The last possibility may be responsible, at least in part, because interferon-γ, which may suppress expression, was detected in the lavage fluids of treated animals.

TABLE 8-1

CFTR EXPERIMENTS

Species	Route	Dose (mg/kg) Lipid	Ratio DNA	Lipid	DNA	Result	Ref.
Mouse	a.s.	25	18.8	DOTMA	CAT	3 week exp.	Stibling et al., 1992
Mouse	i.t.	3	12	DOTMA	CFTR	Expression	Hyde et al., 1993
Mouse	a.s.	175	35	DC-Chol	CFTR	Cl response	Alton et al., 1993
Mouse	i.v.	0.03	0.005	DC-Chol	CFTR	No toxicity	Stewart et al., 1992
Rat	i.t.	1.7	13.3	DMRIE	CFTR, LacZ	Expression	Logan et al., 1995
Rabbit	a.s.	4 * 1.7	4 * 0.3	DOTMA	Antitrypsin	No toxicity	Canonico et al., 1994
Human	nsl	0.0135	—	DC-Chol	CFTR	No toxicity	Middleton et al., 1994
Human	nsl	0.00135	3E-4	DC-Chol	CFTR	CFTR mRNA	Caplen et al., 1995
Human	nsl	0.0135	3E-3	DC-Chol	CFTR	Detected in biopsy	Caplen et al., 1995
Human	nsl	0.04	0.008	DC-Chol	CFTR	Detected in biopsy	Caplen et al., 1995

Note: as, aerosol; i.t., intratracheal instillation; i.v., intravenous injection; nsl, nasal instillation.

Adapted from Schreier, H., Sawyer, S. M., *Adv. Drug Del. Rev.,* 19, 73–87, 1996.

Another recent report shows 100-fold improved CAT gene expression in mice, as compared to the naked DNA, upon intranasal administration when liposomes made from novel lipid, GAP-DLRIE ($\pm$-N-(3-aminopropyl)-N,N-dimethyl-2,3-bis(dodecyloxy)-1-propanaminium bromide) formulated with DOPE (dioleoyl phosphatidyl ethanolamine) were used (Wheeler et al., 1996). Histological immunochemistry revealed that up to 1% of the alveolar epithelial cells expressed the transgene. Expression culminated between days 1 and 3 and then quickly returned to base line with small activity persisting to 3 weeks when a second dose elicited another transient peak of reporter gene expression.

Researchers in both studies used predominantly anionic complexes for gene delivery. The fraction of uncomplexed DNA was not reported but at higher DNA:lipid ratios may be very high. Anecdotal evidence exists that similar formulations in other species, including humans, may not be better than naked DNA. Also, at these high ratios DNA is not protected against nebulization. Some other groups have more success in pulmonary delivery by using cationic complexes and complexes in which the neutral lipid is cholesterol. Also, the same lipids in different laboratories produce different (relative) levels of expression. The operator dependence, especially in intratracheal instillation, as well as in tail vein administration is well recognized. While recent studies solved many artifacts from previous years, when, for instance, expression in the macrophages recruited after lung inflammation due to too large volumes or too toxic lipids were studied, there is still some effort left to understand and optimize these systems. While the synthesis of many novel lipids has not revealed much about structure activity relationships and the mechanism of transfection, it is, I believe, time to concentrate on the physicochemical, colloidal, and biological properties (stability and interaction characteristics) of the complexes and other studies to elucidate the mechanisms involved in the transfection process and improve level, duration, and safety of the process.

Permeability of epithelial cells increases dramatically if skin permeation enhancers, such as myristic acid, sodium cholate, and similar detergents are used. Some of these cationic detergents may have high surface charges and/or weak hydrophobic anchoring, especially if attached to a sterol moiety. Because topical delivery into airways is not subjected to the detrimental interactions in the blood, some of these systems, such as, for instance, polylysine or spermidine attached to cholesterol, can work simply by increasing permeation of membranes onto which the complex did adsorb. Typically, one would expect irritation, reddening, and inflammation at such sites, possibly hemorrhage. Therefore, I urge careful investigations and adequate mechanistic studies to elucidate the exact mechanism which may be much simpler than some of the models proposed. Also, surfactants which prefer micelle over bilayer formation and which may not be suitable for systemic administration may be active in such experiments for a completely different reason, as discussed above.

I am aware of many other studies, but unfortunately the data have not been published yet. It seems that the early enthusiam is being replaced by cautious optimism. Currently, safety of the procedure in humans has been mostly established. We must keep in mind, however, that the doses applied were very low. Also, appropriate controls have to be run. For instance, it was shown that i.t. instillation of naked plasmid in distilled water produced the same expression as DNA complexed with DOTMA/DOPE or DOTAP liposomes. Complexation, however, extended the retention of intact plasmid in the airways. Levels of expression similar to naked plasmid in distilled water were also obtained in isotonic aqueous solutions indicating that hypo-osmotic pressure is not responsible for the uptake (Meyer et al., 1995). The results from aqueous controls have to be carefully evaluated in order to elucidate the exact mechanism. If naked DNA really works as well as cationic lipids and if no physical effects can be associated, it is possible that DNA, perhaps during partial drying, condenses and is taken into a cell by an active internalization mechanism or as a bystander in some other process.

■ OTHER DELIVERY ROUTES

In vivo gene delivery via the intramuscular as well as the oral route was shown with DNA entrapped into cochleates. These are spiral rolls of highly negatively charged bilayers in which Ca^{2+} ions bridge negatively charged surfaces together. The easiest way to imagine these structures, which were discovered by Papahadjopoulos in 1975, is to roll a thin disk into a cigar. They can very efficiently encapsulate DNA which becomes resistant to nuclease degradation. Induction of antigen-specific spleeno-cyte T-helper cell proliferation was observed following intramuscular and, surprisingly, also oral administration of these formulations (Zhang et al., 1995). This is the preferable administration route. However, deleterious conditions in the stomach and digestive tract, especially low pH and presence of digestive enzymes and bile salts, quickly dissolve and disin-tegrate lipid particles, liposomes, peptides, proteins, and nucleic acids. If the particles can pass through these conditions undamaged, they, or the active ingredients, can be adsorbed by Payer's patch which consists of phagocytic epithelial cells. Actually, transfection through mucosal surfaces is becoming increasingly interesting as an alternate route to gain entry into the cells.

The oral route offers also the possibility of transfecting bacteria in the human digestive tract to secrete various proteins which could get adsorbed through the intragastric tract. In line with the induction of fusion as an important step in gene expression we can say that cochleates may represent "frozen fusion intermediates" (Zhang et al., 1995).

The topical route is also a very interesting one. Despite the fact that cationic detergents are known to irritate skin, cationic lipids can act as penetration enhancers and systems for prolonged localization at the application site. If cationic lipids mix well with skin lipids, some enhancement in skin penetration can be achieved. Formulations, which claim increased penetration into skin, such as transfersomes, may be tried as well. A simple thing is to coat cationic genosomes with neutral or anionic lipids and follow penetration and gene expression. Hair follicles are probably an easy target with several potential applications. Another possibility is to condense DNA and complex this with anionic lipids (such as egg lecithin to myristic acid, 1:1) containing penetration enhancers via polyvalent cations.

Using conventional liposomes and encapsulated DNA the expression of reporter gene in the hair matrix cells of hair follicle bulb in mice was reported (Li and Hoffmann, 1995). DOTAP:DNA complex with reporter gene was shown to rapidly penetrate the skin and expression was found in the epidermis, dermis, and hair follicles (Alexander and Akhurst, 1995). These results indicate the possibility of topical route for several gene therapy applications, from skin disorders to a delivery system with a systemical effect. Examples include genetic and other skin disorders, epidermal synthesis, and release of factor IX and apolipoprotein E, as well as treatment of baldness. However, before the cure for hair loss will be found, many well controlled experiments will have to be performed, as well as the gene itself will have to be discovered.

Transfection through mucosal membranes (all exterior surfaces of the body except skin, such as in mouth, sublingual, in gastrointestinal tract, genital organs, etc. and through which most of the infections occur) may be even more important port of entry than through the skin.

In contrast to a number of studies on transfection efficacy under various conditions, not much is known about the mechanism of transfection. As in the case of *in vitro* work, not only the physicochemical characteristics of genosomes but also their biological fate, such as stability in plasma, pharmacokinetics, and biodistribution, have not been investigated. There is no doubt that these studies will have to be performed to optimize systems and understand the mechanism of transfection.

A question of which cells can be transfected arises. For systemic administration this seems to be mostly vascular endothelial cells, mostly in the lung, fixed macrophages, in the liver (Kupffer cells) and spleen, and, if genosome size is below 100 nm, hepatocytes in the liver. Intramuscular injection obviously transfects mostly muscle cells. The mechanism is still not understood. It is well known that the localization of injection can greatly affect the extent and pattern of gene expression. Although the mechanism of the entry of DNA into cells is not known, it is not too unlikely that simple reversible mechanical poking of the membranes of these large cells can explain big differences between horizontal and vertical injection into the muscle, for instance. Along these lines, including that some may get entrapped during the subsequent trauma or its biological repair process, the observed intake of naked DNA can be understood. At present, it is still not known if the expression in all these tissues does not simply reflect the expression from the macrophages in these tissues because normally not many cells are phago-cytic. Alternatively, some still unknown internalization process may be at work, as indicated by Martin and MacDonald (1976), who have shown that erythrocytes, which are absolutely not phagocytic, could take in cationic liposomes. Similarly, Levy et al. (1996) showed that muscle uptake of DNA is saturable (*in vitro*) indicating possibly an active, still undis-covered entry mechanism. Other transfected cells include lung epithelial cells upon pulmonary application and epidermal cells in hair follicles upon topical application. Some of these cells may have a very specific intake mechanism.

The fact that after 10 years of research not much is known about the mechanism of cell entry definitively stresses the importance of basic research in the studies of gene transfection.

Very recent results, however, as reviewed by Felgner (1996), are more promising. In a decade *in vitro* gene expression in COS-7 cells increased approximately 1000-fold, as measured by µg of transgene produce per million cells (from 0.02 to 20), µg per gram of packed cells (5.5 to 5520) or % of total cellular protein (0.006 to 5.5%). This is due to much more effective plasmids. Novel expression constructs can be thousand fold more potent than the early ones, as well as emergence of more potent lipids for transfection. Nature of lipid and charge ratio of the complex has to be optimized for each cell line as well as route of administration for experiments in laboratory animals. Recent *in vivo* data from transfec-tion in the lung (Lee et al., 1996) show also a hundred thousand-fold improvement over the early experiments. The transgene expression of 2.5 µg/g of tissue in the lung equals roughly 10% of the expression of naked DNA in muscle or 0.05% of the expression in the cell culture (Felgner, 1996). The transfection may be even compared to adenoviruses. However, we must be aware that the same expression level in the lung or in the cell culture is achieved by approximately 10,000-fold smaller concentration of viral construct. Typically adenoviruses are added at multiplicity of infection (moi) around 100, meaning that the majority of the cells which are exposed to approximately 100 viral particles per cell, become infected. Comparable levels of genosome expression are achieved when million copies of the plasmid (ca 5 µg/million cells *in vitro*) are used. Along these lines is also a report that 15-fold higher expression in arteries upon catheter-mediated gene transfer into porcine arteries using a novel lipid, *N*-(3-aminopropyl)-*N,N*-dimethyl-2,3-*bis*(dodecyloxy)-1-pro-paniminium bromide (GAP-DLRIE), was achieved (Stephan et al., 1996). Expression was observed in intimal and medial cells at a level of 5% of adenoviral infection.

At present, with respect to *in vivo* testing, from safety to the origin of *in vivo* activity, we must say that rigorous mechanistic, pharmacokinetic and biodistribution as well as toxicity tests have yet to be performed. Additionally, for rigorous measurements of *in vivo* expression, time and dose dependence of the injected genosomes has to be performed. Dose should be increased 3 and 10 fold, if possible, as well as reduced at least for the same amounts and expression measured, with appropriate standard controls, in ≥4 animals at least on day 1, 3 and 7. In the measurements of CAT protein upon systemic administration, levels of CAT should be determined also in the blood, because its presence there would indicate slow death of transfected cells, because CAT is a non-secretable protein. For this reason as well as possible gene expression in blood cells, each measured tissue must be exsanguinated. Time dependence of expression may rule out the death of transfected cells, as for instance, large decrease of transfection between day 1 and 2 may be due to this cause. Immune response needs at least 2 weeks to develop, with only the strongest responses commencing, possibly, after 7 to 10 days. In this respect, genetically engineered mice offer many valuable models. Obviously, contamination of samples with live bacteria, fungi, and other microorganisms has to be checked. Although in normal concentrations, these cannot be responsible for dramatic effects during the first day. On the other hand, appreciable levels of endotoxins can be observed rather quickly because animals shiver, are fibrile and can even die within hours. We have already mentioned that the presence of endotoxins reduces gene expression.

Behavior and appearance of animals should be followed and anatomical changes determined by histological examinations. We have warned of possible artifacts in the transfection, such as capillary blockade or even reversible breakage of thin capillaries upon bolus injection of these large volumes of genosomes (often 20 to 25% of the blood volume in <1 second) and not all capillaries may be elastic enough to withstand this stress and upon reversible, ruptured genosomes may lodge into blood vessel wall cells or other cells underneath. This indicates that transfection may be a function of the injection rate and volume as well. Another possible artifact of intravenous administration is blockage of small capillaries by large (aggregated) complexes which may cause local transfection due to physical, chemical, or biological damage (inflammation) in the area. Similarly, flooding of lungs upon localized instillations should be avoided. Too large volume applied or too toxic lipid may cause local inflammation and transient expression as a result of recruited macrophages (Gromkowski, personal communication). Maximal doses, if applied carefully, are 0.2 mL in mice (preferably <0.1 mL; 0.6 to 1 mL in rats) for intravenous administration and 0.1 mL (mouse) and 0.3 to 0.6 mL (rat) for intratracheal instillation.

Experiments involving breathing aerosol of genosome particles are probably the most difficult to perform with smaller animals in which face masks cannot be applied. Geometry and diameters of lung bronchia and bronchiolli should be correlated with appropriate nebulizer to assure droplets which can pass through those constrictions. Additionally, degradation of DNA and aggregation of genosomes in such systems should be carefully checked. Aerosol experiments should be performed at times when the animals are the most agile, so in the presence of light, food, free movement as opposed to motionally restricted animals in darkness (Gromkowski, personal communication).

We have already stated that the above-mentioned volumes (and lipid concentrations) cannot be scaled up for administration to higher species.

■ GENOSOME ADMINISTRATION INTO HUMANS

Following antitumor response and safety studies, phase I clinical study in humans showed that the treatment with DC-Chol:DOPE liposomes is safe and partial response in melanoma patients was observed. Five HLA B7 negative patients with advanced melanoma using the *HLA B7* gene complexed with DC-Chol liposomes at a ratio of were enrolled into a phase I/II study. Three injections of formulations were applied in one cutaneous lesion of each patient. Biopsies from all five patients showed expressed *HLA B7* gene. B7-specific and CTL cells were detected in two patients with one response: the injected lesion as well as distant ones showed regression. DNA antibodies or plasmid in the blood were not detected. The study, which was the first *in vivo* gene therapy protocol in humans as well as the first nonviral gene transfer study, established the feasibility, safety, and therapeutic potential of the treatment (Nabel et al., 1993).

A similar study is being conducted using DMRIE/DOPE liposomes which were shown to complex higher DNA concentrations at smaller particle sizes and therefore offer larger quantities of plasmids to be delivered to the tumor (San et al., 1993).

Following preclinical studies and six viral protocols, the first liposomal cystic fibrosis trial was conducted in London's Royal Brompton Hospital. The CFTR-DC-Chol spray (pSV-CFTR plasmid: DC-Chol/DOPE at 5/1 w/w ratio) was aimed at the nostrils of 15 patients. In the phase I trial patients received varying doses of the formulation (20, 200, or 600 µg of DNA complexed to fivefold excess of lipid in 4 mL) or liposome-only placebo. No adverse clinical effects were seen. Gene transfer efficacy was difficult to assess. Nevertheless, plasmid-derived mRNA and DNA were observed (only qualitatively at day 4) in most of the patients, and only in the patients who received the CFTR cDNA was 20% improvement in chloride secretion observed. However, no correlation between dose and electrophysiological response was found, indicating possibly too small a sample size, dosing out of the therapeutic window, or some other artifact. Response lasted 1 week. This trial established the safety of the treatment while efficacy is probably too low for a therapeutic application. Obviously in the subsequent studies formulations will have to be applied as an aerosol. Also, the problem of mucus-coated surfaces will have to be addressed and the question of what fraction of the cells have to be transfected in order to effectively treat the disorder answered. Safety of these systems will be discussed below while regulatory aspects have been described by Caplen et al. (1994).

Overall, as of June 1995 already a dozen liposomal gene therapy clinical trials in humans have been undertaken. This compares to 3 other nonviral (two naked plasmids, one gene gun) and 92 viral (76 retrovirus vector, 15 adenovirus, and 1 adeno-associated virus) gene therapy studies in humans approved by federal agencies. In those 107 investigations 597 patients were treated (Ross et al., 1996). These studies conducted in US involve 85% of the gene therapy patients/volunteers worldwide. Most of the studies involves cancer [51 protocols, mostly immunotherapy *ex vivo* and *in vivo* (23+7), pro-drug (11), and tumor suppressor, chemoprotection and antisense], followed by genetic diseases by replacement strategy (20, 11 of those cystic fibrosis) and infectious diseases (9 dealing with immunotherapy and replication inhibition of HIV). Despite importance of the rapid development, however, one cannot escape the feeling, after careful reading of the protocols and their rationale, that some of these studies were conducted prematurely.

With respect to results it is still too early to judge. No clear conclusions have been reached regarding if and when gene therapy will lead to novel medical cures. Cautious optimism and a clear message that more basic scientific work is still required are the main conclusions.

SUMMARY

Gene expression *in vitro* and *in vivo* upon administration of DNA–lipid complexes was reviewed. Efficient transfection was observed in cell culture studies and in animals while preliminary results in humans offer very cautious optimism. Despite some encouraging data, a much more systematic approach and better characterization of preparations and analyses of results are needed. Also, transfection and expression efficiencies and duration of expression will have to be significantly improved in order to produce efficient therapeutic products.

ADDITIONAL READING

Gao, X., Huang, L., Cationic liposome-mediated gene transfer, *Gene Ther.*, 2, 710–722, 1995.

Felgner, P. L., Ed., Issue on cationic lipids, *J. Liposome Res.*, 3, 3–106, 1993.

Lasic, D. D., Barenholz, Y., *Liposomes: From Gene Delivery to Diagnostics and Ecology*, CRC Press, Boca Raton, FL, 1996; chapters by Farhood and Huang, Felgner et al., Maccarone.

Schreier, H., Sawyer, S. M., Liposomal DNA vectors for cystic fibrosis gene therapy. Current applications, limitations, and future directions, *Adv. Drug Del. Rev.*, 19, 73–87, 1996.

9 STRUCTURE–ACTIVITY RELATIONSHIPS

DNA–liposome complexes, as discussed in Chapters 7 to 9, have been shown to be effective in *in vitro* transfection of various cells. It was estimated that in the case of transfection by Ca-precipitation, approximately one out of a million plasmids reaches the cell nucleus and initiates protein synthesis. In the case of liposome-aided transfection, the fraction may be 1 in 10,000 or even less (Felgner and Ringold, 1989). Because the lipid-delivered DNA in general does not incorporate into the chromosome, the longevity of gene expression (i.e., the coded protein synthesis), is, in the absence of special "self-replicating" sequences, at best, a function of the half-life of a particular cell. Despite significant improvements, such efficiencies still cannot be compared with viruses where one can have virtually a 100% efficiency of transfection. A possible improvement might be to include more information, such as nuclear targeting and membrane fusion, from the virus into the plasmid and/or to add a nonimmunogenic, lipid- or polymer-based fusion function on the complex. The ultimate goal — *in vivo* delivery — involves many other hurdles but the options of complex targeting and the use of tissue-specific promoters for gene expression can further improve transfer of DNA into target cells and subsequent protein synthesis.

In vivo transfection, however, is much more difficult to achieve, especially via the systemic route, not to mention the preferred oral one. This is currently a very active area of research in which hundreds of companies and academic groups are engaged. In contrast to mostly trial-and-error work in the last decade, the key to efficient delivery systems will involve gaining an understanding of the transfection process and consequent optimization of the delivery of genes into appropriate cells *in vivo*. As a start, qualitative structure–activity relationships should be established, to be subsequently followed by quantitative structure–activity relationship knowledge. Here, I shall review published information and then speculate on various models and mechanisms.

At present, researchers believe that beneficial effects of cationic lipids may be due to a variety of reasons, including quantitative encapsulation and protection of DNA against degradation, condensation of DNA, increased binding to cells and cellular uptake, endosome disruption, cell membrane destabilization, and eventually targeting of (released) DNA to the nucleus. Additionally, the almost universal use of DOPE as a neutral lipid component is attributed to the phase transition lamellar–hexagonal (II) phase which can release contents from endocytosed complexes trapped in endosomes before lysosomal lysis. All the proposed models describe free diffusion of DNA in the cytoplasm. In reality, however, a complex intracellular traffic may be involved which can depend on the nature of the cells. While several of these possibilities appear likely, a systematic analysis is still lacking. Without going into the details, however, we can conclude that in general the development of an effective *in vivo* transfection system is a much more demanding process than *in vitro* transfection because of the effects of the genosome biological stability, interactions with blood and its components, as well as the pharmacokinetics and biodistribution of the complexes and DNA upon administration.

■ STRUCTURE–ACTIVITY RELATIONSHIPS

To simplify the thought processes I shall define two different cases of structure–transfection activity relationships: molecular structure–activity and colloidal structure–activity relationships. The first encompasses cationic lipid, counterions, and neutral lipids, and the second relates physicochemical properties of genosomes with transfection activity.

Currently, researchers are overwhelmed with the first one and numerous groups are trying to synthesize more-effective and less-toxic cationic lipids. Acknowledging the importance of cationic lipids, I still believe that colloidal characteristics may have an even more important role in the activity because recently it was shown that some "*in vivo*-inactive" cationic lipids (see below) can, if formulated properly, achieve extremely high transfection efficiencies in animal models (Templeton et al., 1996). On the other hand, however, we must also acknowledge that some lipids simply do not work in animal models when they are formulated in exactly the same way as *in vivo*-active lipids. This scientific jargon, at least as of the beginning of 1996, acknowledged lipids such as DOTMA, DODAB, DC-Chol, DOIC, DOGS as being transfection active in (some) animal models and most of the rest, including DOTAP, as inactive. Practically all structure–activity relationship studies, however, have been performed in *in vitro* transfection models and their generality was assessed only in different cell types.

■ STRUCTURE–ACTIVITY RELATIONSHIPS OF CATIONIC LIPIDS ON THE MOLECULAR LEVEL

In the beginning, scientists were simply trying various cationic lipids and liposome compositions complexed with DNA at various ratios *in vitro*. One of the first structure–activity studies was done with cholesterol-anchored positive charges, and because results are rather different from diacyl hydrophobic anchors, we shall discuss the two separately.

Cholesterol-Anchored Cationic Lipids

In contrast to nature but similar to the developments in other lipid bilayer applications, such as complexation of various drugs and rendering anchor for polymer coating of liposome surfaces, the active hydrophilic group can be attached also to sterols to ensure its membrane localization. Leventis and Silvius (1990) investigated, in addition to three different derivatives of DOTAP, quartenary ammonium ion attached to cholesterol on two different spacers, five and seven atoms long, with different spacer hydrophobicity. Lipid mixing upon interaction of cationic liposomes or genosomes with phosphatidylcholine/phosphatidylserine vesicles did not show any correlation with transfection activity. Lipids also showed similar biodegradability in cell monolayers. Comparison with three diacyl cationic lipids showed that optimal transfection efficiency protocols vary with cell lines. When studying the influence of neutral lipid, most of the results showed that DOPE was superior to dioleoylphosphatidyl 2 amino-1-butanol, N-methyl DOPE and 1,2 dioleoylglycerol. Huang and colleagues (Farhood et al., 1992) also studied several different cholesterol derivatives. They dissected cationic lipid in a hydrophobic anchor, linker group, spacer, and positive charge (amine). They also studied cytotoxicity and inhibition of protein kinase C activity. Their conclusions were

> *Transfection activity:* ternary > quaternary, secondary > primary, optimal linker size: 3 to 8 atoms between amino group and the linker group

> *Toxicity:* tertiary < quaternary, ether bonds > amide, carbamoyl > ester

> *Stability:* ether > amide, carbamoyl > ester

> *Neutral lipid:* DOPE $\gg$ DOPC, Chol

From this study it was not difficult to choose, for subsequent studies and applications, tertiary DC-Chol which consists of a hydrolyzable carbamoyl bond, a spacer of three atoms, and a tertiary amino group. The highest stability of liposomes formed was observed in the mixture with DOPE at 3:2 molar ratio. This formulation also showed high transfection efficiency in epithelial cells and fibroblasts and a lower one in macrophages, endothelial cells, and lymphocytes, in line with the well-known dependence of transfection activity on cell line as well as on cell-plating density.

In all these studies only single-charged cholesterol derivatives were used. I am aware of investigators coupling polycations to cholesterol but no reports have been presented. It is likely that at higher charge aqueous solubility of the compound increases which adversely affects bilayer stability. Again, *in vitro* experiments may be less dependent on this effect, as compared with experiments in animals in which constant sample dilution can adversely affect complex structure.

In sterically stabilized systems PEG–cholesterol did not provide efficient formulation as a result of the fact that cholesterol was not a good anchor to retain polymer–lipid in the membrane for prolonged times. One can expect that the fate of the cholesterol anchor is similar especially if linked to multivalent cationic charge. While this may not be a problem for *in vitro* or direct, localized applications, it can certainly reduce association of such molecules in bilayers upon systemic application. What happens to the complexed lipid molecules is still not known, but it is likely that they are associated with complex more strongly. The excess of cationic lipids, however, is toxic and is likely to increase membrane permeabilization. In most cases, however, this excess can be removed by centrifugation which can significantly reduce the toxicity of the preparation. This can be especially true for topical applications, such as inhalation of an aerosol of such particles, intranasal or intratracheal instillation or application on the skin. Analogously, bile salts are known penetration enhancers, and one can imagine the action of molecules such as spermidine–cholesterol as potent penetration enhancers rather than as due to other specific effects. Similarly, increased transfection upon intratracheal instillation can be achieved also by coadministering bile salts.

A recently published study by Genzyme indeed revealed that many of the lipids used were multivalent cholesterol derivatives (Lee et al., 1996). Structurally, most of the lipids used consists of spermine or spermidine linked to diacyl chains and cholesterol. Molecular structure-transfection activity showed that the orientation of polyamine polar head with respect to the backbone is important. Molecules which had spermine or spermidine bound to a secondary amine, resulting in a "T" shaped conformation were much more effective than linear construct s where polycation was bound via terminal primary amine. Such configuration may resemble ligands and facilitate cell entry or interaction with DNA. While the most effective lipid had 3 positive charges attached to the cholesterol anchor, there was no correlation between the number of positive charges and activity. Substitution of cholesterol for dihydro-cholesterol resulted in significant loss of activity. Carbamate bond of polycation to the hydrophobic anchor was found to yield the highest activity which decreased if amide, urea, or amine linkage was used. Polycations linked to the rest of the molecular via nitrogen atom were more effective than the ones linked through carbon atom. *In vivo* data indicated that cholesterol is optimal anchor while *in vitro* assays showed that diacyl chain anchors, especially dilauroyl, are more efficient. Salt derivative was also less efficient than a free base. While these data show the power of systematic approach to gene therapy and allow us to draw some conclusions, they also indicate the complexity of the process and our lack of understanding of the mechanisms involved because not many general conclusions, at least for structure activity relationships, could be reached. However, comparison of these biological data and molecular structures of lipids with physicochemical characteristics of complexes may yield novel clues.

Diacyl Chain Cationic Lipids

Following successful DNA complexation with cationic polymers, cationic lipids were used to coat DNA and complex DNA (Behr, 1986). These techniques were followed by complexation with cationic liposomes and several cationic lipids were introduced (Felgner et al., 1987; Leventis and Silvius, 1990). In the following years hundreds of new cationic lipids were synthesized which showed great differences in transfection activity and toxicity.

Various formulations, containing lipids such as DOTMA, DOGS, DODAB, DOTAP, DOSPA, DC-Chol, resulted in several commercial transfection formulations which showed rather good transfection efficacies in various cell models, but were rather ineffective for *in vivo* applications (see Table 6-1).

Soon after the introduction of DOTMA:DOPE cationic liposomes in DNA transfection several other lipids were shown to be effective in gene transfection. Among many different molecules, which differed in the length and saturation of hydrocarbon chains, presence or absence of the backbone, phosphate on it, spacer length, and nature of the positive charge, not much correlation was found. Mostly quaternary ammonium ions were used, and the general conclusion was that dioleoyl chains, small backbone, and short (few carbon atoms) spacers are preferred. Several structurally different lipids, however, were also shown to be effective, such as synthetic lipid with a phenyl ring in the polar head area (didodecyl N-[p-(2-trimethyl ammonioethoxy)-benzyoyl]-L-glutamate bromide), which was superior to DOTMA in COS cells (Akao et al., 1991). Some lipids with two charges, such as TFX-50, were found to be effective also in the presence of plasma. Otherwise, the number of positive charges did not seem to make much difference. Felgner with collaborators (1994) have studied the effect of various chemical structure changes on the DOTMA molecule. Substitution of methyl in the charged group with hydroxyalkyl, preferably hydroxyethyl, was shown to improve activity of the lipid. In the series of DOTMA-like molecules with respect to the fatty acids the following sequence (decreasing transfection activity) was found: dimyristoyl > dioleoyl > dipalmitoyl > distearoyl. The influence of neutral lipid was studied as well, and most studies agreed that DOPE is the most effective lipid (Farhood et al., 1992). In mixtures with DOTMA-like molecules DOPE was shown to be the most effective neutral lipid, according to the sequence DOPE > oleoyl palmitoyl PE > monomethyl DOPE > dipalmitoyl PE, distearoyl PE, dimethyl DOPE > dimyristoyl PE > dioleoyl phosphatidylcholine (Felgner et al., 1994). Activity as a function of fraction of DOPE in the formulation showed a bell-shaped curve with a maximum at 50 mol%. The use of multilamellar vesicles was found to lead to enhanced expression as compared with SUV. This study established DMRIE as the most-active lipid in this group. Recently, the same group showed that converting the alcohol (hydroxyethyl) into amine increases transfection activity and alters the neutral lipid requirement. It was speculated that hydrogen bonding and possible charging of the amino group on βAE DMRIE (N-(2-aminoethyl)-N,N-dimethyl-2,3-bis(tetradecyloxy)-1-propanaminium bromide) provide this activity. This lipid is an analogue to DMRIE (NH_2 replaces OH) and to DMPE ($-N(CH_3)_2^+-$ replaces $-O-PO_2^--O-$) and this may explain the fact that it does not need DOPE for transfection. Along these lines, I am surprised that "cationic DOPE" (neutralized phosphate charge or eliminated/replaced phosphate) or its close analogue (amino substitution, leading to 2+ lipid) has not yet been synthesized or evaluated in a published report.

Bennet and collaborators (1995) dissected cationic lipid into a hydrophobic domain, a polar domain, and a counterion. With respect to counterions they have concluded that ions with highly delocalized anionic charge improve transfection, and the following anions are listed in order of decreasing transfection activity: bisulfate > trifluoromethylsulfonate > iodide > bromide > chloride > acetate, sulfate. The mechanism was not explained, but the influence of counterion on phase transition (T_c) in the bilayer was noted. Hydrophobic character and effects of these large anions and especially entropic effects (chaotropic–cosmotropic, i.e., structure breaking vs. structure making, which can significantly influence the formation of hydrogen bonds and the structure of the complexes) cannot be ruled out. It is also possible that the ladder indicates pK of the molecules. Studies of the hydrophobic domain showed that dissymmetric fatty acids can enhance transfection. Palmitoyl oleoyl (and vice versa, OP) and myristoyl lauroyl (and LM) chains were found to be more effective than dioleoyl and dimyristoyl. In vivo and in vitro studies were not correlated and no correlation with T_c of the chains was found. The result may not be surprising because mixtures of a long and short (stearoyl and lauroyl) chain effectively substitute dioleoyl chains in lipid bilayers. Polar domain was studied as a function of hydrogen bonding, inductive and steric effects. No clear conclusions could be made.

In the Genzyme study (Lee et al., 1996) diacyl cationic lipids were found to be more effective in vitro (#102 > #89 > #111) while lipids containing cholesterol as hydrophobic anchor were more effective in vivo (#67 > #53 > #75, see Figure 6-8 for molecular structures). While cholesterol-based lipids differ only in the number of positive charges (and size of the polyion), the diacyl lipids differ in hydrocarbon chain lengths (lauroyl is better than stearoyl) and in the spacer between polyamine and chains (propyl is better than bulkier carbamoyl-glycerol). Cholesterol derivatives, however, show no charge dependence because the least active of the three (#75) has 4 charges, the most effective (#67) three and #89 two. This probably indicates that the difference may be in molecular geometry of polycations attached via tertiary amine or solubility properties of these molecules.

The last possibility is consistent with the fact that DOSPA and DOGS, which both contain spermine, presumably do not give rise to the same transfection activity. In these cases, however, spermine is linked to the rest of the molecule via a carbon atom and not nitrogen, resulting in one

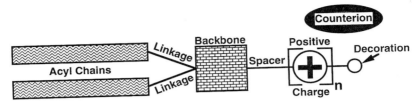

Figure 9-1   Schematic presentation of a hypothetical cationic lipid molecules and its dissection in various parts. (Courtesy of Stan Hansen.)

more charge. The possibility of activity due to the penetration enhancement effect requires thorough studies of the complexes on the colloidal level, their stability upon dilution, and critical micelle concentration of these cationic lipids because of additional toxicity such action may generate.

Following molecular structure more thoroughly, one can dissect cationic lipid into the parts shown in Figure 9-1.

The accumulated knowledge on DNA complexation, condensation, lipid restructuralization, and phase transition may lead to some speculations with respect to optimal activity as a function of chemical structure of various parts:

> *Hydrocarbon chains:* Dioleoyl chains normally preferred over dimyristoyl. Not enough experimental evidence for lauryl–myristoyl or lauryl–stearoyl. Such chains would be preferable due to chemical stability problems (no oxidizable double bonds). Possibly lauryl chains (lauretes are very potent penetration enhancers) and polyunsaturated fatty acids (see Figure 6-5) have not been tried yet. Cholesterol may be a good anchor for *in vitro* applications. Multivalent cholesterol derivatives may reflect nonspecific effects.
>
> *Chain linkage:* From transfection activity data no clear advantages. From the biodegradability and biocompatibility point of view the ester bond is desirable.
>
> *Backbone:* It is not clear yet. It seems that the absence of backbone (DODAB) is not optimal, while too large a backbone may interfere with molecular rearrangements during complexation or possible inversion, such as phosphate-containing backbones (negative charge neutralized phosphatidylcholines).
>
> *Spacer and linkage:* Several atoms to allow charge adjustment and fit to DNA forces. Too long may create a diffuse plane for effective DNA binding and adsorption. For too short spacers electrostatic interaction may compete with intrabilayer dispersion forces.
>
> *Number and nature of positive charge:* Most of the lipids contain a tertiary or quaternary ammonium group. It has a pK above 10 to 11 (normally >12) and is fully ionized at physiological pH and below. Other charges, such as amines on imidazole, aminopyridine

or methylimidazole, may have pK values in a range from 8 to 5, but their benefit to complexation and membrane interactions is not clear. Delocalized (heterocyclic) positive charge may be efficient for binding and effective decondensation. Double positive charge may render increased (colloidal) stability in plasma and blood. Too many charges result in too high aqueous solubility and formation of micellar phases and unstable complexes.

Decoration of polar head: It is still not known how strong DNA binding is optimal. A hydrogen bonding group may be advantageous. Intercalation into DNA has not been shown yet and may be undesirable. In the case of too strong interaction DNA cannot decondense.

Counterion: Chloride is better for liposome preparation. For electrostatic interactions and membrane disruption chaotropic ions may be better. The importance of those for systemic applications may be meaningless due to a fast exchange with the counterions from the milieu. Some data indicate that free bases may be better.

Various metal ions are known to interact with DNA specifically. Perhaps lipid chelators can be incorporated into liposomes and upon chelating a net positive charge may result leading to specific interactions with DNA.

■ STRUCTURE–ACTIVITY RELATIONSHIPS ON THE COLLOIDAL LEVEL

The literature (Sternberg et al., 1995; Gustaffon et al., 1993, 1995; Sternberg, 1996) shows several micrographs of genosomes which were active in *in vitro* transfection. Mostly they are large aggregates containing partially fused liposomes in the range of 200 to 1000 nm. Resolution permitting, some attached fibers can be seen as shown in Figure 7-6. Due to their appearance the structures were described as spaghetti and meatballs, or medusas, and people still discuss which conformation, i.e., spherical aggregates or lipid-coated fibers, are the active structures in transfection. Bangham pointed out that fibrillar structures on the surface of these globular aggregates resemble viral spikes and may serve as attachment points. Indeed, one *in vitro* study concluded that activity could be correlated with structures with high local curvatures, such as pits, spikes, or edges (Xu et al., 1995).

A cryo-EM of a similar complex is shown in Figure 9-2A. This is DNA complexed to commercially available DOTAP liposomes. We could not observe DNA fibers. In contrast to these complexes which were shown to be inactive upon systemic administration (Lasic et al., unpublished), we have studied several complexes which were shown to transfect *in vivo* as measured by expression of CAT protein in the mouse lungs 1 day after tail vein injection. A strikingly different picture was seen. Instead of loose, large, fragile aggregates, smaller dense and compact colloidal particles

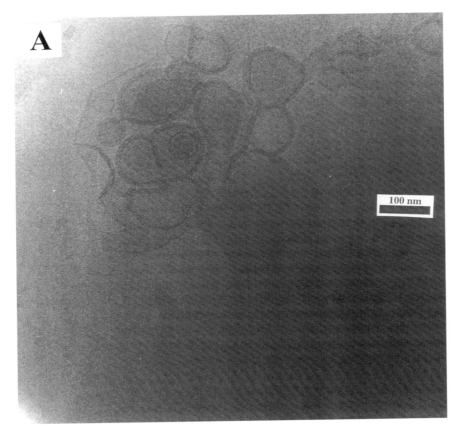

Figure 9-2   Cryo-EM of (A) DOTAP–DNA complex and negative stain EM of (B) DODAB/Chol–DNA complex. (Cryo-EM of this system closely resembles this image and the same periodicity of 6.5 nm can be seen, similarly to Figure 7-10).

   We have noticed that *in vivo* active complex (DODAB/Chol-DNA charge ratio = 1:2, lipid = 1.8 mM) displays two periodicities, while a nonactive complex (DOTAP–DNA, ρ = 0.5, c = 0.7 mM) did not show any periodicity (Lasic et al., 1996a,b). This finding is not unexpected. Systemic delivery requires a certain size window as well tight and protected DNA to prevent physical entrapment and DNA degradation. Analytical ultracentrifuge showed that genosomes are very heterogeneous with respect to their density and sedimentation coefficients from 1000 to 80 s^{-1} were estimated (naked DNA around 5 s^{-1}) (McRorie and Lasic, unpublished). DOTAP:Chol–DNA complexes at higher lipid concentrations (ρ = 0.5) showed compact dark circular structures encapsulated in lipid bilayers.

could be observed (see Figure 7-10A). In some samples locally ordered structures could be seen (Figure 9-2B). Noting two periodicities, a longer one about 5 to 7 nm and a shorter one in the range 3 to 4 nm, we performed small-angle X-ray scattering (SAXS) studies which reproduced EM-determined periodicities completely. As controls, naked DNA, unreacted liposomes, as well as "*in vivo*-inactive" complexes, as shown in Figure 9-2A, did not yield any reflections. Simple tabletop centrifugation

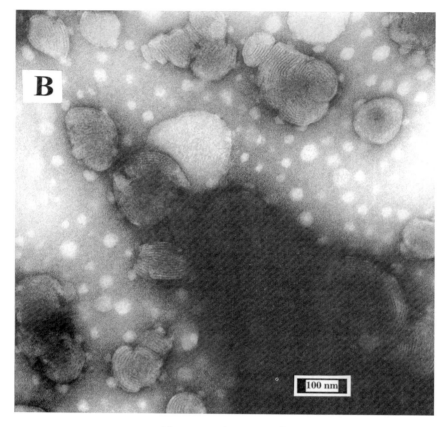

Figure 9-2 (continued)

experiments have shown that the active complexes, containing no visible flocculae can be easily (partially) pelleted, indicating that active complexes contain dense particles and sedimentation coefficients over 500 Sv for that fraction of the sample were calculated from Equation 7-1. Ethidium bromide fluorescence studies also showed that in these complexes DNA was inaccessible for the fluorescent dye intercalation indicating good DNA protection.

These results may indicate that condensed or tightly packed DNA is a necessary condition for efficient gene expression upon systemic administration because large, loose complexes cannot protect DNA in the circulation. It is easy to imagine that a large complex, as shown in Figure 9-2A, can quickly adsorb or disintegrate upon injection. It is known that giant unilamellar or oligolamellar liposomes disintegrate, not only due to mechanical stresses in turbulent circulation, but also because of adsorption and intercalation of plasma components which change the area of outer surface with respect to the inner one and this mismatch causes liposome breakage. It is very likely to expect that in the case of cationic surfaces this plasma-related disintegration is even faster. Upon liposome collapse DNA becomes exposed to DNases in plasma. Additionally, the possibility that DNA in uncondensed form enters into cells is small. Also, large size and possible aggregation would quickly limit free movement of these large particles, even in the absence of immediate adsorption. On the other side, in the case of small, compact complexes it is logical to expect that they have a better chance to achieve a larger volume of biodistribution. Also, DNA seems to be well protected. Smaller particles are also more susceptible for internalization, especially DNA which seems to be too large to become internalized into cells efficiently in a noncondensed form. DNA accessibility studies using ethidium bromide have shown that DNA is well protected and/or condensed because DNA could not intercalate. From the stoichiometry and sizes, it is estimated that a simple complex contains between 5 and 15 DNA plasmids.

Following these experiments and consequent thought analysis, we can state that a necessary condition for effective systemic transfection is small, dense complexes which contain condensed and well-protected DNA plasmids. There are, however, similar complexes which were shown to be ineffective after intravenous administration despite their ability to colloidally suspend high concentrations of DNA. Therefore, the sufficient condition for *in vivo* activity of the complex is, in addition to an active plasmid, stability of complex in plasma, its biodistribution, and internalization ability. With present genosomes we do not have control over the events after internalization or release from endosomes. Obviously, endosomal lysis and nuclear targeting are achieved in some cases, as we can detect from the expression of the encoded protein. With some improvements in plasmid sequences and/or novel genosome components, it may be possible that some control over these events will be gained.

In contrast to *in vitro* experiments, *in vivo* data indicate that the use of cholesterol as a neutral lipid results in significantly better transfection (Zhu et al., 1995; Bennett et al., 1995; Solodin et al., 1995; Templeton et al., 1996). While stability in plasma was shown to differ for various liposomes and genosomes, detailed biodistribution remains to be done. Also, it seems that cholesterol-containing genosomes protect DNA better as can be deduced from complement activation studies and cryo-EM micrographs (Templeton et al., 1996, 1997).

If the structure of small and dense genosomes prepared from cationic SUV are alternate lamellae of bilayer and two-dimensional arrays of ordered DNA, a solid substrate for adsorption seems to be advantageous. This, therefore, prefers cholesterol over DOPE as a bilayer alloying compound and also excludes cationic lipids with several charges which prefer to form micelles. Although stretching elastic moduli of these bilayers have not been measured yet, we can expect from similar lecithin-based systems one order of magnitude increased mechanical stability of bilayers upon replacement of half of the DO chains with cholesterol (Lasic and Needham, 1995). Analogously, cholesterol is known to increase stability of liposomes in the circulation and may have a similar function in the complex.

For still obscure reasons, complexation of DNA with other positively charged colloidal particles, such as cationic micelles, did not result in effective transfection. One of the reasons is increased toxicity of single-chain surfactants, which form micelles. It is also believed that micelles do not provide complexes with cationic surfaces which may be important for adhesion onto cells. One of the reasons may be the absence of DOPE and increased precipitation of the complexes as compared with the use of SUVs. In our hands, phase diagrams with CTAB, CTAC, and DOIC micelles yielded larger solubility gaps (lower concentrations of colloidally suspended DNA) than corresponding SUV containing neutral lipid (at 1:1). The stability of single-chain-surfactant–DNA colloidal systems upon application is much lower. Micellar systems are at thermodynamic equilibrium with the surroundings and this causes instantaneous phase changes upon introduction in biological systems. Micelles and by inference DNA–micelle complexes are less stable upon change in the environment (dilution, presence of proteins) and probably disintegrate and/or flocculate immediately after application onto the plate or injection into the bloodstream. Kinetically trapped systems, such as liposomes and lipid–DNA complexes (genosomes), can be much more robust toward changes in the system, such as dilution (Lasic, 1993a). Another reason may be long-range order of bilayers which can perhaps pack and protect DNA better than isotropic micelles, as well as provide better surfaces for adsorption onto cells. Solid bilayers can also be a better substrate for DNA adsorption, as compared with the ill-defined and ever-changing surface of a micellar aggregate. That may explain why cholesterol, which can form a much stronger bilayer in mixtures with cationic lipids than DOPE, works better *in vivo*. Again, this reasoning does not favor cationic lipids with many positive charges due to their preference for nonbilayered phases.

Other lipid systems, such as mixed micelles, hexasomes, and cubosomes, have not shown significant transfection (possibly due to difficulties in DNA encapsulation and protection and large size of the complexes) while (micro)emulsions are in general not a viable system for the entrapment and delivery of polar substances. Although hydrophobic complexes (Reimer et al., 1995; Bally, personal communication; Huang, personal communication) can be formulated into emulsions, their stability in systemic circulation is not known. In principle, however, by judicious preparation of such a double emulsion (w/o/w) the outer layer may be composed of neutral or anionic lipids. Similarly, by controlled evaporation condensed DNA coated by the bilayer can be produced. Such formulations, however, have not been presented yet. As already mentioned, another way to coat DNA with lipid is by controlled detergent depletion from the cationic lipid–DNA–detergent system. Indeed, stable complexes which were active also in the presence of plasma were prepared by dialyzing DOSPA/DOPE/DNA/octylglucoside mixture (Hofland et al., 1996).

Single-chain surfactants can make liposomes also in mixtures with cholesterol. *In vitro* results show improved transfection as compared with micellar forms (Pinnadawuge et al., 1989) while *in vivo* such systems have not been tried yet.

We have seen that small, dense, tightly packed complexes may be a necessary condition for *in vivo* activity. We are aware, however, of well-condensed and small complexes which are not active *in vivo*. Several laboratories developed ethylated DMPC (DMEPC), which can suspend high concentrations of DNA in small particles, and none of them reported transfection upon systemic administration. Similar dense aggregates were observed in the case of several different cationic liposomes. Although similar in colloidal properties, such as size distribution, turbidity, and density, they are simply not effective upon systemic application.

Physicochemical data indicate that while tightly compacted, condensed, small-sized DNA may be a necessary condition, a sufficient condition for *in vivo* transfection may be in complex stability and interactions in blood which dictate biological fate of the complex. Indeed, preliminary comparison of plasma stability of DMEPC/Chol and DOIC/Chol liposomes and cationic complexes showed that the former ones are rather stable and that it takes hours to flocculate, whereas the latter ones precipitate in plasma in minutes (Leung and Lasic, unpublished). Optical microscopy showed fast growth of "fractal-like" aggregates upon interaction with plasma. Surface charge of genosome–plasma complexes has not been reported yet. In a model system, genosomes should be complexed with albumin and their structure and activity studied. It is possible that relative (in)stability in plasma is a competitve reaction between coating (and stabilization) of genosomes (perhaps with albumin) vs. rapid self-aggregation catalyzed by plasma components.

It is very likely that such interactions determine the pharmacokinetics and biodistribution of particles. Cationic and neutral lipids, as well as other components added, may dictate interactions with cells; cell membranes induce early endosomal release upon endocytosis and improve the yield of transfection. Or, simply, pronounced instability causes partial blockage in the first capillary bed encountered and lipid-mediated poration resulting in transfection. At doses around 0.5 μM of cationic lipids such complexes are not expected to be fatal. At higher lipid doses, however, that may not be true. Doses above 1 μM/mouse (tail vein injection) are normally toxic, and larger concentrations are lethal.

Relatively high expression of marker genes in the lungs after tail vein injection in mice was predominantly reported in the literature (Brigham et al., 1989; Zhu et al., 1993; Solodin et al., 1995; Templeton et al., 1996). This, in the absence of specific receptor-mediated endocytosis, can be understood by either quick adsorption followed by endocytosis or by simple physical trapping of aggregated genosomes and transient cell wall poration induced by the adjacent cationic lipids. The lung also has the largest capillary surface area and is the first capillary bed tail vein–injected genosomes encounter. The next organ that blood flows through is the heart, and therefore it is not surprising that heart muscle has normally the second highest expression. Gene expression in the spleen and liver may reflect the classic particle uptake in these organs as well as clearing of genosome aggregates from capillaries by scavenger cells. Relatively low expression in the organs of the reticuloendothelial system may be due to reduced activity of the same plasmid in those cells and increased DNA digestion in macrophages. It seems that the stability of genosomes in plasma critically depends on the structure of cationic lipid and this may dictate the genosome pharmacokinetics and biodistribution. It is very likely that positively charged particles become immediately coated by albumin and the balance between this adsorption and (self)-aggregation/(co)-flocculation determines their fate and consequently gene expression. In any case, however, it seems that the pharmacokinetics can range from rapid clearance to an extremely rapid uptake. Therefore, the biodistribution of expression follows a first-pass model and correlates with the sequence of passage and volume (surface area of capillaries) of that organ.

The influence of cationic lipids on transfection seems to be in their ability to suspend DNA colloidally, to enhance internalization, and to protect it. High concentrations of small sized DNA particulates seem to be important for effective transfection. Different cationic lipids as well as different liposomal morphologies and solution conditions (temperature, ionic strength, concentration) can suspend DNA to different concentrations. It is not known how the liposome morphology influences interactions with DNA. One can expect that in the case of larger liposomes (MLV) larger particles will result while smaller liposomes form smaller complexes. If complete lipid restructuring occurs and complexes as shown in Figure 7-10 are needed, SUV (below 80 nm) are preferred. They are the least stable and make the smallest and most dispersed building blocks for genosomes. In the case of slightly larger (~100 nm) DOTAP/Chol liposomes, (completely invaginated liposomes, appearing as two lamellar liposomes with an orifice; Figure 7-13) unusual encapsulation of DNA was observed which could be attributed to DNA adsorption which caused liposome inversion and DNA encapsulation (Templeton et al., 1996).

Liposomes and genosomes containing different cationic lipids give rise to different phase behavior, as shown in Figure 9-3. Typically, the phase behavior for a particular cationic lipid scales with charge (i.e., invariant to the presence and nature of neutral lipid) while the difference between cationic lipids is in their ability to suspend DNA; i.e., the size of the solubility gap varies with different lipids. Some of the lipids also cannot make small liposomes, which adversely affects their plasmid solubilization power.

The influence of different cationic lipids on the activity is more difficult to explain. Practically no systematic experiments have been reported. Only with the imidazolinium-derived cationic lipid it was shown that dioleoyl chains are much more active than dimyristoyl and dipalmitoyl chains (Solodin et al., 1995). Polar head group influence is probably

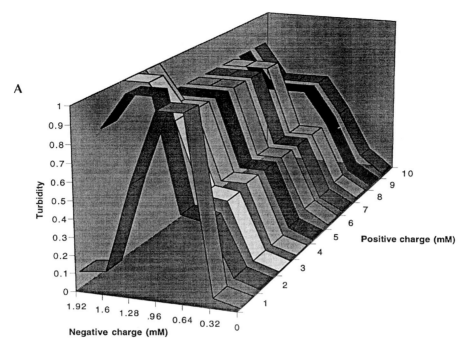

A

Turbidity

Positive charge (mM)

Negative charge (mM)

Figure 9-3 Phase behavior of DODAB/Chol (A) and DOIC/Chol (B) systems complexed to 5-kb DNA. The ability of the latter system to suspend higher concentrations of DNA can be clearly seen. The DOTAP/Chol system was even more effective.

dual — in the stability of bilayer and interactions with DNA. In addition to electrostatic interactions, specific interactions, such as hydrogen bonding, groove binding, or partial intercalation, may occur as well. Some lipids may not mix well with cholesterol and phase separation occurs which destabilizes genosome or comprises its stability and DNA protection in circulation. Some lipids with low/high values of packing parameter form less stable bilayers (P < or > 1) and upon interaction with DNA the liposomal bilayer may change in different ways.

In general, and requiring minimal toxicity, cationic lipid should form a small solubility gap in the phase diagram, form strong bilayer, and confer adequate colloidal stability.

Keeping in mind the above explanation, we can try to explain the influence of neutral lipids on transfection. *In vivo* it seems that cholesterol is a better neutral lipid. This can be due to the formation of more compact genosomes, increased stability in plasma, or forming bilayers which can better protect DNA. It is possible that stronger bilayers present a better support for DNA adhesion and the structure formed is stronger, i.e., more resistant to interactions in plasma. Although the structure of genosomes is different from the structure of liposomes, where the stabilizing effect of cholesterol in plasma is well documented, the outermost genosome

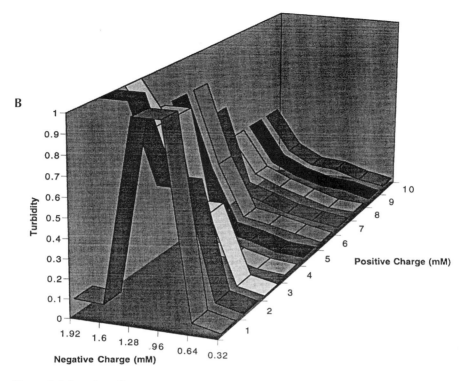

Figure 9-3 (continued)

coating may have a similar effect. Knowing the inability of cationic micelles to form stable complexes, we can now understand the need of (strong) bilayers to support the formation of stable complexes. Continuous bilayers probably present also a better surface for adsorption onto cells.

We must note, however, that these observations argue against well-established endocytotic cell entry in which the presence of DOPE is essential for an early endosomal release. Perhaps some other lipids can also interfere with endosomal membrane or may bypass endosomal entry altogether. In line with this thought, it is well known that some lipids, such as DOTAP, were shown to transfect better without DOPE.

Different lipids give rise to complexes with different transfection activities and the model shown above stresses the importance of colloidal properties on transfection *in vivo*. While subcutaneous, intramuscular, intra-articular, or intracerebral administration may resemble *in vitro* tests, it is plasma stability and pharmacokinetics with biodistribution which determine *in vivo* activity upon systemic application. Topical administrations may have a completely different mechanism of entry. Lipid should provide effective DNA condensation and protection and have appropriate stability and interaction characteristics in plasma. Lastly, the lipid must not bind DNA too strongly so that decondensation is not affected.

Formation of active complex depends more on colloidal phenomena than on the nature of cationic or anionic lipids. Changing reaction conditions, we could make from the same liposomes and DNA very different complexes. For instance, DOTAP and DOTAP/Chol liposomes at low concentrations in high-ionic-strength conditions form large complexes while at higher concentrations (at same charge ratio) and low ionic strengths they can make very compact and dense complexes with high *in vivo* transfection yields. The difference is not only in the size (and shape) of the complexes but also in the concentration of colloidally suspended DNA. While temperature does not seem to have much influence on the complex formation (at higher temperatures slightly smaller and less-turbid complexes were normally prepared) (Lasic, unpublished), reagent concentrations and ionic strength do. Salt concentration should be minimal. In addition to these thermodynamic parameters kinetic effects of reaction, as discussed in Chapter 7, must assure preparation of small particles.

In carefully conducted experiments, dose response was observed (Templeton et al., 1996). This may also explain the relative inefficiency of commerciallly available lipid kits, irrespective of the neutral lipid used. The liposomes concentration in these kits is, due to stability, economic or business reasons, simply too low to allow effective gene expression *in vivo*. Additionally, instructions often recommend the use of electrolyte solutions which results in the formation of larger complexes which are effective *in vitro* but are not expected to achieve sufficient volume of distribution at reasonable DNA levels upon systemic administration as discussed in this chapter.

■ SUMMARY

Some ideas on structure–activity relationships on the molecular and colloidal levels were presented. It was theorized that the nature of cationic lipid, in addition to variable toxicity, is related to the solubility gap in the DNA–lipid phase diagram and reactivity and interactability with plasma components. On the other hand, colloidal characteristics, such as small size (preferably below 500 nm) and effective DNA packaging and protection, seem to be a necessary condition for efficient *in vivo* performance. It was argued that large, loose, and amorphous complexes cannot well protect DNA and achieve reasonable biodistribution. A sufficient condition for effective transfection *in vivo* seems to be appropriate stability in plasma and interactability with cells.

■ ADDITIONAL READING

No reviews exist. Papers by Leventis and Silvius (1990), Farhood et al. (1992), Felgner et al. (1994), Xu and Szoka (1996), and Lasic et al. (1996) discuss some of these topics.

10 MECHANISM OF TRANSFECTION

DNA transfection and gene expression are very complex processes. To date not many studies have dealt with the mechanisms involved. Only some particular steps were studied. Early models, based on rhodamine lipid fluorescence studies which quickly spread to the cell surface, envisioned complex fusion with cell membranes (Felgner et al., 1987), while recently most researchers believe that the complex enters cells by an endocytotic pathway (Zabner et al., 1995; Farhood and Huang, 1996; Friend et al., 1996). In addition, the possibility of decondensation of DNA upon its release from the endosome by anionic lipids from the outer endosome surface was demonstrated (Xu and Szoka, 1996). Anionic (PS/PE/PC 1/2/1) liposomes were shown to rapidly release DNA complexed to DOTAP liposomes at neutral charge ratios. DNA was also released upon incubation with heparin and dextran sulfate while DNA, RNA, poly(glutamic acid), spermidine, spermine, and histones did not induce DNA release. These results suggest that DNA may become decondensed upon release from the endosomes in which the cytosol-facing membrane has similar lipid composition (Xu and Szoka, 1996). Obviously, some still unknown membrane disruption must occur in order that the two systems can interact.

Following this discussion, I would like to comment on the widely perceived opinion that DNA–cationic lipid is an irreversible reaction. It was shown, however, that the presence of high salt, as expected from Manning theory, dissociates the complex (Lasic, unpublished, 1994):

$$\text{DNA} - \text{cationic lipid} \xrightarrow{>1.3 \text{ M NaCl}} \text{DNA} + \text{cationic lipid} \qquad (10\text{-}1)$$

while Xu and Szoka (see above) have also shown reversibility via the following reaction

$$\text{DNA} - \text{cationic lipid} + \text{anionic liposome} =$$
$$\text{DNA} + \text{anionic} - \text{cationic lipid} \qquad (10\text{-}2)$$

In some experiments endosome-disrupting agents could increase gene expression indicating an endocytotic pathway. Endosomal acidification can be reduced by using chloroquine, monesin, or ammonium chloride while colchicine interferes with endosomal uptake. Brefeldin B interferes with endosomal trafficking. These agents, however, were not efficient in all the cases studied (Budker et al., 1996), and the nonpredictable increase or decrease of transfection upon their addition is still not understood.

Although it is very likely that biologically it is the same process, we shall discuss the mechanism of transfection *in vitro* and *in vivo* separately. This is due to the fact that the colloidal properties of genosomes, such as their stability in a deleterious environment, markedly differ between the two cases. We shall try to demonstrate that the two systems are uncorrelated as a result of these interactions. We shall argue that the difference is in the different phagocytic activity of cells in the culture and in the tissue, as well as genosome pharmacokinetics, biodistribution, and stability in plasma.

We shall follow a genosome with given physicochemical characteristics which determine its biological properties during the transfection process. Its stability and interaction characteristics dictate its fate in biological systems, and we shall look at interactions with cells, genosome/DNA entry into the cytoplasm, and interactions in the cytoplasm leading to the entry into the nucleus. Because we can, at present, control mostly behavior up to the DNA release in the cell cytoplasm, we shall concentrate on the first part of the transfection, i.e., transfer of plasmid from the outside of the cell into the cytoplasm. The second part of transfection, consisting of the transfer of the plasmid from cytoplasm into the nucleus, is still very obscure. It is possible that it can be better controlled by special DNA inserts than by delivery vehicles. While there is a constant efflux of nucleic acids from the cell nucleus, there are in nature only viral and spermal DNA which efficiently travel in the opposite direction. There are, however, many proteins which shuttle through the nuclear membrane, including transporters, nucleoporins, and others, which may contain nuclear localization sequences. These are regions rich in basic amino acids and can bind nucleic acids. Such complexes enter nuclei through a nuclear pore complex, a protein which regulates a pore with diameter of approximately 100 nm.

It is therefore possible that by having appropriate DNA stretches or molecular tags, proteins can carry the DNA into the nucleus. It is not known, however, what the optimal DNA conformation for nuclear entry is: in a condensed, supercoiled, or relaxed state. Direct microinjection of cationic lipid–DNA complexes into the cell nucleus resulted in low gene expression (Zabner et al., 1995), indicating that genomic DNA cannot decondense DNA and that it probably enters in a decondensed state which is also likely to shuttle into the nucleus by an active mechanism via a specific recognition mechanism. Also, large amounts of condensed DNA in the cytoplasm did not result in efficient transfection (Stegmann, personal communication). Zabner et al. (1995) reported that despite that, on average, several hundred thousand plasmids were in cells, only 50% of the cells showed transfection activity. Giorgio and colleagues (Tseng et al., 1996) have studied the incorporation of DNA–liposome complexes into murine capillary lung endothelial cells by quantitive flow cytometry. Although they used only 5 mol% cationic lipid, they showed that on average each cell contains 10,000 plasmid molecules covalently labeled by ethidium monoazide. Plasmid uptake showed a typical saturation type behavior with saturation levels reached at approximately 10 h.

■ TRANSFECTION *IN VITRO*

In vitro transfection consists of incubating a cell culture with a genosome dispersion. Interactions between genosomes and cells occur via free diffusion of complexes above the plated cells. Practically all experiments show that positively charged complexes are much more effective for gene expression. This indicates that simple electrostatic binding of the complexes onto cell membranes may improve internalization. Presence of serum, in general, deactivates complexes. This can be explained by the fact that plasma components coat and/or precipitate and therefore inactivate genosomes. There are some indications that two or more valent cationic lipids can increase transfection, possibly because of increased colloidal stability. The size of the complexes that enter into cells is not known.

The occurrence of the endocytotic pathway was inferred from the ability of pH-sensitive and DOPE-containing liposomes, as well as endosome-disrupting agents, to increase transfection. Additionally, electron and fluorescence microscopy have shown electron-dense vacuoles and bright focal spots in the cytoplasm.

Endocytotic cell entry was shown also by extensive EM studies of colloidal gold, as a marker, containing DOTMA:DOPE liposomes and genosomes (Friend et al., 1996). Similar conclusions were also observed for cationic liposomes via a lipid mixing assay (Wrobel and Collins, 1995) which showed that binding to the cell surfaces can result in fusion only after cationic liposome uptake into the endocytotic pathway. No lipid mixing occurred if endocytosis was blocked by ATP depletion or hypertonicity. No fusion was detected at 4°C where endocytosis is also inhibited, while fusion is, according to them, not. The last statement is not exactly true, because fluid bilayers are in most cases a necessary condition for fusion and no one really knows what the fluidity of these bilayers and cell membranes is at that temperature.

It is common knowledge that in *in vitro* assays gene expression increases with increasing concentration of cationic liposomes, even in the case of constant DNA concentration. Proportionally to the lipid concentration, of course, the cytotoxicity of the formulation also increases. Optimal transfection is therefore a result of a delicate balance between the toxicity of lipid and the level of expression. Obviously, toxicity depends on the nature of the cationic lipid, the cell type, and their confluence on the plate. The nature of cationic lipid can be related to its aqueous solubility (cmc), hydrophilic–hydrophobic balance, solubilizing power, affinity for membrane lipids and proteins, and biodegradability. The toxicity of cationic lipids arises mostly from the increasing of cell membrane permeability and creation of transmembrane pores. The dependence of toxicity on the cell confluence can be understood as a fraction of the cell surface exposed to the cationic lipids, i.e., the remaining reservoir of inaccessible membrane lipids which can reseal the pores by lateral diffusion. The creation of membrane pores by single chain cationic surfactants, which were used as pesticides in the 1960s, is well known (Jungerman, 1970). Other mechanisms of toxicity, such as interaction with membrane and cellular components, are also possible.

Presence of larger aggregates does not seem to interfere with the transfection process. These large particles are too big to enter into cells by endocytosis. All the above data may point to the conclusion that in addition to endocytosis another cell entry mechanism may be present. This may not be a cell membrane–genosome bilayer fusion in a classic sense but rather an irregular, "amorphous" process which I will call lipid-mediated poration of cell membrane. Cationic lipids either destabilize membrane and plasmid may become internalized or dissolve part of the membrane and create a transient hole ("burn a hole" mechanism). If there is too much, cationic lipids cells cannot reseal the damaged membrane and cell death results. High local concentrations can be present especially in the case of larger aggregates or in *in vivo* applications upon physical entrapment which will be discussed below. A similar model of translocation of DNA through pores in the membranes, facilitated by the presence of DOPE, was presented by van der Woude et al. (1995).

In conclusion, it is very difficult to determine the internalization pathway which leads to effective transfection, especially because transfection efficiencies are so low. It is also difficult to know what fraction of particles is monitored by a particular assay and if those are responsible for transfection.

■ TRANSFECTION *IN VIVO*

For gene expression *in vivo* we shall distinguish between different administration routes. Intratracheal instillation and inhalation of aerosol may resemble the *in vitro* process with the exception that some macrophages may attack the complexes. Stability and interaction characteristics of genosomes in these "semi-dry" conditions have not been studied yet. They may be important as is their interaction with surface mucus which can block their access to the surfaces of the cells. Intraperitoneal injection and injections in stationary body fluids without large number of macrophages may also be similar to the *in vitro* case.

Localized subcutaneous and intramuscular or other direct injections may resemble either the *in vitro* process or the systemic one if lymph drainage occurs. This suggests that various lipid formulations should be tested, including neutral lipids. A similar situation may also occur in tumor after direct injection, where blood may wash out a portion of genosomes. In these cases, however, some DNA may get injected directly into the cells. Especially muscle cells are very large, and poking at the site of injection may show staining of the marker gene quite far away as a result of their size. This can also explain the difference between horizontal and vertical injections in the muscle, especially in the cases of naked DNA which seems to be highly unlikely to penetrate into cells. Other mechanically induced events such as hydrodynamic or osmotic pressure-related internalization are also possible. After a thorough effort the problem was not solved, indicating the complexity (Dowry and Wolff, 1994). Here, we shall concentrate on systemic administration which is, on one side, the most complex and difficult and, on the other, offers the broadest range of applications.

In the case of similarity with the *in vitro* situation, such as administration into intracerebral fluid or intraperitoneal injection, and in contrast to systemic applications which use mostly cholesterol, DOPE can be tried as a neutral lipid to augment expression. Such data have not been published yet.

Nothing is known about the mechanism of nuclear entry of complexes. If cells divide, DNA may be entrapped during nuclear membrane dissolution and reformation during mytosis. Efficient passive targeting is unlikely, while it is not known if condensed DNA is preferable for the active input. In addition to active trafficking in the cytoplasm, the spatial and temporal localization of DNA decondensation is also still not known. While anecdotal evidence points to the fact that DNA condensation does not help in nuclear entry and targeting, there is no direct experimental evidence that DNA is decondensed in the cytoplasm. And, also, it is very unlikely that in the cytoplasm and nucleus plasmids would not be complexed to endogeneous and natural polycationic species.

In a Gedanken experiment one can think of the various steps in this process which have to occur in order that the encoded protein is expressed: genosome must flow/diffuse to the cell and adhere to its surface, transfer across the cell membrane, escape from the lysosomal degradation of DNA in the endosome after endocytosis, or enter into the cell via direct fusion with the plasma membrane or via (harmless) transient lipid-mediated poration. This must be followed by transfer from the cytoplasm into the cell nucleus, where intact decondensed DNA must be available for transcription. Currently, the integration of genes into chromosomes is undesirable because of the lack of a control on site specificity (efficacious homologous recombination may change that). Nuclear retention can be enhanced by adding specific DNA sequences which can bind plasmid electrostatically to chromatin during cell division. Further improvements include self-replicating plasmids, which divide once per cell cycle due to specific sequence and therefore do not get diluted during cell replication.

Following this model, one can speculate about how various parameters affect the transfection process. Several steps of this model were already proposed and confirmed by experiments (Felgner et al., 1994;

Farhood and Huang, 1996; Xu and Szoka, 1996). Using such a model, one can study the influence of parameters, such as the nature of cationic and neutral lipid (DNA condensation and decondensation, DNA coating and protection, endosomal release, karyophilicity); the solvent system (colloidal stability); and the physical (size, surface charge, shape), chemical (DNA stability in the milieu), and biological properties of genosomes (stability in plasma, pharmacokinetics, biodistribution) and of plasmid (nuclear targeting and retention) (Lasic, 1996) and their influence on transfection. Obviously, plasmids have to be optimized as well and their activity probed in independent *in vitro* experiments.

We shall define optimal genosomes as the ones containing well-condensed and protected DNA in a size range from 50 to 300 nm, depending on the target cells. They should be stable in the biological milieu and be able to induce endocytosis or fusion with cells. Below we shall list some important physicochemical parameters, biological factors, and other requirements in this complex process.

■ FACTORS AND STEPS THAT DETERMINE TRANSFECTION

Factors and steps that determine transfection (Lasic, 1996) can be grouped as follows:

    i.   Physicochemical properties of genosome

        Size (and shape)

        (Surface) charge

        Nature of lipid(s)

        DNA/lipid concentrations and ratio

        Presence of functional groups

        Stability: colloidal, physical, chemical

        Stability of genosome *in vitro*

        • Dictate genosome structure, topology, stability, and interaction characteristics

   ii.   Biological characteristics of genosome

        Stability of genosome *in vitro* and *in vivo*

        Physical stability (thermodynamical and colloidal)

        Chemical stability (DNA protection, lipid toxicity)

        In vivo: pharmacokinetics and biodistribution

        • Dictates pharmacokinetics, biodistribution, and safety/toxicity

iii. Genosome interaction with cells

   Adsorptivity

   Internalizability (endocytosis, fusion or lipid-mediated poration)

   (Targeting ligands, endocytotic receptors)

   • Dictates interaction with cells and cell entry

iv. Genosome entry into cytoplasm

   Endosome disruption

      (Helper polypeptides)

      pH buffering

   Cell membrane fusion, membrane dissolution/disruption

   Plasmid decondensation

   • Dictates cytoplasmic DNA concentration

v. Targeting of cell nucleus and nuclear retention

   DNA (karyotypic sequence), helper molecule, or lipid mediated

   DNA decondensation (and self-replication)

   Free diffusion or specific, cell, DNA and/or lipid-dependent, intracellular trafficking

   • Dictates nuclear localization, level and persistence of expression

This model, which is shown as a cartoon in Figure 10-1, shows that the major difference between *in vitro* and *in vivo* experiments is in the stability of genosomes in biological fluids and their pharmacokinetics and biodistribution. One should also mention large differences between cells in tissue and in the culture where simple changes in cell confluence can dramatically affect their phagocytic behavior.

It is therefore possible that by taking into account these four parameters: (1) stability in blood (PS), (2) pharmacokinetics (PK), (3) biodistribution (BD), and (4) internalization characteristics of cells in the culture, systemic *in vivo* applications can be correlated with *in vitro* results.

$$In\ vitro \xleftrightarrow[\text{phagocytic activity}]{\text{PS, PK, BD}} In\ vivo \tag{10-3}$$

We believe that with improved understanding of all these steps a second generation of genosomes will be developed. These particles may

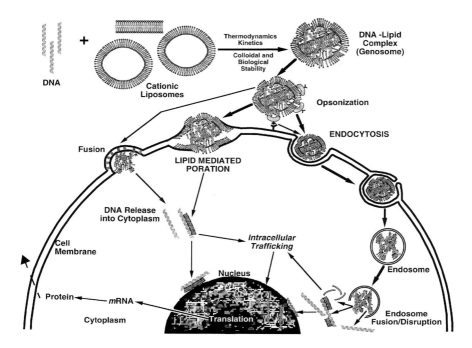

Figure 10-1 A hypothetical model of gene transfection. Three possible methods of cell entry are indicated, including creation of transient pores. (Courtesy of S. Hansen.)

carry special ligands for specific uptake as well as other condensing, fusogenic, lytic, and targeting (cell and nucleus — karyophilicity and nuclear retention) molecules or groups. These molecules may be, in complement and/or in supplement to cationic lipids, polycations, polypeptides, lipopolypeptides, positively charged polyelectrolytes, block copolymers, and so on. Additionally, DNA can also be reengineered to impose cell specificity, nuclear targeting, and duration of expression. Following such improvements, we are sure that further improvements in transfection yields will be obtained and that gene therapy with lipidic vectors will become a viable medical treatment, as gene therapy becomes a recognized therapeutic modality.

■ SUMMARY

In order for gene expression to occur, DNA plasmid has to enter the cell cytoplasm and migrate into the cell nucleus. The exact mechanism of the internalization is still not clear. Several possibilities, including endocytosis, fusion, and lipid-mediated transmembrane translocation (poration) are discussed. Further studies of these processes are needed to optimize gene delivery systems. The same is true for the entry of DNA plasmid from the cytoplasm into the cell nucleus. In addition to active trafficking de- and recomplexation of DNA with endogenous cationic material may be also important.

■ ADDITIONAL READING

This field has not been reviewed yet. Papers by Gao and Huang, 1995; Friend et al., 1995; Xu and Szoka, 1996; and chapters by Lasic, D. D.; Farhood and Huang; and Felgner et al. in Lasic, D. D. and Barenholz, Y. Eds., *Liposomes: from Gene Delivery to Diagnostics and Ecology,* CRC Press, Boca Raton, FL, 1996 review some of these aspects.

11

OTHER CARRIER SYSTEMS AND ARTIFICIAL VIRUS

In this book we have predominantly discussed cationic liposomes and their complexes with DNA as gene delivery systems. We have mentioned potential lipid toxicity and immunogenicity as well as lack of control over the properties of these complexes. The particles are so highly reactive that any kind of targeting or achieving larger volume of biodistribution is practically impossible. Throughout the book we have mentioned that the use of conventional and sterically stabilized liposomes may alleviate some of these problems and after reviewing other colloidal DNA carriers we shall discuss those possibilities in Chapter 13.

POLYELECTROLYTES

In vitro transfection protocols use several cationic polyelectrolytes, such as DEAE dextran or polybrene. While some of the levels of expression are good, to date no data on *in vivo* applications have been published. Similarly, polylysine was shown to be effective *in vitro* if sufficiently long (M_w > 20,000 Da), while systemic applications were not successful. Polyethylenimine, a polyelectrolyte with the highest charge density (+1/44 Da, compared with DOTMA +1/693 Da or DOTMA/DOPE at +1/1450 Da), was shown to effectively transfect cells *in vitro*. At a +/− charge ratio of 13.5 this polymer delivery vehicle was comparable with or better than lipopolyamines. *In vivo* transfection in embryonic neurons showed no toxicity and virtually all the neurons were labeled. Intracerebral luciferase gene expression in newborn mice was comparable with transfection of rat brain endothelial cells in culture. Results were explained by the buffering capacity of the polymer which prevents lowering of pH in the endosomes. Additionally, the swelling of the polymer can rupture endosomes. Polymer, which is highly branched, was compared with a proton sponge because each third atom can be protonated (Boussif et al., 1995).

A similar approach involves dendrimers, which are also known as star-burst or cascade polymers (Service, 1995). These are spherical polymers which originate from an ammonia core by spherical growth in layers. Polymerization attaches on each surface group 2 more monomers, and polyamidoamide spherical polymers grow in shells. For instance, a nine-layered structure has a diameter of 11.4 nm and 2048 terminal amines on the surface. Due to high surface charges these polymers can complex DNA. High transfection activity in several cell lines was reported. The optimal charge ratio was 6/1, terminal amine to phosphate, with a 6.8-nm dendrimer. The high efficiency was attributed also to pK values of amines (3.9 and 6.9) which can buffer endosome and, upon swelling, burst it. In the presence of plasma transfection decreases by a factor of two while covalent attachment of lytic peptide GALA improved transfection efficiency considerably (Hansel and Szoka, 1993).

It is possible that neither PEI nor dendrimers are effective *in vivo* as a result of the fact that the topology of these complexes prevents effective and stable coating of DNA and therefore reduces protection against blood-borne DNases to surface-adsorbed plasmid or knotted coil trapped between loose polymer branches or aggregates of spherical dendrimers. Stability of surface-adsorbed DNA against *in vitro* DNase attack may not automatically be scaled to the *in vivo* case.

■ COMBINATION COMPLEXES

Combination complexes are structures in which DNA is condensed with conjugates having both a ligand for cell attachment/endocytosis and/or an endosomolytic agent such as synthetic peptide, fusogenic protein, or adenovirus.

Many cells can be targeted *in vitro* and *in vivo* using these complexes. Obviously, in addition to specific ligand these constructs react nonspecifically with a variety of other cells and surfaces, due to reactivity of the DNA-condensing agent, mostly polylysine. Ligands asialoorosomucoid, Gal4-peptide, trigalactosylated bisacridine, and lactosylated polylysine target asialoglycoprotein receptor on hepatocytes. Transferrin and insulin ligands can target corresponding receptors in a wide range of cells. Epidermal growth factor can bind to its receptor in epithelial cells while T cells can be targeted via anti CD-X (X = 3,4,7) ligand corresponding to CD-X receptors. Others ligands include anti-thrombomodulin for lung epithelial cells, anti-Ig for B cells, and lung surfactant proteins for pulmonary cells. Ligands trigger endocytosis, and endosome-disrupting agents significantly improve transfection efficiency (Cotton and Wagner, 1993; Wagner, 1994).

Such complexes may contain influenza virus hemagglutinin HA-2 N-terminal fusogenic peptides attached to ligand–polylysine–DNA complex. The fusogenic peptide increases membrane disruption and results in substantial augmentation of gene transfer (Wagner et al., 1992). The whole viral protein is very effective in *in vitro* applications while there is a concern about its immunogenicity for *in vivo* administrations. One possible solution is to trim down all the parts which are not necessary for fusion. Indeed, when endosome-disruptive peptides (amphiphilic peptide of 20 amino acids derived from influenza hemagglutinin) were used with marker plasmid and cationic liposomes, enhanced gene transfer due to induction of membrane fusion was observed (Kamata et al., 1994).

Targetable DNA carrier systems composed of asialooromucoid ligands conjugated to poly-L-lysine (5:1 molar ratio) were also reported. After coupling to DNA, a stable complex was formed. Around a ratio of conjugate to DNA = 2, soluble complexes up to 0.5 mg/mL can be prepared if DNA is smaller than approximately 11 kb (Freese et al., 1994). Selective uptake in the liver was shown by observing 85 to 89% of the injected radioactivity (^{123}I, iodine-labeled ligand and ^{32}P-labeled DNA) in the liver. Following experiments with marker genes (Wu and Wu, 1991), uptake in hepatocytes was proved by correction of a metabolic disorder. Analbuminemic rats were injected with a conjugate containing a plasmid with a structural gene for human serum albumin. This protein was detected in blood 2 days after injection and a level above 30 µg/mL persisted for a month (Frese et al., 1994). When targeting hepatocytes one must be aware that the complex must be smaller than ~100 nm in order to be able to pass through fenestrations in liver sinusoids. Only on such complexes targeting ligands can improve delivery. While most of the approaches to target asialoglycoprotein receptor in mammalian hepatocytes use simple lipids with terminal galactose or lactose, it was shown that three-branched oligosaccharide structures show dramatic improvement in bonding over two- or one-branched constructs. For instance triantennary oligosaccharides can have affinities in the order of 1 to 2 nM while values of K_d around 10 µM characterize diantennary ligands. Single-chain oligosaccharides, such as galactose–glucose–manose have K_d = 283 µM (Lee, 1989). Hepatocyte targeting, including such ligands coupled to small liposomes, genosomes, or polylysine–DNA complexes may be important in delivering a variety of medications in the liver, including clotting factors for hemophiliacs.

Recent studies of hepatic uptake by Scherphof et al. (in preparation) also show that while the presence of various surface ligands on liposomes increases hepatocyte localization in cell culture it actually decreases their targeting *in vivo*. These ligands can also interact, albeit more weakly, with receptors on Kupffer cells, but due to geometric reasons they tend to accumulate there. Simple phosphatidylserine-containing liposomes were shown to achieve the most effective hepatocyte targeting. Certainly, lots of work remains to be done because these experiments are not easy and much of the older literature is very unreliable.

To increase cellular entry, polylysine–DNA complexes were coupled to adenovirus. Polylysine was attached to the virus via an antibody and the whole complex was reacted with DNA. The system showed high-efficiency gene transfer *in vitro* because of the presence of viral entry functions (Curiel et al., 1992). A similar approach was tried also by using cationic liposomes instead of polylysine as the DNA-complexing agent. Adeno-associated virus (AAV) was depleted of *rep* genes, which are needed for viral replication, and capsid genes, and desired DNA fragments

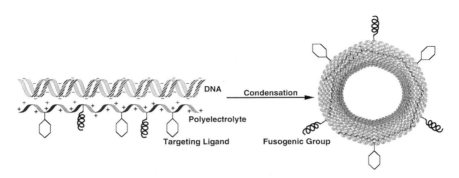

Figure 11-1   Schematic presentation of polymer complex which can have attached various ligands and can contain noncondensed or condensed DNA. (Courtesy of S. Hansen.)

were inserted. When such AAV plasmid is complexed with cationic liposomes (DODAB to DOPE), levels comparable with AAV transduction in cultured tumor cells were observed (Philip et al., 1994). In subsequent studies other cationic liposomes were used in gene therapy of human prostate cancer by delivering IL-2 gene in an AAV-based plasmid (Vieweg et al., 1995). DOSPA to DOPE (3:1) liposomes were the most effective, followed by the same liposomes at a 1:1 ratio, while DODAB to DOPE (1:2 and 1:1) and DMRIE to DOPE (1:1) had approximately tenfold lower IL-2 production. At 37 ng IL-2/24 h/10^6 cells, the expression in the case of DOSPA liposomes was higher than in the case of retroviral transduction.

Chemistry developed in the targeting of liposomes was successfully applied to targeting of lipid–DNA complexes. Asialofetuin is a glycoprotein having triantennary galactose–terminated sugar chains and is an excellent ligand for selective recognition of asilaoglycoprotein receptor of rodent and human hepatocytes. Asialofetuin-labeled liposomes (egg lecithin:trimethylammonioacetyl didodecyl D glutamate chloride to cholesterol 5:2:3) containing encapsulated marker plasmid have shown high activity of β-gal in the primary culture of rat hepatocytes (Hara et al., 1995). The effect was due to the asialoglycoprotein-mediated endocytosis and the efficiency was increased when DOPE was included in the lipid bilayer (Hara et al., 1996).

At present, not many studies are using antibodies or lectins for genosome targeting. Recently, however, a simpler system was introduced. Tumor targeting may be accomplished via receptor for vitamin folic acid, which is often overexpressed on epithelial cancer cells due to their fast growth and large consumption of this intermediate. In the case of doxorubicin delivery, it was shown that folate-labeled liposomes were taken up by KB cells in the culture 45-fold more than the nontargeted liposomes and that their cytotoxicity was 86 times higher. Furthermore, the ligand was coupled to the free end of PEG chain of the PEG–lipid which can improve performance *in vivo* as well (Lee and Low, 1995). This is a much simpler system, and, in addition, the ligand conjugate can be prepared as a crystalline powder and used as a regular lipid, which significantly simplifies liposome preparation. Furthermore, it is very likely that incubation of conventional liposomes with micelles of this reagent can effectively incorporate this lipid into bilayers upon 10 min incubation at 50°C (Uster et al., 1996). In general, sterically stabilized cationic liposomes (^{2000}PEG-DSPE/cationic lipid/neutral lipid = 5–10/50/40–45, mol) do not react with DNA plasmids (Lasic, unpublished) and such "post-stabilization" may be an elegant way to increase the stability of sterically stabilized genosomes. Such liposomes were already tried in the delivery of antisense molecules (Chapter 12), while a variation will be described below.

On several occasions we have mentioned that the use of co-condensing agents to reduce the size of DNA as well as coating of cationic genosomes with anionic lipids may improve gene transfection. Indeed, first results were recently published. Poly(L-lysine) dramatically reduced the size of DNA and upon complexation with cationic liposomes resulted in the complex which protected DNA against nuclease activity. The most active complexes, as measured *in vitro* in CHO cells, were prepared from 40 nM of lipid (DC-Chol to DOPE liposomes), 500 ng of polylysine, and 1 μg of DNA. In the electron microscope they appeared as electron-dense, small (<100 nm) particles, and on some particles a membrane coat could be observed (Gao and Huang, 1995).

A further development was coating of complexed DNA with pH-sensitive, ligand-containing bilayers. Polylysine and DNA were mixed at 0.75:1 w/w and the resulting complex entrapped in anionic liposomes containing a DOPE–cholesterol hemisuccinate (6:4) bilayer which also contained 1% of folate–PEG–lipid conjugate. Coating was a consequence of charge interaction. Transfection of marker genes depended on the overall charge of the complex. For cationic complexes it was independent of the targeting ligand and pH-sensitive bilayer, while for anionic ratios it depended on the ligand and the presence of free folic acid and DOPE. The activity was approximately 30-fold higher for complexes with a lipid:DNA ratio between 10 and 12 than in the case of cationic liposomes (Lee and Huang, 1996). The size of the complexes, as determined by negative stain EM, was around 75 nm.

Serum-mediated inhibition of gene transfer was bypassed by the use of oil-in-water emulsions containing cationic lipid (DC-Chol), DOPE, castor oil, and various detergents, such as Tween 80, Brij, or Pluronics. After formation of emulsions by homogenization of appropriate mixtures (typical ratio cationic lipid to DOPE to oil to detergent = 3:1:1:0.5 w/w) emulsion was incubated with DNA for 1 hour and applied to the cell culture. Expression of luciferase gene in the presence of 20% plasma was typically higher then expression in the absence of plasma in F_0 (murine melanoma), CHO, and human embryonic kidney cells 293 (Liu et al., 1996). Structurally, it seems that DNA is adsorbed on the surface of these particles. On one side, it is possible, that the presence of polymeric head group of detergents (Tween 80 contains 20 poly(ethylene oxide) groups in its polar head) may prevent interaction of these particles with plasmid macromolecules, while on the other it does not prevent adsorption onto the cells.

Another approach is to mimic natural colloidal systems. Erythrocyte ghosts are a well-known system which can entrap very large molecules. Another mimetic system is engineered chylomicron particles which can effectively deliver its cargo to hepatocytes because of glycoproteins with exposed galactose residues which bind to abundant asialoglycoprotein receptors on mammalian hepatic parenchymal cells (Rensen et al., 1995).

In this chapter some novel developments have been presented. It is very likely that the whole field of cationic gene delivery will follow some of these improvements. Most of the data were, however, obtained in *in vitro* tests and more work will be needed before a really effective nonviral gene delivery system is designed. Ultimately, most researchers are trying to assemble an artificial virus in which condensed DNA would be encapsulated, possibly with the addition of endosome-disrupting agents. On the envelope, consisting probably of a noncationic lipid bilayer, various functional groups would be inserted, including targeting and fusogenic entities. Figure 11-2 shows a schematic presentation of such an artificial virus. While, at present, this is still more of a futuristic design than a reality, some of these components are already being tried and in due time undoubtedly some successful *in vivo* applications will result.

■ SUMMARY

Several other systems that can complex DNA into a soluble complex were presented. They can be decorated with a variety of surface ligands and functional groups.

Despite that, the transfection activity of present lipid– and polymer–DNA complexes is still too low for any reasonable application. In this chapter we have shown some other approaches and it is hoped that synergistic overlap of such designs, in addition to potentiated DNA plasmids, will eventually lead to effective, safe, and long-lasting gene expression systems which will benefit humanity. One has to be cautious, however, because even if particular steps can operate, this does not necessarily mean that the assembly of several such steps will work as planned.

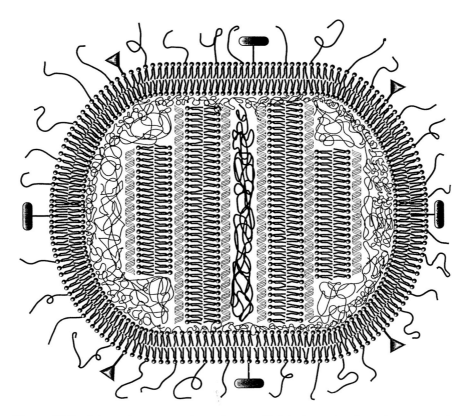

Figure 11-2 Schematic presentation of an artificial virus. Condensed DNA (with cationic lipid, polycation, or polyelectrolyte) is encapsulated in anionic/neutral bilayers with several functions (targeting, fusion) attached to the surface. Endosome-disrupting peptides or polymers can be also encapsulated. Furthermore, steric stabilizing polymer can have preprogrammed release (cleavage) rate to render particles after some time interactive with cells. (Courtesy of S. Hansen.)

■ ADDITIONAL READING

Cotten, M., Wagner, E., Non-viral approaches to gene therapy, *Curr. Op. Biotechnol.,* 4, 705–710, 1993.

Hassan, N., Wu, G. Y., Getting to the core of the matter, *Nature Med.,* 1, 210–211, 1995.

Russell, S. J., Peptide-displaying phages for targeted gene delivery, *Nature Med.,* 2, 276–277, 1996.

Wu, G. Y., Wu, C. H., Delivery system for gene therapy, *Biotherapy,* 3, 87–95, 1991.

12

LIPOSOMES IN THE DELIVERY OF ANTISENSE OLIGONUCLEOTIDES

Delivery of informational molecules encompasses DNA and short single-strand oligonucleotides and to a smaller extent also RNA and ribozymes. In this chapter we shall discuss some aspects of antisense and ribozyme technologies and will briefly mention the delivery of proteins by cationic liposomes.

■ INTRODUCTION

In contrast to DNA therapeutics which turn genes on, some technologies can stop the expression of particular genes. Protein synthesis requires transcription from DNA into mRNA and its translation into a protein. Therefore, expression of a selective gene can be halted on three levels: one can stop transcription by interfering with DNA readout (the so-called triplex strategy), another can impede translation (antisense strategy), or the third can inactivate the synthesized protein with antibodies or some drugs. The so-called aptamer strategy describes inactivation of proteins which bind to DNA and catalyze gene expression by oligonucleotides (Cohen and Hogan, 1994). These possibilities are illustrated in Figure 12-1.

DNA + enzymes -----> mRNA -----> protein
   ↑   ↑   ↑   ↑
triplex aptamer   antisense   antibodies

Figure 12-1 Several ways to stop protein synthesis and cell or viral growth. Factors which can interfere with particular steps

Selective inhibition of transcription and translation can be achieved by binding of appropriate single-strand nucleotides to specific regions of the DNA or mRNA. The former seems to be advantageous because it represents the very first step in protein synthesis. However, as we shall see below, the specificity and affinity for DNA binding is much lower than for mRNA, and to date most of the results are reported for inhibition of translation. Triplex approaches will be briefly mentioned at the end of the chapter.

Antisense oligonucleotides are single-strand DNA molecules typically from 15 to 30 bp long. Because they are chemically rather unstable several chemical modifications were performed, without significantly changing their affinity and specificity for a particular sequence stretch of mRNA (Helene and Toulme, 1990).

There are several diseases that can be treated by controlling viral or cellular genes at various levels. The prime candidates are viral and genetic diseases, for which no effective therapy yet exists, as well as several types of cancer and cardiovascular disorders. Viral or cell growth can be halted by interfering with the replication or with consequent cell proliferation (Wagner, 1994).

Cancer is characterized by an abnormal cell growth. While normal drugs exploit the differences in metabolic processes or try to intervene with DNA randomly and irrespective of the cell phenotype, genetic drugs exploit the differences in genetic properties. Tumors take advantage of either downregulation of some genes or upregulation of others, and the strategies described in this chapter will deal with specific turn off of some of the genes. For instance, aberrant gene expression can result in cell proliferation and by turning off the oncogene the abnormal growth can be stopped. Sequence-specific inhibition of the expression of the activated oncogene can be a truly tumor-specific chemotherapy. The therapy has many possibilities: it can include genes directly involved in the growth, such as proliferation-associated proteins (p120, myc, abl), or genes which are involved indirectly, such as genes responsible for changes in cell adhesion properties, including integrins and CAM (cell adhesion molecules) or genes responsible for conferring drug resistance to cells (MDR genes). The blockage of angiogenesis is another strategy.

Using these terms we can define the sense approach, where single- or double-strand sequences compete for RNA and DNA binding proteins, and the antigene approach, in which a single-strand sequence binds onto DNA forming a triple helix.

Viral proliferation can be stopped by interfering with DNA replication or expression of viral proteins. Examples include HIV, Rous sarcoma, and vesicular stomatitis virus. Restenosis is abnormal growth of vascular smooth muscle cells and accumulation of extracellular matrix (collagen) after balloon angioplasty which occurs in 30 to 50% of patients. Various kinases seem to be the key molecules for proliferation, and experiments are underway to stop this growth by using antisense molecules.

■ ANTISENSE OLIGONUCLEOTIDES: STRUCTURE AND MECHANISM OF ACTION

Oligonucleotides are oligomers in which a linear sequence of alternate sugar (normally deoxyribose) and phosphate groups forms a backbone onto which bases are attached as side groups on C1. The sequence determines the binding properties.

Antisense oligonucleotides form hydrogen bonds with specific, complementary mRNA sequences. For sufficient affinity and specificity at least 15 bases are normally required, while molecules longer than 30 units are difficult to enter the cells, less stable, more difficult to synthesize, but mostly have too slow reaction/binding kinetics and easier to tolerate some mismatches and bind nonspecifically. Affinity constants for binding can reach up to 10^{30} (compared with a typical affinity of drugs for receptors of the order of 10^8) in optimal conditions in the test tube. In physiological conditions they can be much lower and a single mismatch can reduce this constant on the order of 10^3. Specificity is normally measured by measuring the temperature of double-strand denaturation (T_m). The temperature dependence of the absorbance allows the calculation of binding energies which can drop from the range of around −10 to −13 kcal/mol to −9 to −10 kcal/mol upon a single mismatch in the sequence (Crooke, 1992). Obviously, higher values of T_m are necessary for stable binding at 37°C.

In antisense therapy there are predominantly two major problems: quick chemical degradation due to backbone instability and efficient delivery of these molecules into the cells. To reduce the degradation by nucleases inside and outside of the cells the biodegradable phosphodiester linkage is modified. As shown in Figure 12-2 the phosphodiester group ($-O_3PO-$), which spans C3 and C5 carbon atoms on ribose molecules, can be changed into phosphorothioate ($-O_3PS-$), methylphosphonate ($-O_3PCH_3-$), phosphoroamidate ($-O_3PN-$alkyl), and some others. This substitution enhances the resistance of the oligomers to nucleases from minutes to hours and days with tolerable affinity. In fact, affinity of phosphorothioates to RNA and the ability to block the expression of SV40 lathe T antigene increased significantly when the propynepyrimidine group was linked to the C5 position on the base. Similarly, the c-ras protein expression was blocked more efficiently if sugars were modified by 2′-O-methyl or 2′-O-fluoro groups.

In general, however, the chemical modifications of the backbone decrease affinity and specificity. While in some cases these molecules were shown to be toxic, the majority of studies show that toxic levels exceed therapeutic ones. Chemical modifications aimed at improved affinity and specificity have been performed also on the sugar group. Additions on the C2′ carbon in the (deoxy)ribose ring were tried in order to improve the membrane permeability of the molecule. Some modifications also involve capping the 5′ or 3′ end and some others.

There is not much data on *in vitro* and *in vivo* performance of these analogues, and we shall concentrate mostly on phosphorothioates. In general, however, the mechanisms discussed below can be applied to various analogues with a possible exception of methylphosphonates which can be sparsely soluble in water.

These modifications, however, while greatly reducing the degradation rate, did not significantly improve molecular permeability into cells, which represents the major problem in the applications. In order to be active, antisense molecules must be in the cytoplasm or, preferentially, in the nucleus. It was found, however, that oligonucleotides injected into the cell cytoplasm accumulate relatively quickly in the nucleus and the

A

Figure 12-2 Chemical formulae of oligonucleotides and their analogues. Oligonucleotide analogues modified in the backbone are being used for therapeutics. (A) Phosphorothioate, phosphorodithioate, and the neutral methylphosphonate forms of the phosphorus in the backbone of DNA. (B) Stable mixed deoxyribose backbone analogues composed of a chiral methylphosphonate linkage alternating with either a phosphodiester (DE) or a phosphorothioate (PS) linkage. The resulting oligonucleotide has reduced or eliminated sulfur along with a lower charge density by a factor of two providing greatly reduced nonspecific interactions but is not able to activate RNase H cleavage of RNA–oligonucleotide hybridized structures. (C) Stable mixed backbone analogues as in B but with 2′-methoxy on the ribose for situations requiring increased hybridization and stability. (D) Comparison of oligonucleotide constructions showing the change in charge density: A′ and all phosphorothioate oligonucleotide with charges at each linkage between bases, B′ a phosphorothioate core with blocks of alternating neutral methylphosphonate and phosphorus diester or phosphorothioate linkages at either end providing RNase H activity and reduced nonspecific binding, and C′ only alternating neutral and charged linkage which requires 2′-methoxy for sufficiently strong hybridization that steric blocking of the RNA function is effective. (Courtesy of M. Woodle, Genta, Inc., San Diego, CA.)

problem can be reduced to effective delivery of these molecules in an active form into the cytoplasm (Chin et al., 1990).

Therefore, it is believed that antisense technology will become a feasible reality only if efficient delivery systems are found. In some cases sustained release devices, such as osmotic pumps and, potentially, biopolymer- or lipid-based particulate systems, may improve the activity of oligonucleotides but the major issue is the effective intracellular

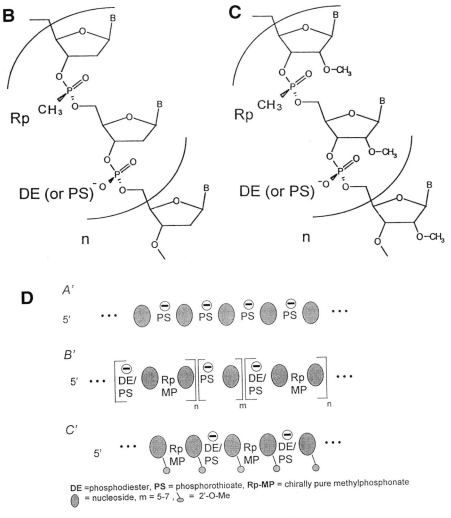

DE = phosphodiester, PS = phosphorothioate, Rp-MP = chirally pure methylphosphonate
= nucleoside, m = 5-7 , = 2'-O-Me

Figure 12-2 (continued)

delivery of these agents. As we have seen in this book, there are not many systems which can enhance intracellular penetration of small molecules safely *in vivo*. Between micro- and nanospheres, various polymeric constructs and emulsion systems, liposomes seem to be the most promising delivery system, and the majority of the researchers have concentrated on various types of liposomes to enhance intracellular accumulation of these oligomers. In addition, liposome encapsulation greatly increases stability of antisense molecules in the extracellular fluids.

Studies with pure compounds have shown that they are taken into cells by endocytosis and were mostly degraded in lysosomes. This prompts the use of pH-sensitive liposomes or immunoliposomes and perhaps fusogenic liposomes. In these systems, however, the encapsulation may be a problem. On the other side, cationic liposomes qualitatively complex these oppositely charged oligomers and offer a very different alternative. Perhaps, the properties of both systems can be combined by encapsulating colloidally concentrated oligomers into normal liposomes. We shall discuss some of these possibilities below.

The main problem remains effective delivery of these molecules in the cell and cell nucleus. Although at the beginning scientists were surprised at the level of cellular internalization, it was shown using fluorescently labeled oligonucleotides that they accumulate in dense granular compartments. This, coupled with their inactivity, indicates endocytosis and the possibility of subsequent degradation in lysosomes. It was reported that in contrast to phosphodiesters and phosphorothioates, the cellular uptake of neutral methylphosphonate oligonucleotides seems to be fluid phase endocytosis rather than passive diffusion (Bennet et al., 1993). When fluorescent oligonucleotides are microinjected into the cell, the fluorescence analysis shows accumulation in the nucleus, with neutral molecules showing somehow different intranuclear distribution. In the case of cationic liposome-mediated cellular entry, in addition to the focal points a diffuse fluorescence in the cytoplasm, followed by nuclear localization, was also observed in 90% of the cells. This indicates that endocytosis is supplemented with a process which gives rise to direct cytoplasmic delivery. Significant differences between cell types and even confluence in a particular well is more in line with the transient lipid-mediated poration than with fusion. The presence of DOTMA–DOPE liposomes increases nuclear localization and could be inhibited by incubation of cells at 4°C and by ionophore monensin while chloroquine or ammonium chloride, agents which interfere with pH in lysosomes and cause disruption of the endocytotic pathway, did not influence the nuclear accumulation (Bennet et al., 1993).

■■ LIPOSOMES FOR THE DELIVERY OF ANTISENSE OLIGONUCLEOTIDES

Liposome structure and surface properties determine several different ways liposomes can interact with oligonucleotides. Oligonucleotides can be encapsulated in the liposome interior, bound onto the liposome surface, and in the case of cationic liposomes they can form an electrostatic complex. Hydrophobic oligonucleotides can be embedded into bilayer. For encapsulation negatively charged and neutral liposomes can be used. Biodistribution can be influenced by addition of targeting ligands and polymer coating.

As we have discussed above, liposome encapsulation of oligomers can improve their passage through the cell membrane as well as protect them in the extracellular milieu. The problem with normal liposomes is that they, along with their contents, become degraded in the endosome after its fusion with the lysosomes. The possible solution is pH-sensitive liposomes which fuse with endosomal membrane upon endocytosis upon lowering of the pH and release the endosomal content into the cytoplasm.

The main problem is the effective encapsulation of these relatively large molecules (molecular weight between 5 and 6 kDa) into liposomes. Mainly, two strategies can be employed. One can work at very high lipid concentrations in which liposomes, if properly formed, encapsulate most of the aqueous phase. The problem with this approach is that often a large contamination with large multilamellar liposomes significantly reduces the fraction of internal aqueous compartments as well as causes heterogeneous vesicle formulations. Another problem is that oligonucleotides are added to preformed lipid film and are therefore not well distributed with respect to the internal/external space of the lipid: in the ideal case of tightly deposited lipid film, without any cracks and pores, no molecules that cannot penetrate hydrating lipid bilayers can become encapsulated. This means that bilayers swell on the internal side only by permeating water molecules, and after the budding and closure no other molecules can become encapsulated. Due to many crystal defects this is not the case, but still the fraction of molecules dissolved in the outer phase largely exceeds the inner one, typically a few times the volume ratio of the phases. This ratio can be increased by freeze-thawing or freeze-drying and rehydration during which bilayers open and close and in the process the asymmetry of the distribution is reduced. Also, if one starts with better dispersed lipid — in the form of SUV — the mixing and asymmetry dissipation can be better. Freezing, however, disrupts liposome structure and large lipid aggregates can be formed. If cryoprotectants are added, however, no structural changes occur and mixing is not effective. In this case one would mix oligomers with preformed SUV and freeze them. After several freeze-drying and rehydration cycles they would be reconstituted with a minimal amount of aqueous phase (creating 5 to 25% lipid dispersion) which would be sized down by an appropriate method, as discussed in Chapter 6. By working at 150 to 100 mM lipid (and preferably high drug concentrations) typically 10 to 40% encapsulation efficiency can be achieved (and oligonucleotide concentration of several milligrams per milliliter).

In reverse phase methods the sequence of steps in the liposome preparation procedure forces asymmetric distribution of dissolved substances in the primary medium. Briefly, in the beginning water-soluble substances are in the core of emulsion droplets in the excess organic solvent. Upon removal of the organic phase, these aqueous droplets become entrapped in a gel structure which upon dilution with water phase disperses into liposomes which largely retain its inner solution. If done properly as much as 70% of the hydrophilic molecules can be retained in the liposome interior. Other demusification methods are used for liposome preparation and even higher encapsulation efficiencies can be achieved (Lasic, 1993).

As the literature can testify, scientists are aware of these problems and use minimum volume or reverse phase methods which can be, I believe, further improved by treatments as discussed above. Some of their approaches will be discussed in the next section.

Some of the chemically modified oligonucleotides are neutral and can bind to the liposome surface via hydrophobic forces. In general, however, such a state of association is not very stable and it is unlikely that these molecules would remain with liposomes after parenteral delivery *in vivo*. *In vitro,* where dilution may not be too large upon application to the cell culture, a part (n) of originally associated molecules (N) may remain on the surface, accordingly to the distribution coefficient and the ratios of volumes

$$n = NKv/V$$

where K is distribution coefficient free/vesicle-bound oligonucleotide and v and V are volumes before and after dilution. In order to assess this dilution-induced release, assays should be performed, as discussed in Chapter 6.

Yet another possibility is electrostatic binding of these negatively charged molecules onto cationic liposomes. Oligonucleotides are not long enough to condense into small particles such as DNA. Therefore, they adsorb onto liposomes and eventually cause their aggregation and fusion. Often this results in very large liposome and/or lamellar precipitates, especially at $\rho = 1$.

Typically, very similar phase diagrams (as in the case of DNA) are observed. When complexing small vesicles with antisense oligonucleotides in the anionic regime, large oligolamellar vesicles were observed, while in the cationic regime oval vesicles were observed. Such a change is expected because upon adsorption the outer surface area changes causing mismatch with respect to the inner monolayer and forcing shape change. Negative stain EM showed some bilayered stacks, but it is not known if they are artifacts of the drying procedure during sample preparation. With the exception of a very weak reflection at 1.9 nm, SAXS did not show any reflection consistent with those stacks. Upon partial drying, however, a weak and diffuse reflection at 5.4 nm was observed (Lasic, Frederik, Podgornik, unpublished).

■ OVERVIEW OF SOME OF THE RESULTS

While chemically modified oligonucleotides showed sufficient stability and binding affinities, the major problem is efficient delivery of these molecules into cell cytoplasm and nucleus where they should inactivate mRNA or pre-mRNA molecules. For *in vivo* applications the particulate drug carriers seem to be the optimal choice and among them liposomes seem to be the most promising. They are widely used delivery systems and applications range from classic encapsulation of oligonucleotides into anionic, neutral, and pH-sensitive liposomes to their complexation with cationic liposomes.

Use of Anionic/Neutral Liposomes for Delivery

The first applications of antisense oligonucleotides made use of bathing cell cultures with free molecules. In light of the large size and high charge (typically from 4000 to 8000 Da and 12 to 30 negative charges) of these molecules and the low permeability of lipid bilayers (Akhtar and Juliano, 1992), it was surprising that some activity was observed at all.

Following the above-mentioned studies of liposome permeability for the encapsulated oligomers, it became apparent that other internalization mechanisms must be at play. Because fusion is a rare phenomenon and because liposomes are known to enter cells via endocytosis, it was a logical next step to encapsulate antisense molecules into liposomes. With the knowledge of the lysosomal degradation of a typical liposome cargo, pH-sensitive liposomes, which can bypass this process, were tried. To target specific cells, antibody-bearing liposomes were also used. Most of the receptors are endocytotic, and therefore the binding of antibody results in the internalization of liposomes, most often via the endocytotic pathway.

In one of the first studies, it was shown that antibody-targeted liposomes containing oligodeoxyribonucleotides complementary to viral RNA selectively inhibit viral replication. While phosphodiester oligonucleotides were inactive, when applied free at a concentration of 50 µM, in the liposome entrapped form, they inhibited viral proliferation at 100-fold lower concentration in a sequence-specific manner. Phosphorothioates inhibited the replication in free and liposome-encapsulated form without sequence specificity in acutely HIV-infected cells while in chronically infected cells the activity was sequence specific. Encapsulation into targeted liposomes increased the efficiency at least 60-fold relative to the same oligonucleotide free in solution. This indicates that the uptake by cell-mediated endocytosis was efficient (Leonetti et al., 1990).

Effective intracellular transport of oligomers encapsulated in negatively charged liposomes (sonicated Cardiolipin to PC to Chol = 1:20:14) was reported. Oligos were encapsulated at high concentration of 60 to 70 µg/mg of lipid using the minimal volume entrapment method. The method consists of adding a small volume of 10 mg/mL oligo solution to dry lipid film, to form at first a 25 wt% lipid suspension. After incubation overnight it was diluted 1:1 with the same solution and the mixture was vigorously vortexed and diluted with aqueous buffer 1:1. After 2 h of swelling this, now 6.25%, suspension was sonicated for 3 min. Nonencapsulated oligos were removed by centrifugation (Thierry and Dritschillo, 1992). After the concept had been tested in leukemia MOLT-3 cells, this delivery system was tried in order to inhibit P-glycoprotein synthesis and reverse multidrug resistance in human tumor cell lines. It was found that liposomal antisense molecules were more effective at reducing doxorubicin resistance than free molecules, both at 5 µM, and that P-glycoprotein synthesis was reduced approximately tenfold when the liposomal preparation was used. As a control, sense oligonucleotide did not have any effect in either form (Thierry et al., 1993).

Inhibition of Friend retrovirus by liposome-encapsulated oligonucle-otides was shown for pH-sensitive liposomes which can protect their cargo against lysosomal degradation. DOPE to oleic acid to cholesterol (5:2.5:1) and control (PC instead of PE) were prepared by the reverse phase evaporation method. The size was around 170 nm, encapsulation was 10%, and final oligo concentration was 12 μM in 18 μM liposomes. The inhibition of the spreading of viral infection was observed, approx-imately twofold better in the case of pH liposomes. It was found that retroviral infection stimulates liposome internalization while in nonin-fected cells liposomes were simply adsorbed onto the cell surface (Ropert et al., 1993).

Some modified analogues exhibit poor aqueous solubility and can be encapsulated into the lipid bilayer. Although the mechanism of action of such complexes as well as the activity of nonsoluble oligos is not understood, it was shown that chronic myelogenous leukemia can be inhibited by blocking the p210[bcr-abl] protein which promotes selective expansion of mature progenitor cells. Hydrophobic drugs to be encap-sulated are normally mixed with lipids in organic phase; in this study they were dissolved in DMSO and mixed with a butanol solution of lipids. After freezing and lyophilization, dry cake was hydrated and sonicated twice for 10 min. Unincorporated oligos were removed by 10% Ficoll centrifugation. Liposomal oligonucleotide (targeted to the *bcr-abl* mRNA) achieved 50% growth inhibition at oligonucleotide concentration of 1 μM. The effect was selective because control cells as well as control oligos did not show this inhibition (Tari et al., 1994).

Constant improvements in the design of conventional liposomes were also used to deliver antisense molecules to KB cells which express epidermal growth factor receptors. The idea is to suppress the expression of this receptor and halt the cell proliferation. In this study not only ligand-bearing liposomes, to enhance specific interaction, but also poly-ethylene-coated liposomes to reduce nonspecific interactions, were used. Furthermore, to optimize binding folate ligand was conjugated to the far end of the polymer. Folate–PEG–DSPE (0.5 mol%) was included in the EPC/Chol (3/2) liposomes. To achieve high encapsulation (30 to 40%) a very high lipid concentration was used (~14%) and 2 mg/mL solution of oligonucleotides. Approximately eightfold improvement of cellular uptake over nonligand-bearing liposomes was observed and the presence of free folate inhibited this specific uptake. A significant inhibitory effect was observed for this system as compared with the controls (Wang et al., 1995).

These studies indicate that various liposome technologies are quickly penetrating this field and we can expect more favorable results. On the other side, however, we must be aware that there are numerous nonspe-cific effects and in many cases seemingly expected results are artifacts of as yet not understood phenomena. Some of those, including nonspecific effects, oligonucleotide and lipid (degradation products) toxicity, and others, will be mentioned before we conclude this chapter. One must be also aware that cells in culture can exhibit specific effects differing from well to well, not to mention from day to day or laboratory to laboratory.

Recent applications of sterically stabilized liposomes were followed also in encapsulation of these molecules. Encapsulation of oligonucleotides in sterically stabilized liposomes resulted in 20-fold increased localization of labeled oligonucleotides in colon C-26 tumors. Blood circulation half-lives increased from 1 h for a free phosphorothioate molecule to 12 and 20 h when encapsulated into fluid and solid liposomes, respectively. As a consequence of long circulation times such liposomes can accumulate in tumors which are characterized by porous blood vessels and malfunctioning lymph drainage (convection process), as can be seen in Figure 12-3B.

Therapeutic studies of antisense sequence to focal adhesion kinase in human tumor lines in nude mice are under investigation (Huang et al., 1996). When 150 mM lipid and 100 mg/mL oligonucleotide solution were used, 10% of molecules were encapsulated. Different sterically stabilized liposomes were tried in order to encapsulate or bind to a partially cationic surface. Targeted liposomes containing Fab′ fragments attached to the far end of the PEG chain were also used. Physicochemical characteristics of complexes and their biological stability and interactability were also followed (Meyer et al. 1996).

Use of Cationic Liposomes in Oligonucleotide Delivery

Despite the fact that this is an ideal area for the studies of physicochemical characteristics, such as binding characteristics, Langmuir isotherm adsorption, Scatchard analyses, lipid aggregation, and lipid fusion and that it is of utmost importance for the understanding of oligonucleotide interactions, not many studies have been performed.

Phase diagram studies, as introduced in DNA–liposome complexing, yielded very similar pattern in the DOIC/Chol–18-mer system (Lasic, unpublished). Mixing cationic liposomes with negatively charged oligonucleotides results in their adsorption onto the liposome surface. Increasing amounts cause liposome aggregation, possibly followed by fusion and precipitation. Often, but not always, complexes with lamellar symmetry can result. A similar sequence was indeed observed by cryo-EM. Lower negative/positive charge ratios (ρ) caused change of liposome shape (at $\rho < 0.4$) into oval, while at high ratios ($\rho > 1.5$) fusion was observed and large and giant uni- and oligolamellar liposomes were observed, typically around 1 to 5 μm. At intermediate ratios precipitation can occur for lipid concentrations above 1 mM. These precipitates resemble aggregated multilamellar vesicles and are therefore characterized by lamellar symmetry. The interaction is electrostatic and ionic strength dependent. At close separation, however, when negatively charged oligonucleotides can bridge vesicles, van der Waals interaction probably dominates (Lasic, Leung, Woodle, Frederik, unpublished). Shape changes upon adsorption are a common observation in liposome systems. If

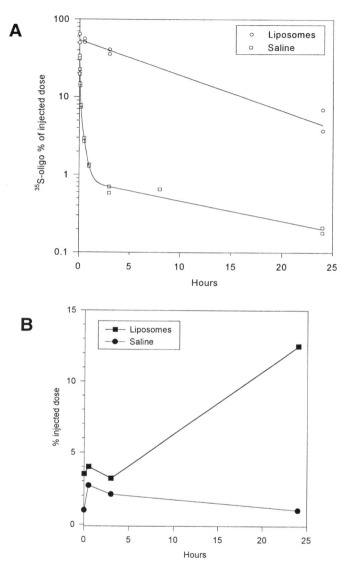

Figure 12-3 Encapsulation of oligonucleotides in sterically stabilized liposomes. (A) Blood levels of free and encapsulated oligonucleotide following intravenous administration to mice of a phosphorothioate oligonucleotide as a free aqueous solution and when encapsulated in sterically stabilized liposomes. The blood levels were determined by radioactivity from 35S-labeled oligonucleotide with two animals per time point. (B) Accumulation in the tumor of the two preparations. Tumor levels were determined from the same samples, animals, and methods as in part A. The tumor is murine B-16 melanoma. (Courtesy of M. Woodle.)

adsorption increases the area of the outer monolayer, larger and larger deviations of sphericity are observed, while strong interaction can reduce the area and lead to negative curvature and invaginations. When the mismatch of the two leaflets reaches around 3 to 5%, the membrane breaks and lipids restructure, normally resulting in fusion.

Titration of DOTAP and DODAB/DOPE liposomes with antisense oligonucleotides showed that the largest size of the formed complex occurred at $\rho = 1$. The destabilizing effect of these complexes on neutral and negatively charged liposomes was used to follow their interaction with lipid bilayers and model interactions with cells. The fluorescent marker calcein was released significantly only from negatively charged or DOPE-containing liposomes, but not from the neutral ones and only for ρ values below 1. The study of the fusion kinetics revealed that second-order reaction of aggregation rate limits fusion, which is a first-order reaction. This indicates concentration dependence and therefore employs kinetic effects. In other words, adding excess oligonucleotides to liposomes may form a stable suspension of negatively charged particles, if done at low concentration, and precipitation, if performed at higher. In general, however, these are complex and heterogeneous systems and often a formation of clusters occurs which makes any theoretical analysis extremely complex. These are the only two studies addressing the interaction between the two systems (Jaasklainen et al., 1994).

Some more information exists in the area of interaction of such complexes with cells and measurements of biological end points. The first study showed up to 1000-fold increased potency of an antisense nucleotide that hybridized the AUG translation initiation codon of human intercellular adhesion molecules (ICAM-1). Qualitative measurements of phosphorothioate oligonucleotide association with cells showed that in the presence of 8 µM DOTMA liposomes, 6- to 15-fold more oligonucleotides in the concentration range from 0.01 to 5 µM associated with cells. Intracellular distribution was assessed by fluorescently labeled oligonucleotide. In the absence of DOTMA, the oligonucleotide was localized mostly in discrete structures in the cytoplasm of the cell, showing a punctuate fluorescence pattern. In the presence of DOTMA–DOPE liposomes the pattern was different; in addition to cytoplasmic foci, the cell nucleus was found to harbor the labeled molecules. In an *in vitro* test the antisense molecule activity was measured. While free molecules added to cell culture in the concentration range 0.01 to 100 µM did not reduce the expression of ICAM-1, addition of 8 µM liposomes practically completely inhibited expression for antisense concentrations above 0.1 µM. It was concluded that cationic liposomes not only enhance the uptake of antisense molecules into the cell, but also markedly alter their subcellular distribution. Agents that interfere with endocytosis, such as chloroquine or ammonium chloride which increase lysosomal pH, did not affect the transfection indicating that part of the molecules could bypass the endocytotic pathway of cell entry. On the other hand, however, a sodium ionophore monensin almost completely eliminated the nuclear uptake of antisense molecules, while a calcium ionophore did not have any effect. This points out the extreme complexity of these interactions and that many similar experiments will have to be performed before these systems are understood (Bennet et al., 1993). Such an entry, however, is consistent with lipid-mediated poration, discussed earlier.

In parallel to the use of commercially available cationic liposome formulations, several groups tried to improve the activity of antisense therapy by synthesizing novel lipids. Two polyaminolipids, prepared by conjugation of spermine and spermidine to cholesterol through a carbamate bond, were used to follow up the uptake and cellular distribution of antisense molecules. Spermine–cholesterol compound was found to be equally efficient as Lipofectin while the spermidine was more efficient. According to the authors, these compounds are relatively nontoxic to mammalian cells and are also effective in the presence of serum. Vero cells were plated at 500 cells/well and after 20 h they were exposed to increasing concentrations of cationic reagents. Cell proliferation measurements showed that none of the agents decreases the growth appreciably (<10%) below 20 μg/mL. The cytotoxicity of DOTMA/DOPE, however, quickly increases at concentration >25 μg/mL while the other two do not. At 40 μg/mL DOTMA/DOPE kills all cells, while in the spermine–cholesterol sample approximately 50% survive and around 80% in the case of spermidine–cholesterol. By doubling the lipid concentration, the numbers fall to ~30% and 75%, respectively. Detailed study of cellular uptake showed that the kinetics of uptake as well as the level is the fastest with spermidine oligonucleotide complex (12 μM at 6 h and 17 at 24 h, compared with 8 and 9 μM for DOTMA/DOPE and 6.5 and 7.5 μM for spermine–cholesterol). By using 36-mers of phosphodiester antisense oligonucleotides, it could be observed that coadministration with polyaminolipids markedly increased chemical stability of oligonucleotides (Guy-Caffey et al., 1996).

This is not the first report where it can be noticed that some lipids with more than one positive charge were effective in the presence of serum. Higher activity of multiple charged cationic lipids can be in direct cell entry because these micelles-forming lipids create (transient) pores in the membranes.

Increased concentration of antisense molecules in cells was shown by flow cytometry when Lipofectamine was used. The uptake time decreased 20-fold to 5 h, and 65 to 75% of the cells showed intrinsic fluorescence as compared with only 2% when naked oligonucleotides were used (Williams et al., 1996).

Throughout this book I argue that we do not understand enough about the delivery of molecules into cytoplasm. Detailed work in this direction entails a study which evaluates different adjuvants for enhancement of oligonucleotide transfer from endosomes into cytosol (Hughes et al., 1996). pH-sensitive polymer (polyethylacrylic acid) and peptide from influenza virus did not interfere with the endocytotic process while addition of fusogenic peptide (GALA), dendrimers, Lipofectin, as well as the liposomal form of pH-sensitive molecule N-dodecylimidazole proprionate (DIP, pK around 6.6) did improve cytoplasmic delivery. The mechanism of DIP was explained by its protonation at lower pH which caused membrane fusion.

In another study, the mechanism of oligonucleotide entry into cells and release from cationic liposomes was recently discussed (Zelphati and Szoka, 1996). Fluorescently labeled oligonucleotides (fluorescein) and lipid (rhodamine) were followed by confocal microscopy. It was shown that the complex dissociates soon after internalization and while oligonucleotide accumulates in the nucleus, the lipid remains in focal spots in the cytoplasm. Test tube studies have also shown that incubation of the complex with anionic lipids releases oligonucleotides. Similarly to their results with DNA, it was shown that the majority of charged agents, such as adenosine triphosphate, polyglutamic acid, DNA, RNA as well as histones, spermine, spermidine, and polylysine did not induce release of oligonucleotides or cationic lipids. Only agents with strong negative linear charge density, such as dextran sulfate or heparin did induce the release, albeit to a smaller extent than anionic (PC:PE:PS 1/1/1) liposomes at charge neutralization. Authors postulated that early release from endosomes upon incubation in the cell culture is due to the mixing of cationic lipids with the cytoplasm-facing monolayer of the endosomal vacuole after membrane perturbation and local destabilization followed by lipid flip-flop. It is not clear, however, why the same process cannot happen on the plasma membrane which has similar, if not identical distribution and asymmetry, as the endosomal membrane which budds off from it. The observation that some biological polyelectrolytes can induce release of nucleic acids from genosomes may be important for *in vivo* delivery. On one side it can neutralize complexes before they reach target cells but on the other it allows coating and stabilization of cationic genosomes with anionic polyelectrolytes which do not release the complex (Zelphati and Szoka, 1996).

The last two sections have shown that recent developments in liposome technology have found their way into antisense oligonucleotide delivery. The next big step is the delivery of these *in vivo*. For many of these applications, when targeting, stability in circulation, as well as escape from the endocytotic vacuole, are required, the field will follow the thorny path led by targeting of liposome encapsulated low-molecular-weight drugs. The most successful application to date makes use of extravasation of small, sterically stabilized liposomes in tumors and sites of infections and inflammations. This provides an opportunity to deliver antisense oligonucleotides to these sites. Because these liposomes are normally not internalized, one can use the time-dependent shedding of polymer coating to increase endocytosis. The bilayer composition can be also pH sensitive. The presence of targeting ligands and if the receptors are endocytotic can further improve delivery. Furthermore, below the unstable PEG coating other active groups can be hidden and activated after a trigger or certain time period. I believe that the use of the above mentioned options and perhaps some new developments may result in effective delivery of these specific molecules.

In conclusion, antisense oligonucleotides have made remarkable progress in recent years. Unfortunately, the delivery of these molecules was rather neglected. Often, sustained-release systems are used to increase activity *in vivo*. It is likely that such treatments, if some improvements are detected, rely on nonspecific effects. Indeed, two recent reviews pointed out numerous nonantisense mechanisms that may explain the observed therapeutic activity. They include nonspecific binding to small molecules, cleavage of target sites, nonspecific binding to proteins, non-specific cellular activation of transcription factors, interference with viral adsorption, penetration, and uncoating, and toxicity of antisense degradation products (Wagner, 1994). Activation of the immune response and binding to growth factors and cell-anchoring proteins (fibronectin, laminin) were also discussed as possible nonspecific effects with therapeutic end points (Gura, 1995).

It is not too likely that these molecules would, alone or upon complexation with some proteins in the circulation, penetrate into appropriate cells. I believe that these systems will work properly only if efficient delivery systems, which will deliver antisense oligonucleotides at least into the cytoplasm of the target cells, are found. And, at present, it seems that there are not any systems available that are better, than the various liposomes discussed above.

■■■ RIBOZYMES

During RNA transcription the intron sequences are spliced out and the ligated exons are translated. In the early 1980s it was discovered that RNA cannot only self-splice (*cis* activity), but can also cleave other RNA in a sequence-specific manner (*trans* activity). These enzymatically active RNA molecules with catalytic activity were termed ribozymes (Cech, 1992). This was the first observation that enzymatic activity was not limited solely to proteins and had profound effects not only on our understanding of cell function but also on the models of the origin of life. Additionally, ribozymes, which may be called molecular scissors, may be effective agents to catalyze splicing of viral or oncogenic mRNA and can therefore be very useful therapeutics. They can be used in plant protection against viruses as well. Furthermore, they enable RNA genetic engineering (Symons, 1994).

Ribozymes are *trans*-acting sequences of RNA, normally from 200 to 1000 bp long, that recognize specific RNA sequences and cleave them after specific binding. Binding arms are around seven nucleotides long. With respect to the conformation of the molecule several different motifs and shapes were recognized. The most widely known are the so-called

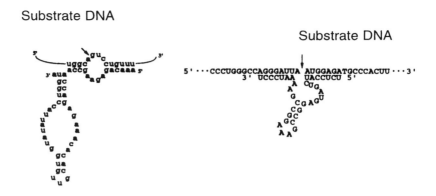

Figure 12-4   Ribozymes can have various structures. The most frequent motifs are hairpin and hammerhead ribozymes. Synthetic ribozymes can be also made much shorter. Typically, 17 bp are for binding on both sides and a similar length sequence can induce the cleavage. The above hammerhead ribosome contains 36 bp (11,800 Da).

hairpin and hammerhead structures (Figure 12-4). Shapes are determined by pairing of some base pairs and short single-stranded sequences inbetween.

Because ribozymes can be designed to bind to specific sites of any target DNA and consequently cleave them, they can be used in human therapy and diagnostics. The sequence specificity potentially offers high specificity and reduced, if not nonexisting, toxic side effects. As with antisense oligonucleotides there is an optimal target site length, in this case of around 15 nucleotides. Shorter matching sequences may have too large nonspecificity, while longer ones may have too high binding affinity and therefore slow enzymatic kinetics.

Ribozymes cleave RNA either by transesterification or hydrolysis between 3′- and 5′-binding sequences. Similarly to antisense oligonucleotides and in addition to chemical synthesis, however, there are two problems associated with their effective applications: chemical instability in the biological milieu and delivery into target cells. Therefore, identical methods as in oligonucleotide applications were employed to enhance the biological stability of their backbone and the stability of an unmodified ribozyme of approximately 6 s (50% degradation in human serum at 37°C) was enhanced several 1000-fold. In parallel, however, the enzymatic activity of these compounds, as measured by cleavage of 50% of the substrate in standard conditions, increased severalfold as well (Marr, 1996). Another possibility to increase their stability against chemical degradation is by flanking the active stretch by DNA sequences.

After all these modifications, however, ribozymes still have to be delivered into appropriate cells in order to be therapeutically active. While in the test tube there is free diffusion, in biological systems there is compartmentalization, and many barriers curtail free diffusion. Currently, there are not many data in the literature besides several proof-of-concept *in vitro* studies in various cell cultures.

Similar methods as were used in the delivery of DNA and antisense oligonucleotides can be used for intracellular delivery of ribozymes. If they are encapsulated into liposomes, complexed with cationic liposomes, or bound to antibodies, they must escape, after endocytosis, from endosomes before they become degraded by nucleases.

To the best of my knowledge, such experiments have not been published yet. One would expect that the same approaches, as discussed elsewhere in this book, will be tried. These include

- Encapsulation in conventional liposomes

- Encapsulation in pH-sensitive liposomes

- Encapsulation in fusogenic liposomes and virosomes

- Complexation with cationic liposomes

and any combination of the above. Also, in the later stages targeting ligands may be attached to these particulates. pH-sensitive, fusogenic liposomes, virosomes, and DOPE-containing cationic liposomes may enhance release from the endosomes and increase therapeutic activity. The problem with virosomes is immunogenicity of viral proteins needed for fusion. Shorter peptides are being tried as fusogens. A purely lipid-based fusion system would be definitively advantageous and liposomes with built-in instability, such as triggered lamellar–micellar and lamellar–hexagonal II phase transition, are being studied. An additional instability can be membrane asymmetry stabilized by a dissipative transmembrane pH gradient. Also, in the case of PEG-lipids the polymer coating can become fusogenic if polymer condensation occurs.

In addition to the delivery of synthesized ribozymes, one can transfect cells with the DNA code for a particular ribozyme. At present, mostly retroviral vectors are used. Obviously, the use of various lipid-based systems can be tried and expression in the cytoplasm with the help of codelivered RNA polymerase may increase the efficiency.

Therapeutic applications include HIV and several other viruses as well as the inhibition of oncogene function. *gag* transcript from HIV, H-*ras* of human bladder carcinoma cells, *bcr/abl* and c-*fos* gene (proto-oncogene which gives cells resistance to antineoplastic drugs) can be targeted as can be positive-strand plant viruses. Some preliminary data are reviewed by Marr (1996).

Only a few examples of liposomal ribozymes were reported. Multidrug resistance, a major obstacle in cancer chemotherapy, was reversed by the use of ribozyme-liposome complex. Ribozyme which cleaves the codon 196 of *MDR* 1 mRNA was complexed with DOTAP and used against 2 P-glycoprotein-producing cell line. Reversal of resistivity to doxorubicin in several cell lines was reported (Masuda et al., 1996).

Therapeutic experiments of ribozymes are only the beginning now. As in the case of antisense oligonucleotides, the main problem seems to be in their effective delivery into appropriate cells. Again, at present I do not see any systems any more efficient than various types of liposomes. Conventional liposomes can deliver their cargo to macrophages in the liver, spleen, bone marrow, and perhaps hepatocytes. Cationic liposome–ribozyme complexes can be used for delivery to vascular endothelium and perhaps to the liver, lung, and spleen. Sterically stabilized liposomes can be used to deliver ribozymes to sites of infections, inflammations, and some tumors. If these systems are endocytosed, pH-sensitive membrane composition may be used. In addition to topical (pulmonary, skin) and localized administrations, targeting with surface-attached ligands is also theoretically possible, and I believe that the field has to move along these lines to achieve therapeutic viability.

■ DELIVERY OF PROTEINS

Delivery of proteins in liposome applications is, in general, a larger problem than researchers admit. These molecules are very large, can interact with bilayers, and in general are difficult to encapsulate in a stable form. Because they often bear many negative charges, it is only logical that cationic liposomes were tried for their delivery as well.

Cationic liposomes can be used also for the delivery of some proteins. Purified recombinant glucocorticoid receptor fragment was effectively delivered into mammalian cells using Lipofectin (Debs et al., 1990). Absence of DOPE in the liposomes also yielded a high efficiency of protein delivery. Several antigens were also introduced into cells by cationic liposome complexation. Herpes simplex virus glycoportein B antigen was delivered to cells after complexation with DOTAP:DOPE liposomes. A peptide fragment of the protein was presented by the class I MHC-restricted specific cytotoxic T lymphocytes (CTL) (Walker et al., 1992). Antigenic ovalbumin protein was complexed with lipopolylysine and a mouse cell line internalized antigen and became sensitized to killing by an ovalbumin-specific CTL (Nair et al., 1992). In another study, DOTAP complexation delivery of ovalbumin protein was shown to be more effective than electroporation and osmotic loading (Chen et al., 1993). Enzyme prostatic acid phosphatase protein was delivered by Lipofectin complexation into human prostate carcinoma cells. Delivery was very fast with 70% of the protein transferred into the cytoplasm within 1 h (Lin et al., 1993). To increase transfection efficiency and induce cytoplasmic expression (see p. 49), Gao and Huang (1993) used DC-Chol liposomes to deliver T7 RNA polymerase into the cytosol.

■ SUMMARY

In this chapter we have seen that cationic liposomes can be used for a variety of other applications and that the specter of their applications may broaden. Also, for the delivery of oligonucleotides and ribozymes the effort must now concentrate on their intracellular delivery, and liposomes seem to be the most promising delivery vehicle.

■ ADDITIONAL READING

Christoffersen, R. E., Marr, J. J., Ribozymes as human therapeutic agents, *J. Med. Chem.,* 38, 2023–2037, 1995.

Crooke, S. T., Therapeutic applications of oligonucleotides, *Annu. Rev. Pharmacol. Toxicol.,* 32, 329–376, 1992.

Farhood, H., Huang, L., Delivery of DNA, RNA and proteins by cationic liposomes, in *Nonmedical Applications of Liposomes, Vol. IV: From Gene Therapy and Diagnostics to Ecology,* Lasic, D. D. and Barenholz, Y., Eds., CRC Press, Boca Raton, FL, 1996, 31–42.

13 PERSPECTIVES AND CONCLUSION

We shall conclude by reviewing various delivery systems and discuss their advantages and disadvantages in the delivery of genetic material into cells. Some possible improvements will also be mentioned. Many of these systems can also be used for the delivery of therapeutic proteins.

First, we shall discuss which tissues can be targeted by various systems. Primarily, these are lungs, liver, spleen, kidney, heart, lymph nodes, and bone marrow upon systemic administration and sites of direct injection. Arterial injections can deliver particles into the next capillary bed, and topical applications include inhalation and instillation into the respiratory tract. In principle, all administration routes can be used.

There is always a question not only as to which tissues but also as to which cells can be transfected. Following systemic administration, I do not believe that many cells that are not in direct physical contact with blood can be targeted. This leaves us with cells of vascular endothelium, fixed and circulating macrophages and monocytes, hepatocytes in the liver, spleen cells, bone marrow cells, cells in the kidney, and cells in the blood, including metastatic cells. In the case of an impaired vascular system, cells at the sites of inflammation, infection, and tumor growth can be targeted. Direct injections can deliver particles into various tissues, from muscle, skin, bone (intra-articular), cells in the neural system and brain, eye, and lung (and airway) epithelial cells upon administration of nebulized formulation. Topical applications are still very questionable, and reports range from enhanced delivery to dermis to the delivery only to hair follicles. Mucosal cells, which form the epithelial surface in the lungs, the digestive tract, as well as the genital tract, are also an attractive target especially for immunization. Tumor cells can be also targeted either systemically or via direct injection. The preferable administration route — oral route — is rather difficult to achieve with lipid-based particles and large molecules. However, the field is improving and oral vaccination was reported for lipid-packed antigens and DNA. In such a case, epithelial cells of the Payer's patch in the intestinal tract can be targeted. Also, the use of osmotic release devices which can precisely control the rate and site of release of the encapsulated agents offers a nice opportunity to target cells in the digestive tract, such as colon cancer cells, for instance.

■ CATIONIC LIPOSOMES

Currently, cationic liposomes are still the most widely used nonviral system for gene transfection. Their major advantage is quantitative DNA encapsulation for $\rho < 0.5$ to 0.8. Another advantage is enhanced internalization which may be due to either positive surfaces or enhanced adsorption of negatively charged proteins. Cell entry may be by endocytosis or direct entry into the cytoplasm via membrane destabilization. DNA seems to be well protected in these complexes if they are prepared correctly. From a pharmaceutical point of view the disadvantages of cationic liposome–DNA complexes are toxicity of cationic lipids and lack of control over their interaction characteristics and stability upon application. These particles are so reactive that it is likely that attachment of special ligands may not change their biodistribution.

On the formulation side, they can be nebulized and lyophilized if prepared in 10% sucrose. If manufactured properly, their stability in liquid form at 4°C can be measured in months. Freezing is another option for increased shelf-life stability. It is less demanding than lyophilization but storage of the sample is more problematic. Instead of sucrose, 5% glucose can be used. Homogeneous size distribution and sterile, pyrogen-free formulations, however, still present a formidable challenge.

Cationic liposome–DNA complexes can be used for direct and systemic injection as well as instillation or aerosolization into airways. Topical administration normally causes skin irritation. Direct injections can deliver DNA into target tissue and DNA internalization can occur. Systemic administration normally results in large uptake in the lung, followed by heart, spleen, liver, and kidney. Nerve cells can be transfected upon direct injection. This is a typical example of the first-pass mechanism and takes into account relative surface areas. Tail vein–injected material first passes through the lung and then through the heart. Expression in RES is relatively low, probably due to effective digestion of DNA by macrophages. Low expression in a variety of tissues indicates spillage of the complexes during the first few passes through the circulation. Blood itself does not contribute much to the transfection, and in general removal of blood results in increased transfection if calculated per weight of tissue.

Upon topical administration mostly lung epithelial cells are transfected, while upon systemic application expression is observed in vascular endothelium, macrophages, and, in the case of small complexes, hepatocytes. I do not think that cells which are not in direct contact with the complexes can be transfected with any efficiency. With respect to the vascular endothelium transfection precise experiments, including FACS analyses of cellularized tissues, remain to be done to evaluate the fraction of macrophages which can contribute to the transfection.

Possible improvements include less-toxic lipids, co-condensing agents, more information on DNA plasmid itself, and improved delivery into cytoplasm. Timely DNA decondensation is also important. At present, however, is still not known when and where it should occur.

Second-generation cationic genosomes may contain coatings containing neutral, anionic, or sterically stabilized lipids with possible active ligands. Simple incubation with anionic liposomes or micelles can reverse surface charge. Again, systems at electrical neutrality tend to precipitate. Another possibility to achieve good coating is by co-dissolving all the components in detergent and dialyzing detergent away. Fusogenic proteins, at present, still elicit an immune response and shorter fragments and polypeptides are being tried. The same is true for targeting ligands where Fab' or even shorter fragments will have to replace large and immunogenic antibodies. We must not forget, however, that targeting of structurally much simpler and better controllable liposomes has not yet produced a promising system.

■ ANIONIC LIPOSOMES

These systems are known to be safe, FDA approved, and can be very stable and reproducibly prepared in large quantities. Insertion of a variety of ligands does not present a problem. Although the encapsulated DNA is well protected, its efficient encapsulation presents the major drawback. Typical DNA is around 2 μm long, and it is difficult to entrap it into a small vesicle with inner diameter from 50 to 200 nm. Dimensions of supercoiled DNA can fit into this cavity. The majority of researchers, however, try to precondense DNA into smaller particles to increase encapsulation efficiency. Ideally, single DNA molecules should condense. In general, however, this is not possible for DNA sizes below 30 kb. Also, this can only happen in very dilute systems while at higher concentrations condensed DNA may precipitate. An additional problem with precondensed DNA is high salt concentration which is normally required to reduce the size in the presence of other condensing agents, such as polylysine. Encapsulation efficiencies may reach several tens of percent, while supercoiled DNA at high concentrations can be encapsulated perhaps with a 10% efficiency. More demanding reverse phase liposome preparation techniques can yield higher efficiencies but at larger liposome sizes and more demanding experimental work.

While, with regard to formulation, anionic liposomes with encapsulated DNA may not be too difficult to prepare, pharmaceutically such particles may be inactive because they are typically endocytosed, which results in DNA degradation in lysosomal endosomes. Therefore, endosome-disrupting agents should be co-encapsulated.

This problem can be tackled also by using pH-sensitive liposomes which disintegrate and fuse with the endosomal envelope upon lowering of pH. Similar escape mechanisms can be obtained by virosomes. They, however, elicit an immune response. Synthetic virosomes, prepared from pure lipids and containing fusogenic peptides, may be less immunogenic. However, no real data on such systems yet exist.

pH-sensitive liposomes may improve delivery of DNA from endosome into the cytoplasm, and sterically stabilized liposomes can improve biodistribution of colloidal DNA.

■ STERICALLY STABILIZED LIPOSOMES

Above we have learned that the optimal system is likely DNA encapsulated in pH-sensitive liposomes. Stealth coating can significantly alter biodistribution of liposomes. Conventional liposomes are predominantly cleared by the cells of the immune system while sterically stabilizing coating reduces interactions with plasma components, resulting in their invisibility to macrophages. After prolonged circulation, however, these liposomes end up in many tissues with a large volume of biodistribution. They accumulate at sites where the vascular system has increased permeability, which often happens to be in tumors and sites of inflammation and infection. While, in the case of normal drugs, delivery to these sites normally brings therapeutic benefit, in the case of encapsulated DNA, oligonucleotide, or ribozyme, liposomes must facilitate entry into the cell. Therefore, polymer coating can be designed to be shed after a preprogrammed rate. PEG–lipid may have either shorter lipid anchors with known dissociation kinetics, or PEG linkage can be degraded with a known (programmed) degradation rate. While the first approach is much easier, the second one is safer and offers better control over kinetics. For instance, in systems where dilution is important, the same formulation may behave completely differently in mice and humans. In the first case bolus injection results in 5-fold dilution and in the second infusion can cause a 5000-fold dilution. This is a consequence of simple thermodynamics but is important to show how animal experiments may be completely misleading due not only to biological factors but also to fundamental laws of physics and chemistry. However, when we have stable particles and stable retention of the agent one can add more chemistry. For instance, on such particles one can attach various ligands and, ultimately, fusogenic and targeting groups.

Recently, it was shown that PEG–lipids can be inserted into preformed liposomes upon incubation with micellar solution (Uster et al., 1996). This process may be used to prepare sterically stabilized genosomes because in general sterically stabilized cationic liposomes do not interact with DNA (Lasic, unpublished).

In a similar way other ligands may be incorporated. The insertion should be performed at higher temperatures (and in mechanically cohesive bilayers) to assure rapid dissociation and diffusion of inserting monomers.

Constant new developments in organic synthesis, physicochemical properties of liposomes, and related areas can give us hope that current problems with gene delivery will be solved in the future.

■ SUMMARY

Although it is possible that some commercial products will result from current generations of cationic lipid–DNA complexes, in the long run, increased control over stability and interaction characteristics may yield advantage to conventional and sterically stabilized liposomes. This potential was discussed in this chapter.

CONCLUSION AND AFTERWORD

In conclusion, delivery of nucleic acids by cationic liposomes has shown extremely rapid development in the last 5 years. Numerous cell types have been transfected, more than half a dozen commercial liposome kits are on the market, and many laboratories which are not involved in any lipid or liposome research are routinely using such liposomes in their work. The field is still rapidly growing and so is our knowledge of the basic science underlying these transfections, cell function, and gene functionality.

From the physicochemical aspect I can remind researchers that they may inadvertently work in the field of supramolecular chemistry. It is well known experimentally and theoretically (see Equation 3-3) that single-valent cations cannot condense DNA because due to entropy they cannot shield the required ≃90% of the DNA charge which induces its self-collapse, i.e., DNA condensation. However, a self-assembly of univalent cations that is not based on covalent forces actually acts as a multivalent species and can effectively condense DNA. Futhermore, due to lipid properties, such as size of molecules and self-organization behavior, this assembly even dictates, over DNA, its own symmetry into the complex, lamellar as opposed to hexagonal or, perhaps, random ("amorphous") self-collapse, as shown in Figure 1.

With respect to gene therapy, however, despite some optimistic outlooks and promising new developments, I shall conclude with a note of caution. Currently, I am not aware of a single gene therapy trial which has shown some absolutely proven benefit. I am aware of some early phase trials which show that certain steps toward the goal were overcome, but I do not think that any of the current formulations will become a commercial success. A lot more basic scientific work will have to be performed before some concepts on paper will be materialized in practice. There is no doubt in my mind that ultimately some of these concepts will work. But, also, there is still a long way to go.

Therefore, the inevitable presentation and publishing of irreproducible, artifactual, and poorly controlled experiments, for which editors can also claim some blame, will not help the field. It will be the good science and not the overwhelming claims of some scientists, businessmen, and venture capitalists which will make the concept work. Titles such as "The genetic revolution: new technology allows us to improve on nature. How

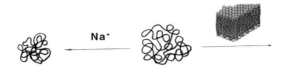

Figure 1 Schematic presentation of DNA condensation. Only a self-organized assembly of univalent
cations can induce phase transition random
coil–collapsed state in DNA.

far should we go?" and "Just what the doctor ordered" in these circum-
stances inevitably cause the appearance of such titles as "Has gene therapy
stalled?," "Promises, promises," "Gene therapy's growing pains," "Antisense has growing pains," and many others.

So, I am asking all the players in this field to act rationally and
through the hard work of basic science without preposterous claims lead
the field to its successful development. I firmly believe that this is the
fastest and easiest way.

■ ADDITIONAL READING

Gura, T., Antisense has growing pains, *Science,* 270, 575–578, 1995.
Lasic, D. D., Liposomes, *Sci. Med. (Sci. Am.),* 3(3), 34–43, May/June 1996.
Marshall, E., Gene therapy's growing pains, *Science,* 269, 1050–1055, 1995.

REFERENCES

Aberle, A. M., Bennet, M. J., Malone, R. W., Nantz, M. H., The counterion influence on cationic lipid-mediated transfection of plasmid DNA, *Biochim. Biophys. Acta,* 1299, 281–283, 1996.

Adams, D. H., Joyce, G., Richardson, V. J., Ryman, B. E., Wisnewski, H. M., Liposome toxicity in the mouse central nervous system, *J. Neurol. Sci.,* 31, 173–179, 1977.

Akao, T., Osaki, T., Motoma, J., Ito, A., Kunitake, T., Correlation between physicochemical characteristics of synthetic cationic amphiphiles and their DNA transfection ability, *Bull. Chem. Soc. Jpn.,* 64, 3677–3681, 1991.

Akhtar, S., Juliano, R. L., Liposome delivery of antisense oligonucleotides: adsorption and efflux characteristics of phosphorothioate oligonucleotides, *J. Contr. Rel.,* 22, 47–56, 1992.

Aksentijevich, I., Pastan, I., Lunardi, Y. I., Gallo, R. C., Gottesman, M. M., Thierry, A. R., *In vitro* and *in vivo* liposome mediated gene transfer leads to human MDR1 expression in mouse bone marrow progenitor cells, *Hum. Gene Ther.,* 7, 1111–1122, 1996.

Alexander, M. Y., Akhurst, L. J., Liposome-mediated gene transfer and expression via the skin, *Human Mol. Genetics,* 4, 2279–2285, 1995.

Alton, E. W. F. W., Middleton, P. G., Caplen, N. J., Smith, S. N., Steel, D. M., Munkonge, F. M., Jeffrey, P. K., Geddes, D. M., Hart, S. L., Williamson, R., Fasold, K., Miller, A. D., Dickinson, P., Stevenson, B. J., MaLahlan, G., Dorin, J. R., Porteous, D. J., Non-invasive liposome-mediated gene delivery can correct the ion transport defect in cystic fibrosis mutant mice, *Nature Genet.,* 5, 135–142, 1993.

Amos, H., Protamine enhancement of RNA uptake by cultured chick cells, *Biochem. Biophys. Res. Commun.,* 5, 1–4, 1961.

Anderson, W. F., Human gene therapy, *Science,* 255, 808–813, 1992.

Balasubramaniam, R. P., Bennet, M. J., Aberle, A. M., Malone, J. G., Nantz, M. H., Malone, R. W., Structural and functional analysis of cationic transfection lipids: the hydrophobic domain, *Gene Therapy,* 3, 163–172, 1996.

Ballas, N., Zakai, N., Sela, I., Loyter, A., Liposomes bearing a quaternary ammonium detergent as an efficient vehicle for functional transfer of TMV-RNA into plant protoplasts, *Biochim. Biophys. Acta,* 939, 8–18, 1988.

Bangham, A. D., Horne, R., Negative staining of phospholipids and their structured modification by surface active agent, *J. Mol. Biol.,* 8, 660–668, 1994.

Barenholz, Y., The role of lipid DNA interaction in amphiphection (amphiphilic lipid based transfection): view through the "lipid eye," in *Artificial Self-Assembling Systems for Gene Transfer,* Book of Abstracts, CHI, Boston, 1995.

Barenholz, Y., Lasic, D. D. (Eds.) *Handbook of Nonmedical Applications of Liposomes,* Vol. III, From Design to Microreactors, CRC Press, Boca Raton, FL, 1996.

Barenholz, Y., Lasic, D. D. (Eds.) *Handbook of Nonmedical Applications of Liposomes,* Vol. IV, Models for Biological Phenomena, CRC Press, Boca Raton, FL, 1996.

Batra, R. K., Wang-Johanning, F., Wagner, E., Garver, R. I., Curiel, D. T., Receptor-mediated gene delivery employing lectin-binding specificity, *Gene Ther.*, 1, 255–260, 1994.

Baumann, C. G., Bloomfield, V. A., Large scale purification of plasmid DNA for biophysical and molecular biology studies, *BioTechniques*, 19, 884–890, 1995.

Behr, J. P., DNA strongly binds to micelles and vesicles containing lipopolyamines or lipointercalants, *Tetrahedron Lett.*, 27, 5861–5864, 1986.

Behr, J. P., Synthetic gene transfer vectors, *Acc. Chem. Res.*, 26, 274–278, 1993.

Behr, J. P., Demeneix, B., Loeffler, J. P., Mutul, J. P., Efficient gene transfer into mammalian primary endocrine cells with lipopolyamine coated DNA, *Proc. Natl. Acad. Sci. U.S.A.* 86, 6982–6986, 1989.

Bennet, C. F., Chiang, M. Y., Chan, H., Shoemaker J. E., Mirabelli, C. K., Cationic lipids enhance cellular uptake and activity of phosphorothioate antisense oligonucleotides, *Mol. Pharmacol.*, 41, 1023–1033, 1992.

Bennet, C. F., Chiang, M. Y., Chan, H., Grimm, S., Use of cationic lipids to enhance the biological activity of antisense oligonucleotides *J. Liposome Res.*, 3, 85–112, 1993.

Bennet, M. J., Malone, R. W., Nantz, M. H., A flexible approach to synthetic lipid ammonium salts for polynucleotide transfection, *Tetrahed. Lett.*, 36, 2207–2210, 1995a.

Bennet, M. J., Nantz, M. H., Balasubramanian, R. P., Gruenert, D. C., Malone, R. W., Cholesterol enhances cationic liposome-mediated DNA transfection of human respiratory epithelial cells, *Biosci. Rep.*, 15, 47–53, 1995b.

Bennet, M. J., Aberle, A. M., Balasubramanian, R. P., Malone, J. G., Nantz, M. H., Malone, R. W., Considerations for the design of improved cationic amphiphiles based on transfection respects, *J. Liposome Res.*, 6, 545–566, 1996.

Benvenisty, N., Reshef, L., Direct introduction of genes into rats and expression of the genes, *Proc. Natl. Acad. Sci. U.S.A.*, 83, 9551–9555, 1986.

Beveridge, D. L., Ravishanker, G., Molecular dynamics studies of DNA, *Curr. Op. Struct. Biol.*, 4, 246–255, 1994.

Bichenikov, E. E., Budker, V. G., Weiner, L. M., Kruppa, A. I., DNA interaction with phosphatidylcholine liposomes (in Russian), *Biol. Membrani*, 5, 501–507, 1988.

Bloomfield, V. A., Condensation of DNA by multivalent cations, *Biopolymers*, 31, 1471–1481, 1991.

Bloomfield, V. A., Crothers, R. M., Tinoco, I., *Physical Chemistry of Nucleic Acids*, Harper & Row, New York, 1974.

Bloomfield, V. A., Ma, C., Arscott, P. G., Role of multivalent cations in condensation of DNA, in *Macroion Characterization*, American Chemical Society, 195–209, 1994, Chap. 15.

Borisov, O., Auroy, P., Auvray, L., Stabilization of colloidal systems by grafted polymers, in *Stealth Liposomes*, Lasic, D. D., Martin, F. J., Eds., CRC Press, Boca Raton, FL, 1995, 31.

Bottega, R., Epand, R. M., Inhibition of protein kinase C by cationic amphiphiles, *Biochemistry*, 31, 9025–9030, 1992.

Boulikas, T., Nuclear envelope and chromatin structure, *Int. Rev. Cytol.*, 17, 493–598, 1987.

Boulikas, T., Function of chromatin in the expression of genes, *Int. Rev. Cytol.*, 17, 599–684, 1987.

Boulikas, T., Phosphorylation of transcription factors and control of the cell cycle, *Crit. Rev. Euk. Gene Expr.*, 5, 1–77, 1995.

Boulikas, T., Nuclear import of protein kinases and cyclines, *J. Cell. Biochem.*, 60, 61–82, 1996.

Boussif, O., Lezoualch, F., Zanta, M. A., Mergny, M., Schermann, D., Demeneix, B., Behr, J. P., A versatile vector for gene and oligonucleotide transfer into cells, *Proc. Natl. Acad. Sci. U.S.A.*, 92, 7297–7301, 1995.

Brigham, K. L., Meyrick, B., Christman, B., Magnuson, M., King, G., Berry, L., *In vivo* transfection of murine lungs with a functioning prokaryotic gene using a liposome vehicle. *Am. J. Med. Sci.*, 298, 278–281, 1989.

Brigham, K. L., Schreier, H., Cationic liposomes and DNA delivery, *J. Liposome Res.*, 3, 31–49, 1993.

Budker, V., Gurevich, V., Hagstrom, J., Bortzov, F., Wolff, J. A., pH sensitive, cationic liposomes: a new synthetic virus-like vector, *Nature Biotechnol.*, 14, 760–764, 1996.

Cabane, B., Duplessix, R., Decoration of semidilute polymer solutions with surfactant micelles, *J. Phys.*, 48, 651–662, 1987.

Canonico, A. E., Conary, J. T., Meyrick, B. O., Brigham, K. L., Aerosol and intravenous transfection of human alpha1-antitripsin gene to lungs of rabbits, *Am. J. Resp. Cell Mol. Biol.*, 10, 24–29, 1994a.

Canonico, A. E., Plitman, J. D., Conary, T. J., Meyrick, B. E., Brigham, K. L., No lung toxicity after repeated aerosol or iv delivery of plasmid-cationic complexes, *J. Appl. Physiol.*, 77, 415–419, 1994b.

Canonico, A. E., Conary, T. J., Meyrick, B. E., Brigham, K. L., Aerosol and iv transfection of human antitrypsin gene to lungs of rabbits, *Am. J. Resp. Cell Mol. Biol.*, 10, 24–29, 1995.

Cantor, C. R., Schimmel, P. R., *Biophysical Chemistry*, W. H. Freeman, New York, 1980.

Caplen, N. J., Gao, X., Hayes, P., Elaswarapu, R., Fisher, G., Kinrade, E., Chakera, A., Schorr, J., Hughes, B., Dorin, J. R., Porteous, D. J., Alton, E. W. F. W., Geddes, D. M., Coutelle, C., Williamson, R., Huang, L., Gilchrist, C., Gene therapy for cystic fibrosis in humans by liposome-mediated DNA transfer: the production of resources and the regulatory process, *Gene Ther.*, 1, 139–147, 1994.

Caplen, N. J., Alton, E. W. F. W., Middleton, P. G., Dorin, J. R., Stevenson, B. J., Gao, X., Durham, S. R., Jeffrey, P. K., Hodson, M. E., Coutelle, C., Huang, L., Porteous, D. J., Williamson, R., Geddes, M., Liposome mediated CFTR gene transfer to the nasal epithelium of patients with cystic fibrosis, *Nature Med.*, 1, 39–46, 1995.

Caplen, N. J., Alton, E. W. F. W., Gene therapy for cystic fibrosis, *Chem. Ind.*, 290–292, 15 April 1996.

Carmona-Ribeiro, A. M., Theoretical and experimental stabilities of amphiphilic vesicles in the presence of NaCl, *J. Phys. Chem.*, 93, 2630–2634, 1989.

Carmona-Ribeiro, A. M., Does the DLVO account for interactions between charged vesicles, *J. Phys. Chem.*, 96, 9555–9557, 1992.

Cech, T. R., Ribozymes and their medical applications, *JAMA*, 260, 3030–3034, 1988.

Cech, T. R., Ribozyme engineering, *Curr. Op. Struct. Biol.*, 2, 605–609, 1992.

Cevc, G., Electrostatic characterization of liposomes, *Chem. Phys. Lipids*, 64, 163–186, 1993.

Challita, P.-M., Kohn, D. B., Lack of expression from a retroviral vector after transduction of murine hematopoietic stem cells is associated with methylation *in vivo*, *Proc. Natl. Acad. Sci. U.S.A.*, 91, 2567–2571, 1994.

Chang, P. L., Shen, N., Westcott, A. J., Delivery of recombinant gene products with microencapsulated cells *in vivo, Hum. Gene Ther.,* 4, 433–440, 1993.

Chen, J., Gamou, S., Takayanagi, A., Shimizu, N., A novel gene delivery system using EGF receptor-mediated endocytosis, *FEBS Lett.,* 338, 167–169, 1994.

Chen, S. G., Development and use of cationic lipids with enhanced gene transfer activity, in *Artificial Self-Assembling Systems for Gene Transfer, Book of Abstracts,* CHI, Boston, 1995.

Chen, W., Carbone, F. R., McCluskey, J., *J. Immunol. Meth.,* 160, 49–57, 1993.

Chen, X., Li, Y., Xiong, K., Wagner, T. E., A self-initiating eukaryotic transient gene expression system based on cotransfection of bacteriophage T7 RNA polymerase and DNA vectors containing a T7 autogene, *Nucleic Acids Res.,* 22, 2114–2120, 1994.

Chiang, M., Chan, H., Zounes, M. A., Freier, S., Loma, W., Bennett, C. F., Antisense oligonucleotides inhibit intercellular adhesion molecule 1 expression by two distinct mechanisms, *J. Biol. Chem.,* 266, 1862–1871, 1991.

Chin, J. D., Gren, G. A., Zon, G., Szoka, F. C., Straubinger, R. M., Rapid nuclear accumulation of injected oligonucleotides, *New Biol.,* 2, 1091–1100, 1990.

Christoffersen, R. E., Marr, J. J., Ribozymes as human therapeutic agents, *J. Med. Chem.,* 38, 2023–2037, 1995.

Cohen, J., Naked DNA points way to vaccines, *Science,* 259, 1691–1692, 1993.

Cohen, J. S., Hogan, M. E., The new genetic medicines, *Sci. Am.,* 76–82, 1994 (Dec.).

Cotton, M., Wagner, E., Non-viral approaches to gene therapy, *Curr. Op. Biotechnol.,* 4, 705–710, 1993.

Crooke, S. T., Therapeutic applications of oligonucleotides, *Annu. Rev. Pharmacol. Toxicol.,* 32, 329–376, 1992.

Culotta, V. C., Hamer, D. H., Fine mapping of a mouse metallothionein gene metal response element, *Mol. Cell. Biol.,* 9, 1376–1380, 1989.

Culver, K. W., Methods for gene transfer, in *Gene Therapy: A Handbook for Physicians,* Mary Ann Liebert, Inc., New York, 1994, 15–31.

Culver, K. W., Blaese, M., Gene therapy for cancer, *TIG,* 10, 174–178, 1994.

Culver, K. W., Ram, Z., Wallbridge, S., Ishii, H., Oldfield, E. H., Blaese, R. M., *In vivo* gene transfer with retroviral vector-producer cells for treatment of experimental brain tumors, *Science,* 256, 1550–1552, 1992.

Curiel, D. T., Agarwal, S., Romer, M. U., Wagner, E., Cotten, M., Birnsteil, M., Boucher, R. C., High efficiency gene transfer to respiratory epithelial cells via receptor mediated endocytosis pathway, *Am. J. Resp. Cell Mol. Biol.,* 6, 247–252, 1992.

Curiel, D. T., Wagner, E., Cotten, M., Birnsteil, M., Agarwal, S., Loechel, S., Hu, P. C., High efficiency gene transfer mediated by adenovirus coupled to DNA-polylysine complex, *Hum. Gene Ther.,* 3, 147–154, 1992.

Curiel, D. T., Wagner, E., Cotten, M., Birnsteil, M. L., Agarwal, S., Li, C. M., Loechel, S., Hu, P. C., Gene transfer to respiratory epithelial cells mediated by adenovirus coupled to DNA-polylysine complexes, *Hum. Gene Ther.,* 3, 147–154, 1992.

Debs, R., Freedman, L. P., Edmunds, S., Gaensler, K. L., Duzgunes, N, Yamamoto, K. R., *J. Biol. Chem.,* 265, 10189–10192, 1990.

Dolar, D., Thermodynamic properties of polyelectrolyte solutions, in *Advanced NATO Study Institute on Charged and Reactive Polymers,* Seligny, E., Ed., D. Reidel, 1974, 97–113.

Durand, D., Doucet, J., Livolant, F., A study of the structure of highly concentrated phase of DNA by X-ray diffraction, *J. Phys. II*, 2, 1769–1783, 1992.

Dwarki, V. J., Malone, R. W., Verma, I. M., Cationic liposome mediated RNA transfection, *Met. Enzym.*, 217, 644–654, 1993.

Eglitis, M. A., Positive selectable markers for use with mammalian cells in culture, *Hum. Gene Ther.*, 2, 195–201, 1991.

Eibl, H., Wooley, P., Electrostatic interactions at charged membrane surfaces. Hydrogen bonds in lipid membrane surfaces, *Biophys. Chem.*, 10, 261–271, 1979.

Eickbush, T. H., Moudrianakis, E. N., The compaction of DNA helices into either continuous supercoils and folded fiber rods and toroids, *Cell*, 13, 295–305, 1978.

Farhood, H., Bottega, R., Epand, R. M., Huang, L., Effect of cholesterol derivatives on gene transfer and protein kinase C activity, *Biochim. Biophys. Acta,* 1111, 239–246, 1992.

Farhood, H., Xiang, G., Son, K.-H., Yang, Y.-Y., Lazo, J. S., Barsoum, J., Bottega, R., Epand, R. M., Huang, L., in *Gene Therapy for Neoplastic Diseases*, B. E. Huber, J. S. Lazo, Eds., New York Academy of Sciences, New York, 1994, 23–35.

Farhood, H., Huang, L., Delivery of DNA, RNA, and proteins by cationic liposomes, in *Liposomes: From Gene Therapy to Diagnostics and Ecology,* Lasic, D. D., Barenholz, Y., Eds., CRC Press, Boca Raton, FL, 1996, 31–42.

Felgner, J. H., Kumar, R., Sridhar, R., Wheeler, C., Tsai, Y. J., Border, R., Ramsay, P., Martin, M., Felgner, P. L., Enhanced gene delivery and mechanism studies with novel series of cationic lipid formulations, *J. Biol. Chem.*, 269, 2550–2561, 1994.

Felgner, P. L., Particulate systems and polymers for *in vitro* and *in vivo* delivery of polynucleotides, *Adv. Drug Del. Rev.,* 5, 163–187, 1990.

Felgner, P. L., Gadek, T. R., Holm, M., Roman, R., Chan, H. S., Wenz, M., Northrop, J. P., Ringold, M., Danielsen, H., Lipofection: a highly efficient lipid-mediated DNA transfection procedure, *Proc. Natl. Acad. Sci. U.S.A.*, 84, 7413–7417, 1987.

Felgner, P. L., Ringold, G. M., Cationic liposome mediated transfection, *Nature,* 337, 387–388, 1989.

Felgner, P. L., Tsai, Y. J., Felgner, J. H., Advances in the design and application of cytofectin formulations, in *Liposomes: From Gene Therapy to Diagnostics and Ecology,* Lasic, D. D., Barenholz, Y., Eds., CRC Press, Boca Raton, FL, 1996, 43–56.

Ferkol, T., Kaetzel, C. S., Davis, P. B., Gene transfer into respiratory epithelial cells by targeting the polymeric immunoglobulin receptor, *J. Clin. Invest.,* 92, 2394–2400, 1993.

Findeis, M. A., Merwin, J. R., Spitalny, G. L., Chiou, H. C., Targeted delivery of DNA for gene therapy via receptors, *Trends Biotechnol.,* 11, 202–205, 1993.

Fraley, R. P., Subramani, S., Berg, P., Papahadjopoulos, D., Introduction of liposome-encapsulated SV40 DNA into cells, *J. Biol. Chem.,* 255, 10431–10435, 1980.

Fraley, R. P., Papahadjopoulos, D., Liposomes: the development of a new carrier system for introducing nucleic acids into plant and animal cells, *Curr. Top. Microbiol. Immunol.,* 96, 171–187, 1982.

Frank-Kamenetskii, M. D., Anshelevich, V. V., Lukashin, A. V., Polyelectrolyte model of DNA, *Sov. Phys. Usp.,* 30, 317–330, 1987.

Frese, J., Wu, C. H., Wu, G. Y., Targeting of genes to the liver with glycoprotein carriers, *Adv. Drug Del. Rev.,* 14, 137–152, 1994.

Friedmann, T., Gene therapy for neurological disorders, *Trends Genet.,* 10, 210–214, 1994.

Friend, D. S., Papahadjopoulos, D., Debs, R. J., Endocytosis and intracellular processing accompanying transfection mediated by cationic liposomes, *Biochim. Biophys. Acta,* 1278, 41–50, 1996.

Fuoss, R. M., Katchalsky, A., Lifson, S., Potential of an infinite rodlike molecule and the distribution of counterions in the solution, *Proc. Natl. Acad. Sci. U.S.A.,* 37, 579–586, 1951.

Gao, X., Huang, L., A novel cationic liposome reagent for efficient transfection of mammalian cells, *Biochem. Biophys. Res. Commun.,* 179, 280–285, 1991.

Gao, X., Huang, L., Cytoplasmic expression of a reporter gene by co-delivery of T7 RNA polymerase and T7 promoter sequence with cationic liposomes, *Nucleic Acids Res.,* 21, 2867–2872, 1993.

Gao, X., Huang, L., Potentiation of cationic liposome-mediated gene delivery by polycations, *Biochemistry,* 35, 1027–1036, 1996.

deGennes, P. G., Polymers at an interface: a simplified view, *Adv. Colloid Sci.,* 27, 189–206, 1987.

Gershon, H., Ghirlando, R., Guttman, S. B., Minsky, A., Mode of formation and structural features of DNA-cationic liposome complexes used for transfection, *Biochemistry,* 32, 7143–7151, 1993.

Ghirlando, R., DNA condensation induced by cationic surfactants, Ph.D. thesis, Weizmann Institute of Science, Israel, 1991.

Ghoumani, A. M., Rixe, O., Yarovoi, S. V., Zerroqui, A., Mouawad, R., Poynard, T., Opolon, P., Khayat, D., Soubrane, C., Gene transfer in hepatocarcinoma cell lines: *in vitro* optimization of a virus-free system, *Gene Ther.,* 3, 483–490, 1996.

Gilboa, E., Smith, C., Gene therapy for infectious diseases: the AIDS model, *TIG,* 10, 139–144, April 1994.

Gluck, R., Combined vaccines — the European contribution, *Biologicals,* 22, 347–351, 1994.

Goldspiel, B. R., Green, L., Calis, K. A., Human gene therapy, *Clin. Pharmacol.,* 12, 488–505, 1993.

Gossen, M., Bujard, H., Tight control of gene expression in mammalian cells by tetracycline-responsive promoters, *Proc. Natl. Acad. Sci. U.S.A.,* 89, 5547–5551, 1992.

Goyal, K., Huang, L., Gene therapy using DC-Chol liposomes, *J. Liposome Res.,* 5, 49–60, 1995.

Grill, L. K., TMV as a gene expression system, *Agro-Food-Ind-High Tech.,* Nov./Dec., 20–23, 1993.

Guo, L. S. S., Radhakrishnan, R., Man, M., The contribution of cationic derivatives of phospholipids and cholesterol to the bioadhesiveness of liposomes and their transfection performance, in *Liposomes: From Gene Therapy to Diagnostics and Ecology,* Lasic, D. D., Barenholz, Y., Eds., CRC Press, Boca Raton, FL, 1996, 67–76.

Gura, T., Antisense has growing pains, *Science,* 270, 575–578, 1995.

Gustaffson, J., Almgrem, M., Arvidson, G., A cryoTEM study of cationic liposomes used for transfection, in *Liposomes, Nineties and Beyond, Book of Abstracts,* No. 82, Gregoriadis, G., Florence, A., Eds., London, 1993.

Gustaffson, J., Almgrem, M., Karlsson, G., Arvidson, G., Complexes between cationic liposomes and DNA visualized by cryoTEM, *Biochim. Biophys. Acta,* 1235, 305–317, 1995.

Guy-Caffey, J. K., Bodepudi, V., Bishop, J., Jayaraman, K., Chaudhary, N., Novel polyaminolipids enhance the cellular uptake of oligonucleotides, *J. Biol. Chem.,* 270, 31,391–31,396, 1995.

Haensler, J., Szoka, F. C., Polyamidoamine cascade polymers mediate efficient transfection of cell in culture, *Bioconjug. Chem.,* 4, 372–379, 1993.

Hannun, Y., Loomis, C. R., Merrill, A. H., Bell, R. M., Sphingosine inhibition of protein kinase C activity and of phorbol dibutyrate binding *in vitro* and in human platelets, *J. Biol. Chem.,* 261, 12604–12609, 1986.

Hansen, S. E., That amazing genetic code: unraveling DNA and RNA. Lecture notes: National Society for Histotechnology, Buffalo, NY, Oct. 1995.

Hara, T., Kuwasawa, H., Aramaki, Y., Takada, S., Koike, K., Ishidate, K., Kato, H., Tsuchiya, S., Effects of fusogenic and DNA-binding amphiphilic compounds on the receptor-mediated gene transfer into hepatic cells by asialoletuin-labeled liposomes, *Biochim. Biophys. Acta,* 1278, 51–58, 1996.

Harding, S. E., On the hydrodynamic analysis of macromolecular conformation, *Biophys. Chem.,* 55, 69–93, 1995.

Hazinski, T. A., Ladd, P. A., DeMateo, C. A., Localization and induced expression of fusion genes in the rat lung, *Am. J. Resp. Cell. Mol. Biol.,* 2, 206–209, 1991.

Helene, C., Toulme, J. J., Specific regulation of gene expression by antisense, sense and antigene nucleic acids, *Biochim. Biophys. Acta,* 1049, 99–125, 1990.

Hershey, A. D., Burgi, E., Molecular homogeneity of the DNA of phage T2, *J. Mol. Biol.,* 2, 143–152, 1960.

Hoffman, R. M., Margolis, L. B., Bergelson, L. D., Binding and entrapment of high molecular weight DNA by lecithin liposomes, *FEBS Lett.,* 93, 365–368, 1978.

Hofland, H. E., Shephard, L., Sullivan, S. M., Formation of stable cationic lipid/DNA complexes for gene transfer, *Proc. Natl. Acad. Sci. U.S.A.,* 93, 7305–7309, 1996.

Holmes, B., Message in a genome?, *New Scientist,* 30–34, Aug. 30, 1995.

Horn, N. A., Meek, J. A., Budahazi, G., Marquet, M., Cancer gene therapy using plasmid DNA: purification of DNA for human clinical trials, *Hum. Gene Ther.,* 6, 565–573, 1995.

Huang, L., in *The Fifth Liposome Days, Book of Abstracts,* Hirota, S., Ed., Shizuoka, July 1996.

Huang, S. K., Quinn, Y., Brown, B. D., Newman, M., Dizik, M., Woodle, M. C., Oligonucleotide encapsulated in stealth liposomes as antisense carriers against solid tumors, *Proc. Am. Assoc. Cancer Res.,* 37, 302, (No. 2053), 1996.

Huber, B. E., Austin, E. A., Richards, C. A., Davis, S. T., Good, S. S., Metabolism of 5-fluorocytosine to 5-fluorouracil in human colorectal tumor cells transduced with the cytosine deaminase gene: significant antitumor effects when only a small percentage of tumor cells express cytosine deaminase, *Proc. Natl. Acad. Sci. U.S.A.,* 91, 8302–8306, 1994.

Hughes, J. A., Bennett, C. F., Cook, D. P., Guinosso, C. J., Mirabelli, C., Juliano, C. R., Lipid permeability of 2′-modified derivatives of phosphorothioate oligonucleotides, *J. Pharmacol. Sci.,* 83, 597–600, 1994.

Hughes, J. A., Aronsohn, A. I., Avratskaya, A. V., Juliano, R. L., Evaluation of adjuvants that enhance the effectiveness of antisense oligonucleotides, *Pharmacol. Res.,* 13, 404–410, 1996.

Hurley, L. H., DNA and associated targets for drug design, *J. Med. Chem.*, 32, 2027–2033, 1989.

Huxley, C., Mammalian artificial chromosomes: a new tool for gene therapy, *Gene Ther.*, 1994.

Hyde, S. C., Gill, D. R., Higgins, F. C., MacVinish, L. J., Cuthbert, A. W., Ratcliff, R., Evans, M. J., Colledge, W. H., Correction of the ion transport defect in cystic fibrosis transgenic mice by gene therapy, *Nature*, 362, 250–255, 1993.

Israelachvili, J. N., *Intermolecular and Surface Forces*, Academic Press, New York, 1985.

Jaaskalainen, I., Monkkonen, J., Urtti, A., Oligonucleotide — cationic liposomes interactions. A physicochemical study, *Biochim. Biophys. Acta*, 1195, 115–123, 1994.

Jolly, D., Viral vector systems for gene therapy, *Cancer Gene Ther.*, 1, 51–64, 1994.

Jungerman, E., *Cationic Surfactants, Surfactant Science Series*, Marcel Dekker, New York, 1970.

Kaler, E. W., Murthy, A. K., Rodriguez, B. E., Zaszadinski, J. A. N., Spontaneous vesicle formation in aqueous mixtures of single-tailed surfactants, *Science*, 245, 1371–1374, 1989.

Kamata, H., Yagisawa, H., Takahashi, S., Hirata, H., Amphiphilic peptides enhance the efficiency of liposome mediated DNA transfection, *Nucleic Acids Res.*, 22, 536–537, 1994.

Katchalsky, A., Biophysics and other topics, selected papers, Academic Press, Orlando, FL, 1976.

Kawabata, K., Takakura, Y., Hashida, M., The fate of plasmid DNA after intravenous administration in mice, *Pharmacol. Res.*, 12, 825–830, 1995.

Kellum, R., Schedl, P., A position-effect assay for boundaries of higher order chromatin domains, *Cell*, 64, 941–950, 1991.

Kirpotin, D., Hong, K., Mullah, N., Papahadjopoulos, D., Zalipsky, S., Liposomes with detachable polymer coating: destabilization and fusion of DOPE vesicles triggered by cleavage of surface grafted PEG, *FEBS Lett.*, 388, 115–118, 1996.

Kossel, A., *The Proteins and Histones*, Longmans, Green, London, 1928.

Kriegler, M., Gene transfer, in *Gene Transfer and Expression: A Laboratory Manual*, W. H. Freeman, New York, 1990, 3–81.

Krysan, P. J., Haase, S. B., Calos, M. P., Isolation of human sequences that replicate autonomously in human cells, *Mol. Cell. Biol.*, 9, 1026–1033, 1989.

Kunitake, K., Okahata, Y., A totally synthetic bilayer membranes, *J. Am. Chem. Soc.*, 99, 3860–3861, 1977.

Kunkel, T., DNA replication fidelity, *J. Biol. Chem.*, 267, 18251–18254, 1992.

Laemmli, U. K., Characterization of DNA condensates induced by poly(ethylene oxide) and polylysine, *Proc. Natl. Acad. Sci. U.S.A.*, 72, 4288–4292, 1975.

Lappalainen, K., Urtti, A., Jaaskalainen, I., Syrjanen, K., Syrjanen, S., Cationic liposome mediated delivery of antisense oligonucleotides targeted to HPV 16 E7 mRNA in CaSki cells, *Antiviral Res.*, 23, 119–130, 1994a.

Lappalainen, K., Urtti, A., Soderling, E., Jaaskalainen, I., Syrjanen, K., Syrjanen, S., Cationic liposomes improve stability and intracellular delivery of antisense oligonucleotides into CaSki cells, *Biochim. Biophys. Acta*, 1196, 201–208, 1994b.

Lasic, D. D., Mixed micelles in drug delivery, *Nature*, 355, 279–280, 1992.

Lasic, D. D., *Liposomes: From Physics to Applications*, Elsevier, Amsterdam, 1993a.

Lasic, D. D., On the formation of inorganic colloidal particles, *Bull. Chem. Soc. Jpn.*, 66, 709–713, 1993b.

Lasic, D. D., Sterically stabilized vesicles, *Angew. Ch. Int. Ed. Engl.,* 33, 1785–1799, 1994.

Lasic, D. D., Liposomes in gene therapy, in *Handbook of Nonmedical Applications of Liposomes,* Vol. IV, Lasic, D. D., Barenholz, Y., Eds., From Gene Delivery and Diagnostics to Ecology, CRC Press, Boca Raton, FL, 1996, pp. 1–6.

Lasic, D. D., Doxorubicin in sterically stabilized liposomes, *Nature,* 380, 561–562, 1996.

Lasic, D. D., Liposomes in Gene Therapy, *Chem. Today/Chim. Oggi,* 13–16, April/May 1996.

Lasic, D. D., Barenholz, Y., Eds., *Liposomes: Theory and Basic Science,* CRC Press, Boca Raton, FL, 1995.

Lasic, D. D., Barenholz, Y., Eds., *Liposomes: From Gene Therapy, Diagnostics to Ecology,* CRC Press, Boca Raton, FL, 1996.

Lasic, D. D., Martin, F., Eds., *Stealth Liposomes,* CRC Press, Boca Raton, FL, 1995.

Lasic, D. D., Papahadjopoulos, D., Liposomes revisited, *Science,* 217, 1245–1246, 1995.

Lasic, D. D., Needham, D., The "Stealth" Liposome: a prototypical biomaterial, *Chem. Rev.,* 95, 2601–2628, 1995.

Lasic, D. D., Strey, H., Podgornik, R., Frederik, P. M., Recent developments in medical applications of liposomes: sterically stabilized and cationic liposomes, *5th European Symp. Control. Drug Del., Book of Abstracts,* Nordwijk aan Zee, April 1996, 61–65.

Lasic, D. D., Templeton, N.S., Liposomes in gene therapy, *Adv. Drug Del. Rev.,* 20, 221–266, 1996.

Lasic, D. D., Strey, H., Stuart, M., Podgornik, R., Frederik, P. M., DNA–liposome complex: structure and structure activity relationships, *J. Am. Chem. Soc.,* in press.

LeBret, M., Zimm, B. H. Monte Carlo determination of the distribution of ions about a cylindrical polyelectrolyte, *Biopolymers,* 23, 271–285,

Lee, R. J., Low, P. S., Folate-mediated tumor cell targeting of liposome entrapped doxorubicin *in vitro, Biochim. Biophys. Acta,* 1233, 134–144, 1995.

Lee, R. J., Huang, L., Folate targeted, anionic liposome entrapped polylysine-condensed DNA for tumor cell specific gene transfer, *J. Biol. Chem.,* 271, 8481–8487, 1996.

Lee, Y. C., Binding modes of mammalian hepatic Gal/GalNAc receptors, in *Carbohydrate Recognition in Cellular Function,* Bock, G., Harnett, S., Eds., J. Wiley & Sons, 1989, 80–95.

Leforestier, A., Livolant, F., Supramolecular ordering of DNA in cholesteric liquid crystalline phases: an ultrastructural review, *Biophys. J.,* 65, 56–72, 1996.

Legendre, J. Y., Szoka, F. C., Delivery of plasmid DNA into mammalian cell lines using pH-sensitive liposomes: comparison with cationic liposomes, *Pharmacol. Res.,* 9, 1235–1242, 1992.

Legendre, J. Y., Szoka, F. C., Cyclic amphiphatic peptide-DNA complexes mediate high efficiency transfection of adherent mammalian cells, *Proc. Natl. Acad. Sci. U.S.A.,* 90, 893–897, 1993.

Leonetti, J. P., Machy, P., Degols, G., Leblue, B., Leeserman, L., Antibody-targeted liposomes containing oligodeoxyribonucleotides complementary to viral RNA selectively inhibit viral replication, *Proc. Natl. Acad. Sci. U.S.A.,* 87, 2448–2452, 1990.

Lerman, L. S., A transition to a compact form of DNA in polymer solutions, *Proc. Natl. Acad. Sci. U.S.A.,* 68, 1886–1890, 1971.

Leventis, R., Silvius, J. R., Interactions of mammalian cells with lipid dispersions containing novel metabolizable cationic amphiphiles, *Biochim. Biophys. Acta,* 1023, 124–132, 1990.

Levine, F., Gene therapy, *AJDC,* 147, 1167–1174, 1993.

Levy, M. Y., Barron, L. G., Meyer, K. B., Szoka, F. C., Characterization of plasmid DNA transfer into mouse skeletal muscle: evaluation of uptake mechanism, expression and secretion of gene products into blood, *Gene Ther.,* 3, 201–211, 1996.

Lewis, J. G., Lin, K. Y., Kothavale, A., Flanagan, W., Matteucci, M. D., DePrince, R. B., Mook, R., Hendren, R., Wagner, R. W., A serum resistant cytofectin for cellular delivery of antisense oligonucleotides and plasmid DNA, *Proc. Natl. Acad. Sci. U.S.A.,* 93, 3176–3181, 1996.

Li, L., Hoffman, R. M., The feasibility of targeted selective gene therapy of the hair follicle, *Nature Genet.,* 1, 705–706, 1995.

Li, Y., Dubin, P. L., Havel, H. A., Edwards, S., Dauntzenberg, H., Complex formation between polyelectrolyte and oppositely charged mixed micelles: soluble complexes vs. coacervation, *Langmuir,* 11, 2486–2492, 1995.

Li, Y., Xia, J., Dubin, P. L., Complex formation between polyelectrolyte and oppositely charged mixed micelles, *Macromolecules,* 27, 7049–7055, 1994.

Liang, X., Hartikka, J., Sukhu, L., Manthorpe, M., Hobart, P., Novel, high expressing and antibiotic-controlled plasmid vectors designed for use in gene therapy, *Gene Ther.,* 3, 350–356, 1996.

Lin, M. F., DaVolio, J., Garcia, R., Cationic liposome-mediated incorporation of prostatic acid phosphate protein into human prostate carcinoma cells, *Biochem. Biophys. Res. Commun.,* 192, 413–419, 1993.

Lindsay, S. M., Lee, S. A., Powell, J. W., Weilich, T., Demarco, C., Luwen, G. D., Tao, N. J., Rupreht, A., The origin of the A to B transition in DNA fibers and films, *Biopolymers,* 27, 1015–1043, 1988.

Litzinger, D. C., Brown, J. F., Wala, I., Kaufman, S., Van, G., Farrell, C., Collins, D., Fate of cationic liposomes and their complex with oligonucleotide *in vivo,* *Biochim. Biophys. Acta,* 1281, 139–149, 1996.

Liu, Y., Liggit, D., Zhou, N., Gaensler, K., Debs, R., Cationic liposome mediated intravenous gene delivery, *J. Biol. Chem.,* 270, 24864–24870, 1995.

Livolant, F., Levelut, A. M., Doucet, J., Benoit, J. P., The highly concentrated liquid crystalline phase of DNA is columnar hexagonal, *Nature,* 339, 724–726, 1989.

Logan, J. J., Bebok, Z., Walker, L. C., Peng, S., Felgner, P. L., Siegal, G. P., Frizzell, R. A., Dong, J., Howard, M., Matalon, S., Lindsay, J. R., DuVall, M., Soecher, E. J., Cationic lipids for reporter gene and CFTR transfer to rat pulmonary epithelium, *Gene Ther.,* 2, 38–49, 1995.

Lurquin, P. F., Incorporation of genetic material into cell liposomes and transfer to cells, in *Liposome Technology II,* Gregoriadis, G., Ed., CRC Press, Boca Raton, FL, 1993, 129–140.

Mahato, R. I., Kawabata, K., Nomura, T., Takakura, Y., Hashida, M., Physicochemical and pharamacokinetic characteristics of plasmid/DNA cationic liposome complexes, J. Pharmacol. Sci., 84, 7–1271, 1995.

Malone, R. W., mRNA transfection of cultured eukaryotic cells and embryos using cationic liposomes, *Focus,* 11, 62–66, 1989.

Malone, R. W., Toxicology of nonviral gene transfer, in *Nonviral Genetic Therapeutics, Book of Abstracts,* International Business Commun., Boston, June 1996.

Malone, R. W., Felgner, P., Verma, I. M., Cationic liposome-mediated RNA transfection, *Proc. Natl. Acad. Sci. U.S.A.*, 88, 6077–6081, 1989.

Manning, G. S., The molecular theory of polyelectrolyte solutions with applications to the electrostatic properties of polynucleotides, *Q. Rev. Biophys.*, 11, 179–246, 1978.

Marr, J. J., Ribozymes as therapeutic agents, *Drug Discovery Today*, 1, 94–102, 1996.

Marsh, D., *Handbook of Lipid Bilayers*, CRC Press, Boca Raton, FL, 1990, 81.

Martin, F. J., MacDonald, R. C., Lipid vesicle–cell interactions, I–III, *J. Cell. Biol.*, 70, 506–526, 1976.

Masuda, Y., Kobayashi, H., Holland, J. F., Ohnuma, T., Reversal of multidrug resistance by a liposome–MDR1 ribozyme complex, *Proc. Am. Assoc. Cancer Res.*, 37, 353 (abst. 2412), 1996.

McQuigg, D. W., Kaplan, J., Dubin, P. L., Critical conditions for binding of polyelectrolytes to small oppositely charged micelles, *J. Phys. Chem.*, 96, 1973–1978, 1992.

Melnikov, S. M., Sergeyev, V., Yoshikawa, K., Discrete coil-globule transition of large DNA induced by cationic surfactant, *J. Am. Chem. Soc.*, 117, 2401–2408, 1995.

McRorie, D., Lasic, D. D., Analytical ultracentrification of anionic and cation genosomes, unpublished.

Meyer, K. B., Thompson, M. M., Levy, M. Y., Barron, L. G., Szoka, F. C., Intratracheal gene delivery to the mouse airway, *Gene Ther.*, 2, 450–460, 1995.

Meyer, O., Kirpotin, D., Hong, K., Woodle, M. C., Papahadjopoulos, D., New liposome formulations of antisense oligonucleotides as efficient delivery systems in cancer therapy, *Proc. Am. Assoc. Cancer Res.*, 37, 304 (abst. 2070), 1996.

Michael, S. I., Curiel, D. T., Strategies to achieve targeted gene delivery via the receptor-mediated endocytosis pathway, *Gene Ther.*, 1, 223–232, 1994.

Middleton, P. G., Caplen, N. J., Gao, X., Huang, L., Gaya, H., Geddes, D. M., Alton, E. W. F. W., Nasal application of cationic liposome Dc-Chol:DOPE does not alter ion transport, lung functions or bacterial growth, *Eur. Respir. J.*, 7, 442–445, 1994.

Miller, A. D., Human gene therapy comes of age, *Nature*, 357, 455–460, 1992.

Miller, N., Vile, R., Targeted vectors for gene therapy, *FASEB J.*, 9, 190–199, 1995.

Minsky, A., Ghirlando, R., Gerhson, H., Structural features of DNA–cationic liposome complexes and their implication for transfection, in *Liposomes: From Gene Therapy to Diagnostics and Ecology*, Lasic, D. D., Barenholz, Y., Eds., CRC Press, Boca Raton, FL, 1996.

Miralles, V. J., Cortes, P., Stone, N., Reinberg, D., The adenovirus inverted terminal repeat functions as an enhancer in a cell-free system, *J. Biol. Chem.*, 264, 10763–10772, 1989.

Monsigny, M., Roche, A. C., Midoux, P., Mayer, R., Glycoconjugates as carriers for specific delivery of therapeutic drugs and genes, *Adv. Drug Del. Rev.*, 14, 1–24, 1994.

Morishita, R., Gibbons, G., Kaneda, Y., Ogihara, T., Dzau, V. J., Novel and effective gene transfer technique for study of vascular renin angiotensin system, *J. Clin. Invest.*, 91, 2580–2585, 1993.

Mulligan, R. C., The basic science of gene therapy, *Science*, 260, 926–932, 1993.

Nabel, E. B., Plautz, G., Nabel, G. J., Site specific gene expression *in vivo* by direct gene transfer into arterial walls, *Science*, 249, 1285–1288, 1990.

Nabel, E. G., Gordon, D., Yang, Z.-Y., Xu, L., San, H., Plautz, G. E., Wu, B.-Y., Gao, X., Huang, L., Nabel, G. J., Gene transfer *in vivo* with DNA-liposome complexes: lack of autoimmunity and gonadal localization, *Hum. Gene Ther.*, 3, 649–656, 1992.

Nabel, E. G., Yang, Z., Muller, D., Chang, A. E., Gao, X., Huang, L., Cho, K., Nabel, G. J., Safety and toxicity of cathethe gene delivery to the pulmonary vasculature in a patient with metastatic melanoma, *Hum. Gene Ther.*, 5, 1089–1094, 1994.

Nabel, G. J., Chang, A., Nabel, E. G., Plautz, G., Fox, B. A., Huang, L., Shu, S., Immunotherapy of malignancy by *in vivo* gene transfer into tumors, *Hum. Gene Ther.*, 3, 399–410, 1992.

Nabel, G. J., Nabel, E. G., Yang, Z.-Y., Fox, B. A., Plautz, G. E., Gao, X., Huang, L., Shu, S., Gordon, D., Chang, A. E., Direct gene transfer with DNA-liposome complexes in melanoma: expression, biologic activity, and lack of toxicity in humans, *Proc. Natl. Acad. Sci. U.S.A.*, 90, 11307–11311, 1993.

Nair, S., Zhou, X., Huang, L., Rouse, B. T., *J. Immunol. Meth.*, 152, 237–243, 1992.

Neidle, S., *DNA Structure and Recognition*, IRL Press, 1995.

Nicolau, C., Cudd, A., Liposomes as carriers of DNA, *Crit. Rev. Ther. Drug Carrier Sys.*, 6, 239–271, 1989.

Olins, D. E., Olins, A. L., Model Nucleohistones: the interaction of F1 and F2a1 histones with native T7 DNA, *J. Mol. Biol.*, 57, 437–455, 1971.

Olmstedt, M., Anderson, C., Record, T. M., Monte Carlo description of oligoelectrolyte properties of DNA oligomers, *Proc. Natl. Acad. Sci. U.S.A.*, 86, 7766–7700, 1989.

Ono, T., Fuyimo, J. T., Tschiya, T., Tsuda, M., Plasmid DNAs directly injected into mice brain with lipofectin can be incorporated and expressed by brain cells, *Neurosci. Lett.*, 117, 259–263, 1990.

Pansu, R., Arrio, B., Rocin, J., Faure, J., Vesicles vs. membrane fragments in DODAC suspensions, *J. Phys. Chem.*, 94, 796–801, 1990.

Parente, R. A., Nadasdi, L., Subbarao, N. K., Szoka, F. C., Association of pH sensitive peptide with membrane vesicles: role of amino acid sequence, *Biochemistry*, 29, 8713–8719, 1990a.

Parente, R. A., Nir, S., Szoka, F. C., Mechanism of leakage of phospholipid vesicle contents induced by the peptide GALA, *Biochemistry*, 29, 8720–8728, 1990b.

Philip, R., Brunette, E., Kilinski, L., Muregesh, D., McNally, M., Ucar, K., Rosenblatt, J., Okarma, T., Lebkowski, J. S., Efficient and sustained gene expression in primary T lymphocytes and primary and cultured tumor cells mediated by adeno-associated virus plasmid DNA complexed to cationic liposomes, *Mol. Cell Biol.*, 14, 2411–2418, 1994.

Pinnaduwage, P., Schmitt, L., Huang, L., Use of quaternary ammonium detergent in liposome mediated DNA transfection of mouse L-cells, *Biochim. Biophys. Acta*, 985, 33–37, 1989.

Plank, C., Mechtler, K., Szoka, F. C., Wagner, E., Activation of the complement system by synthetic DNA complexes: a potential barrier for intravenous gene delivery, *Hum. Gene Ther.*, 7, in press.

Plautz, G. E., Yang, Z. Y., Wu, B. J., Gao, X., Huang, L., Nabel, G. J., Immunotherapy of malignancy by *in vivo* gene transfer into tumors, *Proc. Natl. Acad. Sci. U.S.A.*, 90, 4645–4649, 1993.

Podgornik, R., Jonsson, B., Stretching of polyelectrolyte chains by oppositely charged aggregates, *Europhys. Lett.*, 24, 501–506, 1993.

Podgornik, R., Rau, D. C., Parsegian, V. A., Parametrization of direct and soft steric undulatory forces between DNA double helical polyelectrolytes in solutions of several different anions and cations, *Biophys. J.,* 66, 962–971, 1994.

Podgornik, R., Strey, H. H., Rau, D. C., Parsegian, V. A., Watching molecules crowd: DNA double helices under osmotic stress, *Biophys. Chem.,* 57, 111–121, 1995.

Raz, E., Carson, D. A., Rhodes, G. A., Abai, A., Tsai, Y., Wheeler, C., Morrow, J., Felgner, P. L., Baird, S. M., Cationic lipids inhibit intradermal genetic vaccination, in *Vaccines 94,* Cold Spring Harbor Laboratory Press, p. 71–75.

Reich, Z., Ghirlanod, R., Minsky, A., Secondary conformational polymorphism of nucleic acids as a possible functional link between cellular parameters and DNA packaging process, *Biochemistry,* 30, 7828–7836, 1991.

Reich, Z., Wachtel, E. J., Minsky, A., Liquid crystalline mesophases of plasmid DNA in bacteria, *Science,* 264, 1460–1462, 1994.

Reimer, D. L., Zhang, Y., Kong, S., Wheeler, J. J., Graham, R. W., Bally, M. B., Formation of novel hydrophobic complexes between lipids and plasmid DNA, *Biochemistry,* 34, 12,877–12,883, 1995.

Remy, J. S., Sirlin, C., Vierling, P., Behr, J. P., Gene transfer with series of lipophilic DNA-binding molecules, *Bioconjug. Chem.,* 5, 647–654, 1994.

Remy, J. S., Kichler, A., Mordovinov, V., Schuber, F., Behr, J. P., Targeted gene transfer into hepatoma cells with lipopolyamine-condensed DNA particles presenting galactose ligands: a stage towards artificial viruses, *Proc. Natl. Acad. Sci. U.S.A.,* 92, 1744–1748, 1995.

Roessler, B. J., Davidson, B. L., Direct plasmid mediated transfection of adult micrine brain cells *in vivo* using cationic liposomes, *Neurosci. Lett.,* 167, 5–10, 1994.

Ropert, C., Malvy, C., Couvreur, P., Inhibition of the Frien retrovirus by antisense oligonucleotides encapsulated in liposomes: mechanism of action, *Pharmacol. Res.,* 10, 1427–1433, 1993.

Rosengarten, O., Horowitz, A. T., Tzemach, D., Huang, L., Gabizon, A., *In vitro* cytotoxicity and pharmacokinetics of cationic liposomes in mice, Abstract from the American Cancer Society Meeting, San Diego, CA, Oct. 1994 (abst. in press in *Cancer Gene Ther.*).

Rosenkranz, A. A., Yachmenev, S. V., Jans, D. A., Serebryakova, N. V., Murav'ev, V. I., Peters, R., Sobolev, A. S., Receptor-mediated endocytosis and nuclear transport of a transfecting DNA construct, *Exp. Cell Res.,* 199, 323–329, 1992.

San, H., Yang, Z., Pompili, V., Jaffe, M., Plautz, G., Xu, L., Felgner, J., Wheeler, C., Felgner, P., Gao, X., Huang, L., Gordon, D., Nabel, G., Nabel, E. G., Safety and short term toxicity of a novel cationic lipid formulation for human gene therapy, *Hum. Gene Ther.,* 4, 781–788, 1993.

Schaack, J., Ho, W. Y.-W., Freimuth, P., Shenk, T., Adenovirus terminal protein mediates both nuclear matrix association and efficient transcription of adenovirus DNA, *Genes Devel.,* 4, 1197–1208, 1990.

Schenborn, E., Oler, J., Goiffon, V., Balasubramaniam, R. P., Bennet, M. J., Aberle, A. M., Nantz, M. H., Malone, R. W., Transfection: TFX reagent: a new transfection reagent for eukaryotic cells, *ProMega Notes,* 52, 12–17, 1995.

Schlick, T., Olson, W. K., Trefoil knotting revealed by molecular dynamics simulations of supercoiled DNA, *Science,* 257, 1110–1115, 1992.

Schmitz, K. S., *Macroions in Solution and Colloidal Suspension,* VCH Publishers, New York, 1993.

Schmutz, M., Brisson, A., Liposome polymorphism visualized by cryo electron microscopy, *Proc. 13th International Congress on Electron Microscopy,* Vol. 3B, Jouffray, B., Colliex, C., Eds., ICEM, Paris, 1994, 731–732.

Schreier, H., The new frontier: gene and oligonucleotide therapy, *Acta Pharm. Helv.,* 68, 145–163, 1994.

Schreier, H., Sawyer, S. M., Liposomal DNA vectors for cystic fibrosis gene therapy. Current applications, limitations, and future directions, *Adv. Drug Del. Rev.,* 19, 73–87, 1996.

Schwartz, B., Benoist, C., Abdallah, B., Scherman, D., Behr, J. P., Demeneix, B. A., Lipo-spermine based gene transfer into the newborn mouse brain is optimized by a low lipospermine/DNA charge ratio, *Hum. Gene Ther.,* 6, 1515–1524, 1995.

Seibel, G. L., Singh, U. C., Kollman, P. A., A molecular dynamics simulation of double helical B DNA including counterions and water, *Proc. Natl. Acad. Sci. U.S.A.,* 82, 6537–6540, 1985.

Senior, J. H., Trimble, K. R., Maskiewitz, R., Interaction of positively charged liposomes with blood, *Biochim. Biophys. Acta,* 1070, 163–172, 1991.

Service, R. F., Dendrimers: dream molecules approach real applications, *Science,* 267, 458–459, 1995.

Service, R. F., Just how old is that DNA anyway?, *Science,* 272, 810, 1996.

Shao, Z., Yang, J., Progress in high resolution atomic force microscopy in biology, *Q. Rev. Biophys.,* 28(2), 295–321, 1995.

Smith, J. G., Walzem, R. M., German, B. J., Liposomes as agents of DNA transfer, *Biochim. Biophys. Acta,* 1154, 327–340, 1993.

Smithies, O., Gregg, R. G., Boggs, S. S., Koralewski, M. A., Kucherlapati, R. S., Insertion of DNA sequences into the human chromosomal beta-globin locus by homologous recombination, *Nature,* 317, 230–234, 1985.

Solodin, I., Brown, C. S., Bruno, M. S., Chow, C. Y., Jang, E. H., Debs, R. J., Heath, T. D., A novel series of amphiphilic imidazolinium compounds for in vitro and in vivo gene delivery, *Biochemistry,* 34, 13,537–13,544, 1995.

Soriano, P., Dijkstra, J., Legrand, A., Spanjer, H., Londos, D., Roerdink, F., Scherphoff, G., Nicolau, C., Targeted and nontargeted liposomes for *in vivo* transfer to rat liver cells of a plasmid containing the preproinsulin I gene, *Proc. Natl. Acad. Sci. U.S.A.,* 80, 7128–7131, 1983.

Sternberg, B., Sorgi, F., Huang, L., New structures in complex formation between DNA and cationic liposomes visualized by freeze-fracture electron microscopy, *FEBS Lett.,* 356, 361–366, 1994.

Sternberg, B., Liposomes as model for membrane structures and structural transformations, in *Handbook of Nonmedical Applications of Liposomes,* Vol. IV, Lasic, D. D., Barenholz, Y., Eds., From Gene Delivery and Diagnostics to Ecology, CRC Press, Boca Raton, FL, 1996, pp. 271–298.

Stewart, M., K., Plautz, G., Buono, L., Yang, Z., Xu, L., Gao, X., Huang, L., Nabel, E. G., Nabel, G. J., Gene transfer *in vivo* with DNA-lipid complexes: safety and acute toxicity in mice, *Hum. Gene Ther.,* 3, 267–275, 1992.

Strauss, J., Maher, J. L., DNA bending by asymmetric phosphate neutralization, *Science,* 266, 1929–1934, 1995.

Stribling, R., Brunette, E., Liggit, D., Gaensler, K., Debs, R., Aerosol gene delivery *in vivo, Proc. Natl. Acad. Sci. U.S.A.,* 89, 11,277–11,281, 1992.

Strick, T. R., Allemand, J. F., Bensimon, D., Bensimon, A., Croquette, V., The elasticity of a single supercoiled DNA molecules, *Science,* 271, 1835–1837, 1996.

Sun, W. H., Burkholder, J. K., Sun, J., Culp, J., Turner, J., Lu, X. G., Pugh, T. D., Ershler, W. B., Yang, N. S., *In vivo* cytokine gene transfer by gene gun reduces tumor growth in mice, *Proc. Natl. Acad. Sci. U.S.A.*, 92, 2889–2893, 1995.

Symons, R. H., Ribozymes, *Curr. Op. Struct. Biol.*, 4, 322–420, 1994.

Tai, I. T., Sun, A. M., Microencapsulation of recombinant cells: a new delivery system for gene therapy, *FASEB J.*, 7, 1061–1069, 1993.

Tang, M., Redemann, C. T., Szoka, F. C., *In vitro* gene delivery by polyamido-amine branched polymers, in *Artificial Self-Assembling Systems for Gene Transfer, Book of Abstracts*, CHI, Boston, 1995.

Tari, A. M., Tucker, S. D., Deisseroth, A., Lopez-Berestein, G., Liposomal delivery of methylphosphonate antisense oligonucleotides in chronic myelogenous leukemia, *Blood*, 84, 601–607, 1994.

Templeton, S. N., Lasic, D. D., Roberts, D. D., Frederik, P. M., Pavlakis, G., Novel DNA:liposome complexes for increased systemic delivery and gene expression, submitted.

Templeton, S. N., Pavlakis, G., Roberts, D. D., Strey, H., Jin, Y., Szebeni, J., Benarsky, M., Frederik, P. M., Lasic, D. D., in preparation.

Templeton, N. S., Roberts, D. D., Schloss, D. J., Safer, B., High absolute frequency of homologous recombination in mouse embryonic stem cells, *J. Biol. Chem.*, submitted.

Thalberg, K., Lindman, B., Polyelectrolyte — ionic surfactant systems: phase behavior and interactions, in *Surfactants in Solution*, Mittal, K., Shah, D. O., Eds. Plenum Press, New York, 243–260, 1991.

Thierry, A. R., Dritschillo, A., Intracellular availabilty of unmodified, phospho-rothioated and liposomally encapsulated oligonucleotides for antisense activity, *Nucleic Acids Res.*, 20, 5691–5698, 1992.

Thierry, A. R., Rahman, A., Dritschillo, A., Overcoming MDR in human tumor cell lines using free and liposomally encapsulated antisense oligonucleotides, *Biochem. Biophys. Res. Commun.*, 190, 951–960, 1993.

Thierry, A. R., Iskandar, Y. L., Bryant, J., Rabinovich, P., Gallo, R. C., Mahan, L. C., Systemic gene therapy: biodistribution and long-term expression of a transgenic mice, *Proc. Natl. Acad. Sci. U.S.A.*, 92, 9742–9746, 1995.

Tomita, N., Morishita, R., Higaki, Tomita, S., Aoki, M., Ogihara, T., Kaneda, Y., *In vivo* gene transfer of insulin gene into neonatal rats by the HVJ-liposome method resulted in sustained transgene expression, *Gene Ther.*, 3, 477–482, 1996.

Tomlinson, E., Controllable gene therapy using non-viral systems, in *Artificial Self-Assembling Systems for Gene Transfer, Book of Abstracts*, CHI, Boston, 1995.

Trifonov, E. N., DNA in profile, *TIBS*, 16, 467–470, 1991.

Trewavas, A., A new method for counting labeled nucleic acids by scintillation, *Anal. Biochem.*, 21, 324–329, 1967.

Tseng, W., Purvis, N. B., Haselton, F., Giorgio, T. D., Cationic liposomal delivery of plasmid to endothelial cells measured by quantitative flow cytometry, *Biotechnol. Bioeng.*, 50, 548–554, 1996.

Tsukamoto, M., Ochiya, T., Yoshida, S., Sugimura, T., Terada, M., Gene transfer and expression in progeny after intravenous DNA injection into pregnant mice, *Nature Genet.*, 9, 243–248, 1995.

Ulmer, J. B., Donnelly, J. J., Parher, S., Rhodes, G., Felgner, P., Dwarki, V., Gromkowski, S. H., Deck, R., DeWitt, C. M., Friedman, A., Hawe, L., Leander, K., Martinez, D., Perry, H., Shiver, J., Montgomery, D. L., Liu, M. A., Heterologous protection against influenza by injection of DNA encoding a viral protein, *Science*, 259, 1745–1749, 1993.

Uster, P. S., Allen, T. M., Daniel, B. E., Mendez, C. J., Newman, Zhu, G., Insertion of PEG derivatized phospholipid into pre-formed liposomes results in the prolongation of blood circulation time, *FEBS Lett.,* 386, 243–246, 1996.

Venanzi, F. M., Zhdanov, R., Petrelli, C., Moretti, P., Amici, A., Petrelli, F., Entrapment of supercoiled DNA into preformed amphiphilic lipid vesicles, in *Liposomes, Nineties and Beyond, Book of Abstracts,* Nos. 122 and 123, Gregoriadis, G., Florence, A., Eds., London, 1993.

Vieweg, J., Boczkowski, D., Robertson, K., Edwards, D., Philip, M., Philip, R., Rudoll, T., Smith, C., Robertson, C., Gilboa, E., Efficient gene transfer with adeno associated virus based plasmids complexed to cationic liposomes for gene therapy of human prostate cancer, *Cancer Res.,* 55, 2366–2372, 1995.

Ville, R. G., Gene therapy for treating cancer–hope or hype?, *Chem. Ind.,* 285–289, 1996 (April 15).

Verwey, E. J., Overbeek, J. Th. G., The Theory of Stability of Lyophobic Colloids, Elsevier, Amsterdam, 1948.

Wagner, E., Zenke, M., Cotten, M., Beug, H., Birnsteil, M. L., Transferrin-polycation conjugates as carriers for DNA uptake into cells, *Proc. Natl. Acad. Sci. U.S.A.,* 87, 3410–3414, 1990.

Wagner, E., Plank, C., Zatloukal, C., Cotten, M., Birnsteil, M. L., Influenza virus hemagglutinin HA 2N terminal peptides augment gene transfer by transferrin-polylysine-DNA complexes: toward a synthetic virus-like gene transfer vehicle, *Proc. Natl. Acad. Sci. U.S.A.,* 89, 7934–7938, 1992.

Wagner, R. W., Gene inhibition using antisense oligonucleotides, *Nature,* 372, 333–335, 1994.

Walker, C., Selby, M., Erickson, A., Cataldo, V., Valesi, J. P., Nest, G. V., *Proc. Natl. Acad. Sci. U.S.A.,* 89, 7915–7918, 1992.

Wang, S., Lee, R. J., Cauchon, G., Gorenstein, D. G., Low, P. S., Delivery of antisense oligodeoxyribonucleotides against the human epidermal growth factor receptor into cultured KB cells with liposomes conjugate to folate via polyethyelene glycol, *Proc. Natl. Acad. Sci. U.S.A.,* 92, 3318–3322, 1995.

Wang, Y., O'Malley, B. W., Tsai, S. Y., O'Malley, B. W., A regulatory system for use in gene transfer, *Proc. Natl. Acad. Sci. U.S.A.,* 91, 8180–8184, 1994.

Wasan, E. K., Reimer, D. L., Bally, M. B., Plasmid DNA is protected against ultrasonic cavitation induced damage when complexed to cationic liposomes, *J. Pharm. Sci.,* 85, 427–433, 1996.

Weber, M., Moller, K., Welzcak, M., Schorr, J., Effects of lipopolysaccharide on transfection efficiency in eukaryotic cells, *BioTechniques,* 19, 930–939, 1995.

Wheeler, C. J., Sukhu, L., Yang, G., Tsai, Y., Bustamante, C., Felgner, P., Norman, J., Manthorpe, M., Converting an alcohol to an amine in a cationic lipid dramatically alters the co-lipid requirement, cellular transfection activity and the ultrastructure of DNA-cytofectin complexes, *Biochim. Biophys. Acta,* 1280, 1–11, 1996.

Willems, L., Portetelle, D., Kerkhofs, P., Chen, G., Burny, A., Mammerickx, M., Kettmann, R., *In vivo* transfection of bovine leukemia provirus into sheep, *Virology,* 189, 775–777, 1992.

Williams, S. A., Herbst, T., Chang, L., Seth, T., Cairo, M. S., Cationic lipid delivery speeds internalization of c-*myc* antisense oligonucleotides: anti CD 77 and nested PCR to monitor *ex vivo* purging of Burkitt's lymphoma, *Proc. Am. Assoc. Cancer Res.,* 37, 353 (No. 2408), 1996.

Winterhalter, M., Helfrich, W., Bending elasticity of electrically charged bilayers, coupled monolayers, neutral surfaces, and balancing stresses, *J. Phys. Chem.*, 96, 327–334, 1992.

Winterhalter, M., Lasic, D. D., Liposome stability and formation: experimental parameters and theories on size distribution, *Chem.Phys. Lipids*, 64, 35–43, 1993.

Wolff, J. A., Malone, R. W., Williams, P., Chong, W., Acsadi, G., Jani, G., Felgner, P. L., Direct gene transfer into mouse muscle *in vivo*, *Science*, 247, 1465–1468, 1990.

Wollfe, A. P., Genetic effects of DNA packaging, *Sci. Am. Sci. Med.*, 2, 68–77, 1995.

Wong, F. M. P., Reimer, D. L., Bally, M. B., Cationic lipid binding to DNA: characterization of complex formation, *Biochemistry*, 35, 5756–5763, 1996.

Woude, I. van den, Visser, H. W., ter Beest, M. B. A., Wagenaar, A., Ruiters, M. H. J., Engberts, J. B. F. N., Hoekstra, D., Parameters influencing the introduction of plasmid DNA into cells by the use of synthetic amphiphiles as a carrier system, *Biochim. Biophys. Acta*, 1240, 34–40, 1995.

Wrobel, I., Collins, D., Fusion of cationic liposomes with mammalian cells occurs after endocytosis, *Biochim. Biophys. Acta*, 1235, 296–304, 1995.

Wu, G. Y., Wu, C. H., Receptor-mediated *in vitro* gene transformation by a soluble DNA carrier system, *J. Biol. Chem.*, 262, 4429–4432, 1987.

Wu, G. Y., Wu, C. H., Delivery systems for gene therapy, *Biotherapy*, 3, 87–95, 1991.

Wu, G. Y., Wilson, J. M., Shalaby, F., Grossman, M., Shafitz, D. A., Wu, C. H., Receptor mediated gene delivery *in vivo*. Partial correction of genetic albuminemia in nagase rats, *J. Biol. Chem.*, 266, 14338–14342, 1991.

Xu, Y., Hui, S. K., Szoka, F. C., Effect of lipid composition and lipid-DNA charge ratios on physical properties and transfection activity of cationic lipid-DNA complexes, *Biophys. J.*, A432, 1995.

Xu, Y., Szoka, F. C., Mechanism of DNA release from cationic liposome/DNA complexes used in cell transfection, *Biochemistry*, 35, 5616–5623, 1996.

Yanagihara, I., Inui, K., Dickson, G., Turner, G., Piper, T., Kaneda, Y., Okada, S., Expression of full length human dystophin cDNA in mdx mouse muscle by HVJ-liposome injection, *Gene Ther.*, 3, 549–553, 1996.

Yang, J. P., Huang, L., Direct gene transfer to mouse melanoma by intratumor injection of free DNA, *Gene Ther.*, 3, 542–548, 1996.

Yang, N. S., De Luna, C., Cheng, L., in *Gene Therapeutics: Methods and Applications of Direct Gene Transfer*, J. A. Wolff, Ed., Birkhäuser, Boston, 193–209, 1994.

Yates, J. L., Warren, N., Sugden, B., Stable replication of plasmids derived from Epstein Barr virus in various mammalian cells, *Nature*, 313, 812–815, 1985.

Yoshikara, E., Nakae, T., Cytolytic activity of liposomes containing stearylamine, *Biochim. Biophys. Acta*, 854, 93–101, 1986.

Yoshikawa, Y., Yoshikawa, K., Diaminoalkanes with an odd number of carbon atoms induce compaction of a single double stranded DNA chain, *FEBS Lett.*, 361, 277–281, 1995.

Zabner, J., Fasbender, A. J., Moninger, T., Poellinger, K. A., Welsh, M., Cellular and molecular barriers to gene transfer by a cationic lipids, *J. Biol. Chem.*, 270, 18,997–19,007, 1995.

Zalipsky, S., Mullah, N., Harding, J., Gittelman, J., Guo, L., Poly(ethylene glycol)-grafted liposomes with oligopeptide or oligosaccharide ligands appended to the terminal of the polymer chains, *Bioconjugate Chem.*, in press.

Zelphati, O., Szoka, F. C., Mechanism of oligonucleotide release from cationic liposomes, *Proc. Natl. Acad. Sci. U.S.A.*, 93, 11,493–11,498, 1996.

Zenke, M., Steinlein, P., Wagner, E., Cotten, M., Beug, H., Birnstiel, M. L., Receptor-mediated endocytosis of transferrin-polycation conjugates: an efficient way to introduce DNA into hematopoietic cells, *Proc. Natl. Acad. Sci. U.S.A.*, 87, 3655–3659, 1990.

Zhang, F., Feketeova, E., Gould-Fogerite, Mannino, R. J., DNA cochleates as mediators of *in vivo* gene expression, in *Artificial Self-Assembling Systems for Gene Transfer, Book of Abstracts,* CHI, Boston, 1995.

Zhou, X., Huang, L., DNA transfection mediated by cationic liposomes containing lipopolylysine: characterization and mechanism of action, *Biochim. Biophys. Acta,* 1189, 195–203, 1989.

Zhu, J., Zhang, L., Hanisch, U. K., Felgner, P. L., Reszka, R., A continuous intracerebral gene delivery system for *in vivo* liposome mediated gene therapy, *Gene Ther.,* 3, 472–476, 1996.

Zhu, N., Liggitt, D., Liu, Y., Debs, R., Systemic gene expression after intravenous DNA delivery in adult mice, *Science,* 261, 209–211, 1993.

APPENDICES

APPENDIX A:
SOME FUNDAMENTAL
CONSTANTS

Speed of light in a vacuum	$c_0 = 2.9979 \times 10^8$ m/s
Electronic charge	$e = 1.6022 \times 10^{-19}$ C
Gravitational acceleration	$g = 9.806$ m/s^2
Gravitational constant	$g = 6.67 \times 10^{-11}$ Nm^2/kg
Planck's constant	$h = 6.6262 \times 10^{-34}$ J s
Boltzmann constant	$k = 1.3806 \times 10^{-23}$ J/K
Electron rest mass	$m_e = 9.1096 \times 10^{-31}$ kg
Proton rest mass	$m_p = 1.6726 \times 10^{-27}$ kg
Atomic mass unit	$m_{au} = 6600 \times 10^{-27}$ kg
Classical electron radius	$r_0 = 2.8179 \times 10^{-15}$ m
Electronvolt	1 eV $= 1.6022 \times 10^{-19}$ J $= 23.06$ kcal/mol $= 39.61$ kT
Temperature associated with 1 eV	1 eV/k $= 11{,}605$ K
Ionization potential of hydrogen atom	13,606 eV
Avogadro's number	$N_a = 6.023 \times 10^{26}$/particles/kmol
Faraday constant	$F = 96{,}486.7$ C/mol
Universal gas constant	$R = 8.3144$ kJ/kmol/K $= 0.082057$ 1 atm/gmol/K $= 1.986$ kcal/kmol/K
Molar volume	$V = 22.4138$, m^3/kmol at 273.15 K, 760 torr
Permeability of vacuum	$\mu_0 = 1.2566 \times 10^{-6}$ H/m
Permittivity of vacuum	$\epsilon_0 = 8.8541 \times 10^{-12}$ F/m
Bohr magneton	$\mu_e = 9.2741 \times 10^{-24}$ J/T
Stefan constant	$\sigma = 5.6703 \times 10^{-8}$ W/m^2/K^4
π	$\pi = 3.1415926$
e	$e = 2.7182818$

APPENDIX B: PERIODIC SYSTEM OF ELEMENTS

Group I	Group II		Transition Elements											Group III	Group IV	Group V	Group VI	Group VII	Group VIII
1 H 1.00797																			2 He 4.0026
3 Li 6.939	4 Be 9.0122													5 B 10.811	6 C 12.01115	7 N 14.0067	8 O 15.9994	9 F 18.9984	10 Ne 20.183
11 Na 22.9898	12 Mg 24.312													13 Al 26.9815	14 Si 28.086	15 P 30.9738	16 S 32.064	17 Cl 35.453	18 Ar 39.948
19 K 39.102	20 Ca 40.08	21 Sc 44.956	22 Ti 47.90	23 V 50.942	24 Cr 51.996	25 Mn 54.9380	26 Fe 55.847	27 Co 58.9332	28 Ni 58.71	29 Cu 63.54	30 Zn 65.37			31 Ga 69.72	32 Ge 72.59	33 As 74.9216	34 Se 78.96	35 Br 79.909	36 Kr 83.80
37 Rb 85.47	38 Sr 87.62	39 Y 88.905	40 Zr 91.22	41 Nb 92.906	42 Mo 95.94	43 Tc (99)	44 Ru 101.07	45 Rh 102.905	46 Pd 106.4	47 Ag 107.870	48 Cd 112.40			49 In 114.82	50 Sn 118.69	51 Sb 121.75	52 Te 127.60	53 I 126.9044	54 Xe 131.30
55 Cs 132.905	56 Ba 137.34	57 La* 138.91	72 Hf 178.49	73 Ta 180.948	74 W 183.85	75 Re 186.2	76 Os 190.2	77 Ir 192.2	78 Pt 195.09	79 Au 196.967	80 Hg 200.59			81 Tl 204.37	82 Pb 207.19	83 Bi 208.980	84 Po (210)	85 At (210)	86 Rn (222)
87 Fr (223)	88 Ra (226)	89 Ac# (227)																	

*Lanthanide Series

58 Ce 140.12	59 Pr 140.907	60 Nd 144.24	61 Pm (147)	62 Sm 150.35	63 Eu 151.96	64 Gd 157.25	65 Tb 158.924	66 Dy 162.50	67 Ho 164.930	68 Er 167.26	69 Tm 168.934	70 Yb 173.04	71 Lu 174.97

#Actinide Series

90 Th 232.038	91 Pa (231)	92 U 238.03	93 Np (237)	94 Pu (242)	95 Am (243)	96 Cm (247)	97 Bk (247)	98 Cf (249)	99 Es (254)	100 Fm (253)	101 Md (256)	102 No (253)	103 Lw (257)

APPENDIX C:
A SHORT TUTORIAL
ON DIFFERENT UNITS

There is a considerable confusion in the units used to describe concentration of DNA and liposomes in the literature. Often I have noticed that some people have trouble converting between various units; therefore, I'll solve few typical problems.

Many researchers list DNA either as $\mu g/ml$ or, in *in vivo* studies, as μg DNA per animal. Because mice are mostly used and injected volumes are 0.2 ml, this concentration is simply multiplied by 5 to get $\mu g/ml$. The data can be best normalized if one defines concentration of DNA in molar charge. For this one has to express DNA as molarity in base pairs. Average molecular weight of a base pair is around 660 Da (g/mol) and one simply has for the concentration of DNA, C_{DNA}

$$C_{DNA}\left(\mu g/ml\right) * 1000 \ ml/l * 0.001 \ g/\mu g/660 \ \left(g/mol\right) =$$

$$C_{DNA}\left(\mu g/ml \ \text{or} \ g/l\right)/660 \ g/mol$$

or, for instance, 1 mg/ml DNA solution is 1.6×10^{-3} M or 1.6 mM in base pairs. Because each base pair has two negative charges this gives 3.2 mM concentration of negative charge.

Liposome concentration is normally given as mM (or $\mu mol/ml$) of cationic lipid. If neutral lipid is present this doubles total lipid concentrations for the most frequently used equimolar compositions. In order to calculate liposome concentration in mg/ml one has to calculate molecular weight of an "average lipid" in liposome. For a single-component liposome, such as DOTAP, this is its molecular weight. For a lipid mixture one calculates average molecular weight from

$$\langle M \rangle = \Sigma_i \ x_i \ M_i$$

where x are mole fractions of constituent lipids and M their respective molecular weight. For instance, for equimolar DOTAP:Chol liposome this is

$$\langle M \rangle = 0.5 * 732 + 0.5 * 386 = 559 \ Da$$

257

Therefore, 1 mM DOTAP:Chol liposome solution is 559×10^{-3} g/l or 0.559 mg/ml. If the concentration refers only to cationic lipid, concentration becomes $(732 + 386)$ g/l (or mg/ml) and this yields 1.118 mg/ml.

To calculate the molar concentration of 1 mg/ml DOTAP solution one gets 1 mg/ml * 1000 ml/l * 0.001 mg/g/732 (g/mol) = 1.37×10^{-3} M. Similarly, 1 mg/ml equimolar DOTAP:DOPE liposome ($\langle M \rangle = 0.5 * 732 + 0.5 * 804 = 768$ Da) is 1.3 mM.

The charge molarity of univalent cationic liposomes equals the molarity of cationic lipid. So, we can see that negative charge density per molecular weight is several times higher for negative charge, so we can roughly estimate that in terms of volume there is also 2 to 5 times more lipid material than DNA for a negative/positive charge ratio = 0.5. For the DOTAP:Chol–DNA system there is one negative charge per approximately 330 Da and one positive charge per 1118 Da.

APPENDIX D: GEOMETRIC PARAMETERS OF LIPIDS AND NUCLEIC ACIDS

Often simple geometric calculations are very useful for various estimations. Here we shall define the very simplest geometry and estimate the number of molecules in various complexes.

We shall treat a liposome as a 4-nm-thick shell. The approximate surface area can be calculated from $2 * 4\pi R^2$ (or if vesicle size, D, is given, as $2\pi D^2$) because it has two surfaces. Surface area is also Na, where N is the number of lipid molecules with cross-sectional area a. For cationic lipids the area is around 0.6 to 0.7 nm^2, for DOPE around 0.55 nm^2; and for cholesterol around 0.4 nm^2. From these two equations one can calculate the number of molecules in a liposome with radius R as

$$N = 8\pi R^2/\langle a \rangle$$

where $\langle a \rangle$ is the average surface area in the case of mixed bilayer (for equimolar DOTAP:DOPE liposomes it would be $0.5 * 0.7 + 0.5 * 0.55 = 0.625$ nm^2, for equimolar DOTAP:Chol analogously 0.55 nm^2, and for plain DOTAP liposomes, of course, 0.7 nm^2).

Now we shall calculate how much DNA (length L) can be adsorbed on a 100-nm liposome. We shall simply take DNA as d = 2.5-nm-thick rod and match the surface areas to calculate the length. From $4\pi R^2 = d * L$ one gets L = 12.56 μm. Knowing that 1 bp is 0.34 nm, we can calculate around 36 kb. It was shown, however, that tightly adsorbed DNA is around 4 to 5 nm apart, so the real number would be more like 23 kb, giving rise to 46,000 negative charges. If we compare the number of charges, we have for DOTAP liposome $4\pi R^2/0.7 = 44,800$ molecules and positive charges. Obviously, only approximately half of the charges are on the bilayer side of the helix, and therefore such a system tends to adsorb another lipid bilayer/liposome.

As another example, let us calculate the number of plasmids (5 kb) and liposomes when 1 ml DNA at 0.5 mg/ml is mixed with 100-nm DOTAP:Chol liposomes at charge ratio $-/+ = 0.5$.

$$0.5 \text{ mg/ml} = 0.5 \text{ g/l} \rightarrow 0.5/660 \text{ (g/mol)} = 8 \times 10^{-4} \text{ M in base pairs}$$

Dividing by 5000 bp/molecule, one gets $8 \times 10^{-4}/5000 = 1.6 \times 10^{-7}$ M plasmid solution. We must mix this with double excess of cationic lipid. Number of negative charges is double the concentration in base pairs (2 phosphates per base pair), i.e., 1.6×10^{-3} M negative charge. We need 3.2×10^{-3} mol of cationic lipid. If we have liposomes at 10 mM we need for 1 ml of 1.6×10^{-3} M negative charge (= 1.6 μmol) 3.2 μmol of cationic lipid. If we have 10 mM solution of DOTAP liposomes (10 μmol/ml), we need 320 μl of this solution.

Now, let us calculate how many plasmids and cationic liposomes (all 100 nm) are in this mixture. Plasmid solution is 1.6×10^{-7} M. We have 1 ml of it and therein there are 1.6×10^{-10} mol of plasmids. Multiplying by 6×10^{23} molecules/mol we get around 10^{14} plasmid molecules.

We have 3.2×10^{-6} mol of cationic lipid. Multiplying by Avogadro's number, 6×10^{23}, we get the number of DOTAP molecules of 2×10^{18}. Each liposome contains double surface area/DOTAP cross-section area molecules, so

$$8\pi(50)^2/0.7 = {\sim}90,000 \text{ molecules}$$

Dividing all molecules with the number of molecules in a 100-nm liposome we get the number of liposomes

$$2 \times 10^{18}/90,000 = 2.2 \times 10^{13}$$

And we see that at this size there are approximately five plasmids per liposome. If liposomes were smaller, 50 nm in diameter, the number of particles and macromolecules would be roughly the same.

This may indicate that theoretically there may be an optimal liposome size for each plasmid length. However, I do not think that it is possible to make single liposome-single plasmid complexes in solutions with nonlimiting concentrations.

APPENDIX E:
ABBREVIATIONS

A: adenine

ADP: adenosin diphosphate

AFM: atomic force microsocpy

AIDS: acquired immunodeficiency syndrome

ATP: adenosin triphosphate

BisHOP: 2,3-dihyexadecyloxyl-propyl-N,N,N-trimethylammonium chloride

C: cytosine

C14GluCN: dimyristoyl N-[p-(2-trimethylammonio ethoxy)]-L-glutamate bromide

$C_{14}GluC_nN^+$: dimyristoyl N-[p-(2-trimethylammonioethoxy)]-ʟ glutamate bromide

C14GluPhCN: dimyristoyl N-[p-(2-trimethylammonio ethoxy)]-benzoyl-L-glutamate bromide

$C_{14}GluPhC_nN^+$: dimyristoyl N-[p-(2-trimethylammonioethoxy)-benzoyl-ʟ glutamate bromide

C8GlySper: octyl-glycyl spermine

$C_8GlySper^{3+}$: octyl-glycyl spermine

$(C18)_2Sper$: distearoyl spermidine

$(C_{18})_2Sper^{3+}$: distearoyl spermine

CAT: chloramphenicol transferase

CEA: carcino embrionic antigen

CF: cystic fibrosis

CFTR: cystic fibrosis transregulatory (protein)

Chol: cholesterol

CMV: cytomegalovirus

CNS: central nervous system

CTAB: cetyl trimethyl ammonium bromide

CTAB/CTAC: cetyl trimethyl ammonium bromide/chloride

CTL: cytotoxic T lymphocytes

DC-Chol: 3β[N-(n′,N′-dimethylaminoethane)-carbamoyl]cholesterol, dioleoyl)

DDAB: dodecylammonium bromide

DEAE: diethylaminoethyl

DLS: dynamic light scattering

DLVO: Derjaguin, Landau, Verwey, Overbeek

DMEPC: dimyristoyl ethyl phosphatidylcholine

DMRIE: dimyristooxypropyl dimethyl hydroxyethyl ammonium bromide

DNA: deoxyribonucleic acid

DODAB/C: dioctadecyl diammonium bromide/chloride

DODAB/DODAC: dioctadecyl dimethyl ammonium bromide/chloride (DO can be also

DODAP: 1, 2-diacyl-3-dimethyl ammonium propane

DOGS: dioctadecyl amido glycyl spermine

DOIC: 1-[2-(oleoyloxy)-ethyl]-2-oleoyl-3-(2-hydroxyethyl) imidazolinium chloride

DOPC: dioleoyl phosphatidylcholine

DOPE: dioleoyl phosphatidylethanolamine

DORIE: dioleoyl oxy propy dimethyl hydroxyethyl ammonium bromide

DOSPA: 2, 3 dioleoyloxy-N-[sperminecarboxamino)ethyl]-N,N-dimethyl-1-propanaminium

DOSPER: 1,3-Di-oleoyloxy-2 (6-carboxy-spermyl)-propylamid {four acetate}

DOTAP: 1, 2-diacyl-3-trimethylammonium propane

DOTMA: [2, 3-bis(oleoyl)propyl] trimethyl ammonium chloride

DPG: cardiolipin

DPPES: dipalmitoyl phosphatidylethanolamyl spermine

DSC: differential scanning calorimetry

DSPC: distearoyl phosphatidyl choline

EDTA: ethylene diamino acetic acid

EM: electron microscopy

ESR: electron spin resonance

FDA: Federal Drug Administration

FTIR: Fourier transfer infrared spectroscopy

G: guanine

GAP-DLRIE: (±)-N-(3-aminopropyl)-N,N-dimethyl-*bis* (dodecyloxy)-1-propanamonium bromide

GC: gas chromatography

GMCSF: granulocyte/macrophage-stimulating factor

GOV: giant oligolamellar vesicle

GTPase: guanosine-5′-triphosphate

GUV: giant unilamellar vesicle

HIV: human immunodeficiency virus

HPLC: high pressure liquid chromatography

HSV: herpes simplex virus

ICAM: intercellular adhesion molecules

IL: interleukin

IRES: internal ribosome entry site

LAK: lymphokine-activated killer cells

LDL: low-density lipoproteins

LMV: large multilamellar vesicle

LPLL: lipophilic polylysine

LUV: large unilamellar vesicle

MDR: multidrug resistance

MHC: major histocompatibility complex

MLV: multilamellar vesicle

MVL: multivesicular liposome

NK: natural killer cells

NMR: nuclear magnetic resonance

OM: optical microscopy

ORI: origin of replication

PC: phosphatidylcholine

PCR: polymerase chain reaction

PCS: photon correlation spectroscopy

PE: phosphatidylethanolamine

PEG: poly(ethylene) glycol

PEG-DSPE: poly(ethylene oxide) distearoyl phosphatidyl ethanolamine

PEI: polyethyline imide

PG: phosphatidyl glycerol

PI: phosphatidyl inositole

PL: phospholipid

PS: phosphatidylserine

RNA: ribodeoxy nucleic acid

RS: Raman spectroscopy

SAXS: small-angle X-ray scattering

SDS: sodium dodecyl sulfate

Sper–Chol: spermine–cholesterol

SUV: small unilamellar vesicle

SV: simian virus

Sv: Svedberg, unit for sedimentation coefficient ($\cong 10^{13}$ s)

T: thymine

TDAB: tetradecylammonium bromide

TE: Tris-EDTA buffer

TIL: tumor-infiltrating lymphocytes

TLC: thin layer chromatography

TMAG: lipophilic esther of glutamic acid
   triflurocetate,

TTAB: tetradecyl ammonium bromide

U: uracil

VEGF: vascular endothelial growth factor

APPENDIX F: GLOSSARY

adeno-associated virus (AAV): a small, nonpathogenic virus used for gene delivery, which cannot replicate without adenovirus or herpes virus.

adenosine deaminase deficiency (ADA): disorder in immune system.

adenovirus: virus of the upper respiratory system used for gene delivery.

allele: different forms of the same gene in identical locations on the chromosome.

amino acids: organic acids containing nitrogen; building blocks of proteins.

amphiphile: molecule which contains "water-loving" (hydrophilic) and "water-hating" (hydrophobic) group on the same molecule. Examples: soaps, detergents, lipids.

antibody: modified soluble protein with a specific amino acid sequence which enables it to react with the antigen that induced its synthesis. Immunoglobulin proteins.

anticodon: a specific sequence of three nucleotides in a transfer RNA, complementary to a codon for an amino acid in mRNA.

antigen: a substance that causes an immune response and induces the formation of antibodies. They may be toxins, foreign proteins, particulates, bacterias, cells.

antiparallel: the 5' and 3' ends are reversed in relation to each other.

antisense: a short stretch of nucleic acids (15 to 25 mer) designed to bind to mRNA and block protein expression.

apoptosis: cell self-programmed death upon a specific stimulus.

bacteria: microscopic unicellular mechanisms.

bacteriophage lambda: virus that infects bacteria. Cloning vectors for DNA studies.

base: in nucleic acids part of the molecule which makes up the informational content.

base pairing: formation of hydrogen bonds between adenine and thymine and guanine and cytosine. In RNA uracil replaces thymine.

bile salts: steroid detergents participating in digestion of lipids.

biodistribution: the distribution of a substance (drug, gene) in the body.

biotechnology: the use of microorganisms, plant, and animal cells to produce medicine, food, and chemicals.

biotin: a small vitamin used to link labels on DNA or lipid molecules via avidin or streptavidin binding.

capsid: the protein coat of a virion or a virus particle.

carbohydrates: essential molecules consisting of carbon, hydrogen, and oxygen.

carcinoma: cancerous tumor covering outer and inner surfaces in the body. It can spread into surrounding tissues and throughout the body.

cationic: positively charged.

cDNA: DNA synthesized *in vitro* from an mRNA template by reverse transcription. Complementary DNAs are important for isolating genes.

chaotropic: structure breaking. Chaotropic agents can lyse membranes and break water structure (H bonds). Examples: guanine, thyocianate, sulfate.

chemotherapy: medical treatment using drugs which act by inhibition of cell growth.

chimeric: composed from parts from two different species (recombinant DNA).

chromatin: complex of genomic DNA and protein.

chromosome: a structure in the cell nucleus containing genes. Carries the inheritable characteristics of an organism.

cloning: laboratory technique to produce multiple copies asexually.

codon: a sequence of three base pairs coding for an amino acid.

colloid: a suspension of microscopic particles in a different phase.

colloidal solution: a suspension/dispersion of small solid, semisolid, or liquid (immiscible) particles (10 nm to 10 μm) in a liquid phase.

condensation: in polyelectrolytes binding of counterions around polymer; in DNA decrease in its size due to tight packing.

cosmotropic: ions which form structured water around them. Examples: chloride, sodium.

cytokine: chemical messenger released by the immune system.

cytosol: the continuous aqueous phase of cytoplasm containing various solutes.

dalton: unit of molecular weight ($\sim 1.6 \times 10^{-24}$ g).

deamination: removal of amino groups in amino acids.

differentiation: biochemical and structural changes by which cells become specialized.

diploid: having two complete sets of chromosomes (in humans 23 pairs, i.e., 46 chromosomes).

DLVO: Derjaguin–Landau–Verwey–Overbeek model of colloid stability. System is stable if electrostatic repulsion is larger than van der Waals attraction.

DNA: deoxyribonucleic acid — molecule which is the substance of heredity.

DNA denaturation: separation of the two strands.

DNA polymerase I: a prokaryotic enzyme capable of synthetizing DNA from the DNA template.

DNA sequencing: a technology used to determine the order of nucleotides.

downstream: sequences further in 3′ direction.

drug delivery system: systems which change pharmacokinetics and biodistribution of drugs in the body. Can be mechanical (pumps, capsules, patches) or particulate, such as liposomes, microspheres, etc.

electrolyte: salt which upon dissociation in water yields cations and anions.

electroporation: the process of using electrical current to transiently open pores in cell membranes.

ELISA: enzyme-linked immunosorbent assay: an assay that detects an antigen–antibody complex via an enzyme reaction.

encapsulation: entrapment of molecules into the liposome interior.

endocytosis: a cellular process which transports extracytoplasmic material into cells.

endosome: a compartment-vacuole in the cell where influxed material is concentrated and broken down by digestive enzymes.

enhancer: a short regulatory DNA sequence which can potentiate the utilization of some promoters resulting in elevated levels of RNA transcription.

enzyme: a protein catalyst which accelerates chemical reactions.

episome: a stretch of DNA which is not incorporated in the chromosome.

Escherichia coli: a common bacteria found in the small intestine of vertebrates.

eukaryote: cells which contain a membrane-surrounded nucleus; includes yeast, higher plants, and mammals.

exon: any segment of an interrupted gene that is represented in the mature mRNA. May or may not be translated.

ex vivo: outside of the body.

free energy: the part of the total energy of a system that can do work at constant pressure and temperature.

fusion: a process in which two membranes merge and the contents are mixed.

fusion protein: membrane protein which facilitates fusion between membranes by insertion into the other one upon a trigger.

gene: a small section of chromosome, a defined segment of DNA which codes for one protein.

gene cloning: isolation and propagation of a gene fragment by insertion into a suitable vector.

gene expression: manifestation of genetic material in the form of a protein or polypeptide.

gene mapping: determination of the relative locations of genes on chromosomes.

gene regulation: control of the synthesis or suppression of gene products.

gene splicing: joining pieces of DNA from different genes.

gene therapy: set of methods for introduction of functional genes into appropriate cells in which the original gene is defective. The gene for protein, not the protein itself, is delivered into the cell.

gene transfection: transfer of DNA onto cytoplasm and cell nucleus.

gene transfer: artificial introduction of foreign genes into recipient cells.

genetic code: genetic repertoire of an organism.

genetic switches: technology which permits turning gene expression on or off.

germ cells: ova and sperm.

glycoprotein: protein containing carbohydrate groups. Surface-located glycoproteins play a role in cell recognition but also include antigens, enzymes, and hormones.

haploid: having half the usual number of chromosomes.

herpes: a large virus which can be used in gene therapy as a vector.

HIV: human immunodeficiency virus which causes AIDS.

human papilloma virus: a virus that causes genital warts and cervical cancer.

hybridization: the formation of hydrogen bonds between two complementary single strands. DNA and RNA probes detect specific sequences.

hydrogen bonding: attraction of protons with electronegative elements.

hydrolysis: reaction with water resulting in the cleaving of a molecule.

hydrophilic: water loving, water soluble.

hydrophobic: water hating, immiscible with water.

immune: protected from disease.

immunogenicity: the ability of a substance to induce antibodies against it.

immunoglobulin: protein of the immune cascade.

immunotherapy: a therapy which stimulates or regulates the immune system to accelerate or inhibit immune response.

insertional mutagenesis: a cancer-causing mutation resulting from an insertion of a gene.

intron: a DNA sequence that interrupts the coding sequences (exons) for a gene product. Introns are spliced out before heterogeneous nuclear RNA is transferred into mature mRNA.

in vitro: reaction in the test tube or petri dish with biological sample.

in vivo: in the body.

knockout mice: animals engineered to lack a specific gene; they can be used to study the function of a gene or the efficacy of various drugs.

ligand: a chemical moiety which interacts with surface receptors. Can be immunoglobulin, part of it, lectin, oligosaccharide, or monosaccharide.

lipid: fatlike molecules. Polar lipids form ordered structures in water which are used to transfect DNA.

lipid bilayer: a thin sheet of ordered lipid molecules organized in two opposed leaflets. The nonpolar part of the molecules is hidden in the plane interior. On the surface are polar heads.

lipid-mediated poration: entry of lipid-associated material into cell cytoplasm due to membrane destabilization and/or creation of transient pores.

lipid monolayer: one leaflet of the bilayer.

liposome: hollow colloidal structure in which lipid bilayer encapsulates part of the solvent.

LMV: large multilamellar vesicle (new terminology).

locus: the position on a chromosome.

LUV: large unilamellar vesicle.

lymphoma: a tumor of lymphoid tissue that is usually cancerous.

lysosome: vacuole in the cell cytoplasm where digestive enzymes are located. Also low pH.

macrophage: a phagocytic cell which circulates in the bloodstream or is fixed in some organs, mostly liver, spleen, and bone marrow, and acts as a first-line defense.

malignant: tumor that is cancerous.

marker: easily detectable genetic variant.

meiosis: nuclear division with daughter cells having only half the original number of chromosomes.

membrane: a thin sheath encapsulating a closed space.

Mendelian inheritance: inheritance patterns, such as dominant or recessive, that apply to single genetic traits.

micelle: a small amphiphilic colloidal particle.

mitosis: a process whereby the cell nucleus divides into two daughter nuclei and cells having the same number of chromosomes.

MLV: large multilamellar vesicle.

molecular genetics: the study of genetic mechanism in favor of the denaturation option whenever possible.

monoclonal antibody: moleule which strongly binds to selective, specific antigen. Single species antibody which are produced by hybridoma.

mRNA (messenger RNA): the ribonucleic acid molecule that transmits the genetic information from genomic DNA to the translation machinery where it directs protein synthesis.

neuroblastoma: cancer made up of primitive tissues from life in the womb. Tumor begins in the nervous system and is most common in the adrenal glands.

neurotoxicity: poisonous to the nervous system.

neutrophils: infection-fighting white blood cells.

nick: a break in a strand of circular double helix.

nick translation: an enzyme method for generating continuously labeled DNA probes.

Northern blotting: a technique for transferring electrophoretically chromatographed RNA from a gel matrix to a filter paper for subsequent immobilization and hybridization.

nucleases: enzymes that cleave nucleic acids.

nucleic acid: DNA or RNA formed by polymerization of nucleotides.

nucleoside: a compound consisting of a purine or pyrimidime base covalently linked to a pentose.

nucleotide: a nucleoside phosphorylated at one of its pentose hydroxyl groups.

oligonucleotide: a short, artificially synthesized single strand of DNA.

oncogene: a gene which may be carried by a virus that affects the normal metabolic control and metabolism causing cancer.

osmolarity: concentration of solutes which gives certain osmotic pressure.

palindrome: a segment of duplex DNA in which the base sequences of the two strands exhibit a twofold symmetry about the central axis. Restriction endonucleases often recognize and cut DNA on different palindromic sites.

pathogen: a microorganism causing disease.

PCR (polymerase chain reaction): a systematic, primer-mediated enzymatic process for the amplification of a target DNA sequence.

In ideal conditions a single DNA molecule can be reassembled into numerous copies.

pentose: a simple sugar whose backbone consists of five C atoms.

peptide: a fragment of protein.

permeability: a property of lipid bilayer to allow diffusion across the membrane.

pH: measure of acidity/basicity of a solution. proportional to proton (hydrogen ion) concentration.

pharmacokinetics: study of the quantitive activity of drugs. Temporal and spatial distribution of active agents.

phosphorylation: formation of a phosphate derivative of a biomolecule. Normally enzymatically from ATP.

plasmid: a small self-replicating molecule of DNA that is separate from the main chromosome in bacteria, yeast, and some plant and eukaryotic cells.

platelets: small cells involved in blood clotting.

polyadenylation: the enzymatic addition of a tract of adenosine residues to the 3′-OH of precursor RNA.

polyelectrolyte: charged polymer.

polyethylene oxide: synthetic polymer which is hydrophilic and hydrophobic.

polymer: a string of subunits creating long macromolecules.

polymorphism: variation of the genetic code for the same protein. In lipids, different structures formed by the same system. In liposomes, particles which can change their structure upon an internal or external trigger.

poration: creating transient pores and crossing the membrane.

primer: a short nucleic acid sequence which on base pairing with a complementary sequence provides a free 3′-OH for any of a variety of primer extension-dependent reactions.

prokaryote: a microorganism which has no nucleus and other organelles.

promoter: a DNA sequence preceding the gene at the 5′ end to which RNA polymerase binds. This region contains several regulatory elements intricately involved in initiation, regulation, and efficiency of RNA transcription.

protein: a large polymeric molecule consisting of a linear sequence of amino acids.

purine: a basic nitrogenous heterocyclic compound. It contains fused pyrimidine and imidazole rings.

pyrimidine: a nitrogenous heterocyclic (aromatic ring with at least one atom different from carbon) compound.

radionuclide: unstable isotope that decays spontaneously and emits radiation.

receptor: organ, cell, or part of the cell initiating response upon external trigger. Example: endocytosis of bound particle.

recombinant DNA: the hybrid DNA produced in the laboratory by joining pieces together, frequently from different organisms.

recombinant vaccines: consisting of cloned pieces of an infectious organism.

renaturation: reassociation of denatured, complementary single strands.

reperfusion injury: tissue damage caused by the reinitiation of blood flow to an organ.

replication: formation of an exact copy. DNA replication occurs when each strand acts as a template for a new, complementary strand, formed according to base-pairing rules.

RES: reticuloendothelial system: proteins and phagocytic cells involved in clearance of foreign particulates from the body. Also called mononuclear phagocytic system, MPS.

restriction endonuclease: a class of enzymes which recognize specific sequences in a double-stranded DNA and cut both strands at each site where this sequence occurs.

restriction fragments: fragments of DNA produced by enzymatic cuts.

retrovirus: viral class with the RNA genome that integrate their DNA into that of their host and is used as a gene therapy vector.

reverse transcriptase: a class of enzymes which catalyze the formation of DNA strands from RNA templates.

RNA (ribonucleic acid): a single-stranded nucleic acid. Common forms are messenger (mRNA), transfer (tRNA), and ribosomal (rRNA).

ribonuclease: a family of enzymes which rapidly degrade RNA molecules. Control of RNase activity is a key consideration in all manipulations involving RNA.

ribozyme: an enzyme made from RNA rather than protein.

sarcoma: a highly malignant type of tumor that arises in connective tissue as a solid mass of cells.

sedimentation coefficient: physical constant specifying the rate of sedimentation in a centrifugal field.

somatic cells: all cells other than sperm and ova.

Southern blotting: a procedure for transferring DNA fragments of electrophoretically chromatographed DNA on a filter paper for subsequent immobilization and hybridization.

splicing: ligation of two fragments of DNA/RNA end to end.

stealth liposome: liposome invisible to the immune system.

stem cells: cells in bone marrow which differentiate into blood and immune cells.

steric stabilization: surface coating with polymers to increase colloidal stability.

sterol: lipid molecules found in biomembranes (cholesterol).

supercoiling: the alteration of normal numbers of turns in a DNA helix. Can be positive or negative.

SUV: small unilamellar vesicle (<100 nm).

targeting: labeling particles with antibodies, their fragments (Fab′), lectins, or oligosaccharides to target particles to specific cells.

T_c: temperature at which solid bilayers melt into liquid phase.

template: information blueprint for the synthesis of macromolecules.

termination codon: codons which signal the termination of the synthesis of a polypeptide chain (UAA, UAG, UGA).

T_m: temperature at which 50% of the duplexes are dissociated into single strands.

transcription: the transfer of information from DNA to RNA.

transduction: transfer of genetic material into different cells using viral vectors.

transfection: delivery of genes by nonviral vectors.

transgenic mice: mice who carry on modified genes.

translation: synthesis of protein using information in mRNA.

tumor: abnormal swelling caused by the growth of new tissues which differ in structure from the part of the body where they are growing.

upstream: sequences in the 5′ direction.

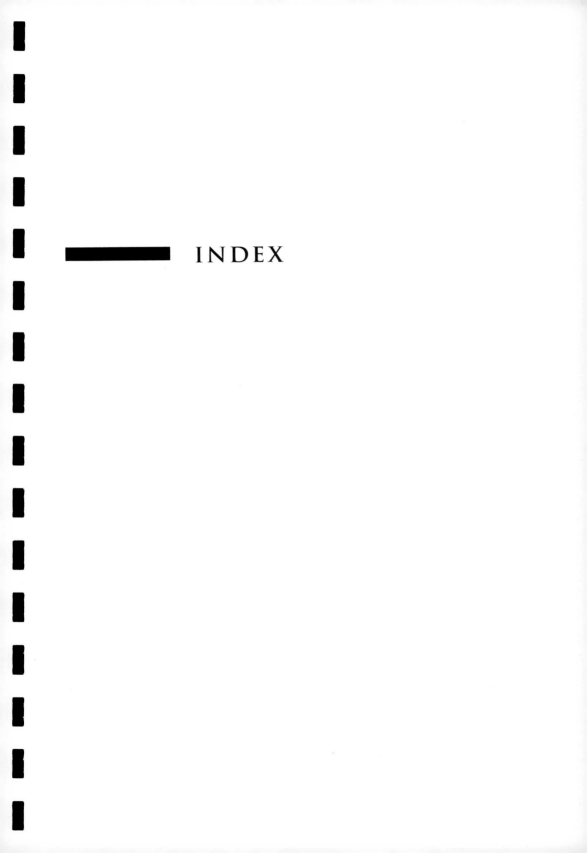

INDEX

INDEX

C